Short Notes for Dental PG Entrance Examinations

Second Edition

Including Review for UG Students

Clinical Sciences Volume 4

- Operative Dentistry
- Endodontics
- Oral Surgery
- Local Anaesthesia
- Orthodontics
- Pedodontics

Volumes in the Series

Short Notes for **Dental PG Entrance Examinations**

Second Edition

Basic Sciences

- **Volume 1 BDS I**
- **Volume 2 BDS II**
- **Volume 3 BDS III**

Clinical Sciences

- **Volume 4** Operative Dentistry, Endodontics, Oral Surgery, Local Anaesthesia, Orthodontics, Pedodontics
- **Volume 5** Periodontics, Prosthodontics, Basic Radiology Self-Assessment Paper, Model Test Papers

Short Notes for Dental PG Entrance Examinations

Second Edition

Including Review for UG Students

Clinical Sciences Volume 4

SANDEEP GOYAL MDS (Orthodontics)
Professor
Department of Orthodontics and Dentofacial Orthopedics
ITS College of Dental Sciences and Research
Murad Nagar, UP

Edited by
Sonia Goyal MDS (Oral and Maxillofacial Surgery)
Associate Professor, Department of Oral and Maxillofacial Surgery,
ITS College of Dental Sciences and Research, Murad Nagar, UP

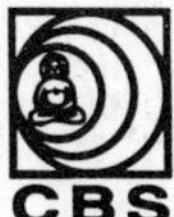

CBS Publishers & Distributors Pvt Ltd
New Delhi • Bangalore • Pune • Cochin • Chennai

Second Edition

Short Notes for Dental PG Entrance Examinations

Volume 4

First Edition : 2006
Second Edition : 2010

ISBN : 978-81-239-1801-3

Published by Satish Kumar Jain and produced by Vinod K. Jain for
CBS Publishers & Distributors Pvt Ltd
4819/XI Prahlad Street, 24 Ansari Road, Daryaganj,
New Delhi 110 002, India.
Fax: 011-23243014 e-mail: cbspubs@vsnl.com; delhi@cbspd.com
Website: www.cbspd.com

Branches

- **Bangalore:** Seema House 2975, 17th Cross, K.R. Road, Banasankari 2nd Stage, Bangalore 560 070
  Fax: 080-26771680 e-mail: cbsbng@gmail.com
- **Pune:** Shaan Brahmha Complex, Basement, Appa Balwant Chowk,
  Budhwar Peth, next to Ratan Talkies, Pune 411 002
  Fax: 020-24464059 e-mail: pune@cbspd.com
- **Cochin:** 36/14 Kalluvilakam, Lissie Hospital Road, Cochin-682018, Kerala.
  e-mail: cochin@cbspd.com
- **Chennai:** 20, West Park Road, Shenoy Nagar, Chennai 600030.
  email: chennai@cbspd.com

Printed at Somya Printers, Delhi-110053

dedicated
to
Ma Vaishno Devi,
my parents
and
my teachers

Acknowledgments

At the very outset, I bow my head to the Almighty God and my Guruji for all the grace showered on me to compile the second edition of the book. I am also thankful to my parents for their unforgettable sacrifices and choicest blessings.

I acknowledge the words of advice given to me by Dr Prof. Hari Parkash, Director General, ITS College of Dental Sciences and Research, Murad Nagar.

I place on record my deep gratitude towards my mentors and guides, my respected teachers during my postgraduation, Dr D N Kapoor, the then Professor and Head; Dr V P Sharma, Professor; Dr Pradeep Tandon, Professor, Department of Orthodontics and Dentofacial Orthopedics, Faculty of Dental Sciences, KGMC, Lucknow, for all their blessings, ideas and inspiration.

Prof P B Sood, Principal, ITS College of Dental Sciences and Research, Murad Nagar, has always been a constant source of insipiration and advice.

Dr Sanjay Tiwari, Professor and Head, Department of Endodontics, and Principal, GDC, PGIMS, Rohtak, for all his good wishes, the support, stimulating criticism and magnanimous help during my UG/PG days and afterwards.

My wife Dr Sonia Goyal MDS (oral and maxillofacial surgery), for her support, constant advice, contribution and editing the text, and all the pains she took during the compilation of the project.

Mr S K Jain and Mr Y N Arjuna of CBS Publishers & Distributors Pvt Ltd and their team of professionals for their best suggestions and help in getting this work published in the present form.

Last but not the least, I acknowledge all my family members and friends for their best wishes to boost my morale.

Sandeep Goyal MDS

Preface to the Second Edition

We thank all our readers for their overwhelming support and inputs for the first edition of our series **Short Notes for PG Dental Entrance Examinations**. However, with the increasing competition and increasing base of knowledge, a strong requirement for the improvement has been felt.

In the second edition, we have tried to incorporate a few new topics which will be helpful to postgraduate aspirants. We have now compiled the basic subjects and clinical subjects separately. This will help those undergraduate students also who aspire to compete for postgraduate entrance examination in the future. This edition will help and guide them to build their knowledge base from the very beginning of their dental career and will be helpful in their regular BDS examinations and also *viva voce* examinations.

We have included MCQs in this new edition for the side-by-side exercise and testing the skills and growth of their knowledge base. The book in the second edition has now been split into five volumes, considering the valuable additions made in the text as well new sections of MCQs which have been selectively added to strengthen the inherent appeal of this title amongst the potential readers. Basic Sciences are covered in Vols 1–3 and Clinical Sciences in Vols 4 and 5.

We request our readers to continue sending their suggestions to us for future improvements for the benefit of their friends, juniors and other future dental surgeons.

In the end, we again emphasize that all the aspirants should synergize their knowledge by reading standard theory books to smoothly sail through the ocean of entrance examination, since our volumes may not be complete in every aspect.

Sandeep Goyal MDS
Sonia Goyal MDS
goyalsandeep2000@rediffmail.com
goyalsandeep2000@gmail.com

Preface to the First Edition

There has been a marked increase in competition in dental PG entrance examinations, which have become tougher in recent times. A proper guidance to the aspirants is, therefore, necessary for making their preparations.

The trend of today being MCQ-based, the aspirants just memorise the MCQs from the books available in the market without going into the depth of the statement, leading to errors during the examination. Also, a series of MCQs currently available in the market unfortunately contain 50 to 60% repetition of the questions, and the answers to many questions given in the answer key are also misleading and confusing for the students.

Most of the students do not want to undertake a detailed study of the subjects for their preparation and hence look for the easiest method to get through in the examinations which they consider to be present in the MCQ books.

In my view, MCQ books are for practice only. Your basic knowledge is tested through MCQs and they help to churn your mind, but you should not read them blindly thinking that they will be repeated in the examinations as such. The paper setters change the statements and options of the MCQs for better judgement of the student, therefore, only those students who have a strong basic knowledge can easily analyze and correlate the statement and the option. Also, for some of those students who read the textbooks and do not make notes but rather underline the text or write in the textbooks only, revision becomes very confusing and time-consuming.

This book has been compiled with an idea in mind to provide handy information in the form of a ready-reckoner to the aspirants. This volume covers eight important subjects, and other subjects will be included in the latter volume(s). The motive of compiling information in this manner is to bring important points of each topic together so that a student while reading the topics can revise all the key points immediately and at one stretch.

I have tried with the best possible efforts to tabulate and alphabetically arrange most of the important information so as to make it easy for the students to search for the required topic. The book speaks about the points to be stressed in the form of lists, like the most common terms, syndromes, synonyms, etc.

This book gives the students the guidelines and information about the topics most often asked in the examinations. However, they are advised to go for **further detailed reading from standard textbooks to supplement and reinforce their knowledge.**

I have attempted my best to include almost 80 to 90% of the important information on the covered subjects. However, the readers must study additionally and add their own points on the topics for their benefit.

No project can be completed and improved upon without **feedback**, constructive criticism and healthy suggestions. It is my humble request to all the readers and students to send me their suggestions and points/ topics to be added in further editions of the book, to make it more informative and useful for their younger friends and students. It is promised that these suggestions will be suitably incorporated in the future editions and all the contributors will be suitably acknowledged. My e–mail address is goyalsandeep2000@sify.com. Wishing you all the success in your examinations.

Sandeep Goyal MDS

Suggested Readings

Since we do not claim this book to be complete in all the respects, we advise the students to further supplement their information by going through other standard textbooks on particular topics. We are providing below a list of some books for reference for the students.

	Author	Textbook on
1.	Monheim's	Local anesthesia
2.	Malamed's	Local anesthesia
3.	Graber's	Orthodontics – an art or science
4.	Profitt's	Orthodontics
5.	Grossman's	Endodontics
6.	Cohen's	Endodontics, i.e. pathways to the pulp
7.	Ingle's	Endodontics
8.	Gupta	Removable Partial Prosthodontics
9.	Orban's	Dental and oral histology
10.	Ten cate's	Oral histology
11.	Shafer's	Oral pathology
12.	Stone's	Oral pathology
13.	Burkitt's	Oral medicine
14.	Sikri	Dental Radiology, 4/e
15.	Sikri	Conservative Dentistry
16.	Goaz /White	Radiology
17.	Singh	Embryology
18.	Garg	Histology, 4/e

Standard books of MCQs which should be read definitely:

- Series of NDBs, i.e. national dental board papers, available upto L – series in I and II volumes.
- Rudman's
- Boucher's
- Steele's
- Gardiner's
- Cawson's
- Reed's Vols I & II
- Arco's Vols I & II

Besides these books, the students should always refer to the MCQ books available in the market for practice but they should not get confused.

Contents of Volume 4

Contents of Volume 5

CLINICAL SCIENCES
Volume 5

Abbreviations Used in the Book

AD	autosomal dominant
A.	artery
Ag/Ab/	antigen/antibody
Aka	also known as
Alv.	alveolar
Ant./post.	anterior/posterior
As	arsenic
Ass.	associated
B/W	between
Bact.	bacteria
BCC	basal cell ca.
C/E	clinical exam.
Ca.	carcinoma
Ch.	chronic/characteristics
Chr.	chromosomes
Cp.	compared
CT	connective tissue
Def.	deficiency
Dev.	develop/developmental
Dis	disease/distance as per the case
D/D	differential diagnosis
Enz.	enzyme
Epith.	epithelium/-al
ECA/ICA	external/internal carotid A
H/E	histology examination
IU	intrauterine
LAP	lymphadenopathy
LN	lymph nodes
LO	lateral oblique
M.	muscles
Mm	mucous membrane
MO/m.o.	malocclusion
Md/mand	mandibular
Memb.	membrane
MNGC	multinucleated giant cells
MNP/LNP	median/lateral nasal process
Mo.	months
Mx/max	maxillary
n.m.	neuromuscular
O/F	oral features
Org./orgs.	organisms
OTM	orthodontic tooth movement
OMV	occipito-mental view
OFD	object – film dis.
PO	presence of
PA	periapical/posteroanterior
PNS	para nasal sinus
Pt.	patient
PDL	periodontal ligament
R/G	radiograph
R/L	radiolucent
R/O	radiopaque
REE	reduced enamel epith
Reqd.	required
SCC	squamous cell ca.
SG	salivary gland
S/S	signs and symptoms
SMV	submento-vertex view
Synd	syndrome
TFD	target-film distance
TOD	target – object dis.
Vit.	vitamin

How to Prepare for the Entrance Examinations

This is my personal experience for PG entrance preparation and a time-tested method as many of my friends who have followed this method have been successful in the exams.

1. You have to believe in that hard work and luck go side by side.
2. Keep at least 6–8 months for preparation, which should be free from any sort of disturbance and forget about your surroundings.
3. Devote at least 8–10 hrs/day for the studies.
4. Divide your time and make a time bound schedule.
5. Pick important subjects first depending on the numbers of questions asked in the examinations. The subjects to be studied and stressed during entrance preparation are : general anatomy; dental materials; dental histology; pharmacology; oral pathology; fluorides; endodontics; periodontology; local anaesthesia; pedodontics; basics of all the clinical subjects.
6. Make your daily routine and diligently follow it.
7. Read MCQs two times from NDBs and any other standard book available on a particular subject. This will give you an idea about the style of MCQs and the part of the topic from which the question has been picked from the text, e.g. many MCQs are taken from the legends written below the figures in the book especially dental histology, periodontology, orthodontics.
8. Pick up a standard textbook which you have read during UG days. Read the topics and make notes separately and underline the important points. This will help you to strengthen your knowledge on that topic. Then take other subjects and follow the same pattern.
9. Read only relevant parts of the non-clinical subjects. Stress on anatomy, embryology, dental histology, pharmacology and physiology during the preparation.

10. All the topics and subjects should be covered in the time that at least two months are left for revision before the examination which you are preparing for.
11. When you have finished all the subjects, pick the MCQs books and read the 2–3 times. Any problem can be referred to your notes/textbooks.
12. Mark difficult MCQs in the book with different colors and read them carefully everytime.
13. 15 days before exams, read the notes on all the subjects, followed by one more revision of MCQs.
14. Discussion with your friends is a very important part of preparation. It gives an insight into the topics and more informations.
15. Take all the exams as far as possible; it tells you the trend; your standing and reshuffles your knowledge.

If you follow these rules, I can guarantee you 100% success in the examinations.

Syllabus

Given below is brief outline of the syllabus and topics the students should follow during preparation which should be supplemented by other topics for better knowledge.

Subjects	Topics	Books advised
Anatomy	♦ Head and neck — complete ♦ Brain — basics	Chaurasia's
Embryology	♦ Basics ♦ Pharyngeal arches ♦ Fetal circulation ♦ Fate of germ layers ♦ Development of oral cavity and face	I B Singh
Histology	♦ Basics ♦ Cell structure, cell division ♦ All glands and appendages, spleen, liver, etc. ♦ Skin, epithelium, A, V, N, M, CT	I B Singh
Dental materials	Complete	Skinners
Physiology	♦ Basics ♦ Blood, GIT, CVS, respiration, endocrinology	Chatterjee
Biochemistry	Basic concepts, enzymes, DNA/RNA, Krebs's cycle, HMP, etc. cycles carbohydrate/ lipid/ protein structure and metabolism, vitamins, minerals, energy requirements, etc.	Rama Rao, Harper's

Subjects	**Topics**	**Books advised**
Dental histology	Complete	Orbans
Dental anatomy	Basics, difference in morphology of molars, premolars, canines, mand lateral incisors, etc., occlusion, TMJ, alveolar bone	Wheeler's
Microbiology	Basics, sterilisation, structure of bacteria and virus, immunity, Ag–Ab reactions, *Strept.*, *Staph.*, *Clostridia*, *Mycobacterium*, HIV, Hepatitis virus	Ananthnarayan
Pathology	Basics only, neoplasia definitions, blood pathology (Do not waste much time on it.)	Robins
Pharmacology	Basic concepts, pharmacokinetics and dynamics, dental pharmacology, antibiotics, analgesics, LA/GA, sympathomimetic/lytic drugs, cholinergics/adrenergic, etc., briefly about CVS, CNS, antiepileptic, etc. Mechanism of action of all the drugs, MCQs	K D Tripathi
Oral pathology	Complete	Shafer's
Surgery/ medicine	Basics only, HT, TB, DM, infections, etc.	Any book
PCD	Fluorides, epidemiology, definitions, indices;	
Orthodontics	Basics, growth, ceph, diagnosis, appliances, wire properties, tissue reactions, forces, anchorage, tooth movements	Graber's, Proffit's

Subjects	Topics	Books advised
Local anesthesia	Complete	Monheim's, Malamed
Oral surgery	Basics; sterilisation, sutures, grafts, fascial infections, maxillary sinus, TMJ, salivary glands, fractures and x-rays	Kruger's, Killey's
Operative	Basics, cavity preparation, classification, cariolgy, instruments, cements and restorative materials, differences between cavity of silver, gold, porcelain, etc.	Sturdevant, Marzouk
Endodontics	Complete book	Grossman, Weine
Pedodontics	Complete book	Mcdonald's, Finn's
Periodontics	Complete book	Glickmann's
Radiography	Brief, basics	Any standard book
Prosthodontics	Basics of CD/impressions; materials, occlusions, jaw relations, implants, TMJ, movements, immediate dentures, etc. Basics of FPD preparations, finish lines, crown preparations, principles, gingival retraction, impression, casting, etc. Basics of RPD, DR, IR, connectors, classification of RPDs, diagnosis and Rx plan, surveyor, etc.	Boucher's Fenn Winkler's Shillinburg Dykema McCracken's Steward

Clinical Sciences

Volume 4

- Operative Dentistry
- Endodontics
- Oral Surgery
- Local Anaesthesia
- Orthodontics
- Pedodontics

1 Operative Dentistry

- **Operative** dentistry is defined as the diagnosis, prevention and Rx of defects of natural teeth. These defects can be dental decay, erosion, abrasion, attrition, hypoplasia, trauma, etc.
- **Diagnosis** = it is the statement of the nature of the disease or other conditions made after correlating the history of patient; signs and symptoms; clinical examination and the lab tests.
- **Prognosis** = it is an advanced indication or forecast of the course of the disease. It is the prediction of the duration, course and termination of a disease and patient's response to the Rx.
- **Signs** = are the conditions related to the disease, which are observed by the doctor.
- **Symptoms** = are those conditions related to the disease, which are observed by the patient and told to the doctor.
- **Treatment planning** = it is the blue print of the case management. It is a carefully sequenced series of cvents or services designed to eliminate or control the etiological factors, repair the existing defects and create a functional maintainable environment.
- **Dental emergencies** = are those events in which, the patient is in dental related pain or in immediate threat of damage to the dentition or its supporting tissues, e.g. trauma.
- **Dental URGENCIES** = those incidents in which the patient is not experiencing pain nor is there immediate threat of sustaining damage to the dentition or supporting tissues. They do not require immediate attention.

- **Post-op. complications** = are related to previously performed dental procedures, arising especially shortly after treatment. These are related to ______________.

RECENT RESTORATIVE TREATMENT

- **Chief complaint** = is a symptom described related in the patients own words.
- **Cavity** = it is any defect in enamel/dentin due to pathologic process of dental caries.
- **Cavity preparation** = it is the performance of those dental surgical procedures required to expose the carious lesions, permit removal of affected tissues and so shape the remaining enamel and dentin as to contribute to a biologically and mechanically sound restoration.

4. **Fundamental aims** of operative dentistry are:

- Prevention
- Interception
- Preservation
- Restoration

Different systems of tooth designation:

1. **Universal system/American system** of tooth numbering (By ADA–CDA)

	(R)	(L)	
(1)	ABCDE	FGHIJ	Primary teeth
	TSRQP	ONMLK	
(2)	1 – 8	9 – 16	Permanent teeth
	32 – 25	24 – 17	

2. **Zsigmondy/Palmer system**–1861

- **Oldest system**, most widely used.
- Also known as Angular/**grid** system/Chevron or set/square system.

8 – 1	1 – 8
8 – 1	1 – 8

E – A	A – E
E – A	A – E

3. 2–Digit system (FDI) system–1971

- First digit indicates quadrant.
- Second digit indicates tooth.
- Quadrants = 1–4 in permanent dentition.

  5–8 in primary dentition.
- Quadrants are allotted in clockwise sequence and start from upper right.
- Digits should be pronounced separately.

18 – 14 13 12 11	21 22 – 28
48 – 41	31 – 38

4. European system: for permanent teeth

8+ 7+6+5+4+3+2+1+ \\+1+2+3+4+5+6+7+8
8-7-6-5-4-3-2-1- \\-1-2-3-4-5-6-7-8

for primary teeth

05+04+03+02+01+ \\+01+02+03+04+05
05-04-03-02-01-\\-01-02-03-04-05

DIAGNOSIS OF DIFFERENT CONDITIONS

Vitality Tests (Refer to pedo/endo sections also.)

- Vitality tests indicate whether a viable nerve supply exists.
- Percussion verifies whether there is PDL inflammation.
- Electric pulp testing relies on direct electrical stimulation of sensory Ns of pulp.
- Lack reproductibility; depends on subjective nature of pain.

RADIOGRAPHY

VERTICAL ANGULATIONS

Teeth	Incisor	Canine	Premolar	Molar
Upper	+ 40 (50–60)	+ 45 (45–50)	+ 20 (35–40)	+ 10 (20–30)
Lower	– 15	– 20	– 10	– 5

- For incisors = the rays are through the nose to the extension of ala–tragus line.
- For canine = ala of nose along the inter-dental space b/w canine and first PM.
- Where the perpendicular from mid point of the infraorbital margin crosses the line of concentration/ala–tragal line or above the corner of mouth.
- Perpendicular 1 cm behind the outer canthus of eye crosses ala–tragus line.
- Anode film distance = 20 cm.
- Buccal object/SLOB/Clark's rule: it is also known as tube shift technique.

Entry point of rays

Teeth	Incisors	Canines	Premolars	Molars
Upper	Tip of nose	Ala tragus line	Zygomatic buttress	Zygomatic arch
Lower	Mid point of chin/symphysis 1 cm above the mandibular lower border	Corner of mouth	B/w para-symphysis and body of mandible	Angle of jaw

- For Mandible = Tragus–corner of mouth line should be parallel to floor.

- For Maxilla = ala-tragus line parallel to floor.
- Parallel cone technique = also know as 16″ technique.

Size of films

No.	Use	Size	
0	Pedofilm	22 × 35 mm	
1	Only 2 anteriors (less projection)	24 × 40 mm	
2	Adult film	32 × 41 mm	Mostly commonly used
3	Occlusal	57 × 76 mm	

Prevention from 2° radiations

1. 6 feet distance in a zone of 90°–135° from x-ray source.
2. 3 feet brick wall.
3. 1 feet concrete.
4. Gypsum boards on wall = 8–12 mm thick.
5. Lead point.
6. Lead shield.
7. Lead apron = 0.5–1.0 mm; mostly 1.0 mm.
   *Why lead? Due to its high atomic no. and compact crystal lattice, the x-rays cannot pass.

Types of lead aprons: Type 1, 2, 3 or heavy/medium/low; heavy is used for the patient, medium by operator.

- IOPA x-ray shooting requires time = 0.4 sec.
- Radiograph is C/I in pregnancy esp in 1st trimester and in untreated thyrotoxicosis/hyperthyroidism.
- **Inherent filter** = occurs due to glass tube and mineral oil; is approx 0.7 mm Al.
- Total filter = 2 mm Al.
- Mineral oil = to dissipate heat generated; so rest of the filter, i.e. 1.3 mm Al; by Al filter, etc.
- **Machine** = 70 kvp × 8 mA.

R/G

- Bite wing R/G help determine the proximal carious lesions.
- By the time, the proximal lesion can first be seen on enamel, the demineralization has often extended into dentin.
- Surface lesions without cavitation can get remineralized by fluorides.
- B/W, R/G are taken every 2 years because the carious progress is slow.
- Enamel, sclerotic dentin, primary dentin have descending order of radiopacity.
- 4 B/W R/G are required for the posterior segments of both arches.
- B/W R/G is exposed at 8° vertical angulation to minimize vertical overlapping.
- A devital posterior tooth usually requires a minimum of an MOD —protected cusp or only cast gold restorations because of susceptibility of fracture of tooth.
- Teeth of older patients require CUSP protection, because of increased friability with age.

Electric pulp tester: different types of responses are noted as follows.

No response	Either tooth is not vital or cusps are highly calcified; apical periodontitis
Moderately transient	Vital pulp
Painful transient	Hyperemia; reversible pulpitis
Painful lingering	Irreversible pulpitis

- The EPT and ultrasonic scaling are absolutely contra-indicated in patients having pacemakers.
- If moderate transient response, it means the tooth is vital.
- A current of 5–20 mA is sufficient to modify the normal pacemaker function.
- False +ve readings = tooth is non-vital; it may be due to the factors, i.e. pulp tester touching the metallic restoration; improper

isolation; anxiety of the patient; liquefaction necrosis; coagulation; moist gangrenous pulp.

- Periapical lesions do not respond to pulp vitality tests except liquefaction necrosis and tooth having more than one root canals.
- False negative response = is due to heavily pre-medicated patients.
- In internal resorption = EPT is normal.
- Reversible pulpitis = sensitive to cold stimulus; relieved by hot stimulus.

ODONTALGIA is defined as pain in a tooth.

Referred pain = pain is often not well–localized within the oral region.

- Spontaneous pain and sensitivity to percussion are clinical s/s, which correlate with pulpal/PA response.
- Spontaneous pain is related to IRREVERSIBLE PULPITIS while sensitivity to percussion is related to PA inflammation.
- A single evoking stimulus of cold/sweets/biting pressure = implies reversible pulpitis.
- Spontaneous pain/prolonged sensitivity to heat, which is not relieved by cold–implies irreversible pulpitis.
- **Dentinal pain** = sharp, jabbing pain of short duration (< 1–3 min) upon removal of stimulus is a sign of reversible pulpitis.
- **Pulpal pain** = dull aching/throbbing pain of longer duration (> 5 min) indicates irreversible pulpitis.

DENTINAL PAIN (Also refer to section of endodontics in Vol. I.)

- Is a sharp lancinating pain.
- Easily localised.
- Immediately initiated by specific stimuli, e.g. heat/cold.
- Lasts for a few seconds to a few minutes after removal of stimulus.

PULPAL PAIN

- Dull, throbbing ache.
- Pulp does not contain proprioceptive nerve endings, so ***pain is poorly localized***.

- Not associated with a stimulus.
- Slowly responds to heat.
- Reaction continues for a minute to hours.
- Sensitivity to heat checked by placing WARM impression compound for 5 sec.
- Ice/metal instrument chilled with ETHYLENE CHLORIDE spray is placed for 5 sec. to test sensitivity to COLD.
- Ability of pulp to recover from injury depends on its blood supply and not on the nerve supply.
- Pain of reversible pulpitis = subsides after removal of stimulus.
- Pain of irreversible pulpitis = lasts for several hours; pulsatile in nature; worse at night; cold helps in decreasing the pain; pain remains after removal of stimulus.

Erosion

- It is the loss of E/D from slow dissolution.
- Is a form of **chemical reduction** of hard tissues.
- Incisors have the greatest degree of erosion.
- It is generally seen in patients taking acidic drinks, having hyper-acidity, etc.
- Lesion is of sharp V-shape.
- Lesion is most sensitive in initial stages, gradually becomes less sensitive as 2° dentin is deposited.

Abrasion = is a **mechanical reduction** of hard tissues usually occurring over a long period of time.

Cervical abrasion = occurs mainly from ***faulty total brushing***.

Attrition = loss of occlusal and incisal enamel, which occurs throughout life. Due to Aging/Stress. It is also a form of **mechanical reduction** of hard tissues.

Bruxism = is diagnosed by the p.o. atypical wear facets on the teeth, which are generally outside the general range of masticatory functions.

Fractured cusp = most commonly are the lingual cusps, mandibular molars and cusps of maxillary premolars.

Cracked tooth syndrome = it is due to incomplete fracture of tooth. There is sensitivity to cold.

- Sharp pain on RELEASE of pressure during mastication.
- Symptoms gradually intensify with time.
- Diagnosis by asking the patient to bite on a wooden stick.

Cracked tooth syndrome = diagnosis is done by asking the patient to bite gently on small rubber polishing wheels or an orange wood stick.

- ♦ Its best treatment is CAST RESTORATION.

REVERSIBLE PULPITIS

- ♦ Most common form of ODONTALGIA associated with reversible pulpitis is POST-OPERATIVE HYPERSENSITIVITY.
- ♦ Cavity preparation may lead to REVERSIBLE pulpitis, so should be made with adequate coolant, with sharp bur and with intermittent pressure.
- ♦ Gold has more thermal conductivity than amalgam and so gold castings have a potential for greater thermal sensitivity.
- ♦ Formation of reparative dentin and occlusion of dentin may result in decrease in sensitivity due to increased thickness of remaining dentin.

IRREVERSIBLE PULPITIS

- ♦ Electric pulp testing = NIL response.
- ♦ Tooth may feel elongated and sensitive to percussion.
- ♦ R/G = widened PDL.

  Periapical pain = PDL has proprioceptors and so patient can localize the affected tooth.
- ♦ Acute periapical abscess = severe pain; tender tooth; drain pus and relieve the occlusion for its treatment.

MAXILLARY SINUSITIS

- ♦ Throbbing pain in all maxillary posterior teeth.
- ♦ May be result of common cold also.

- Is due to that the apices of teeth closely approximate the wall of sinus.

DISPLACED TEETH

- Intruded teeth usually re-erupt within 6 mos. in a young patient with no root fracture.
- EPT will normally give NO RESPONSE for at least 1 month after trauma.

Avulsed teeth: permanent anterior teeth of young adult = should be REPLANTED AS SOON AS POSSIBLE; tooth should be free in all excursive movements; RCT should be done within 2 weeks.

Root fracture: refer to section of pedo also

- **If in apical 3rd**—should be stabilized by splinting with adjacent teeth; successful in young teeth due to wide open apices.
- Prognosis is poorest if fracture is in gingival 3rd root.
- Most difficult to treatment = if fracture is in mid 3rd of root.
- **Union/healing**—refer to section on pedo also.

VERTICAL ROOT fracture—Poorest prognosis.

- **Attrition** = is loss of surface tooth structure due to direct frictional forces b/w contacting teeth. It is a **physiological** process.
- **Abrasion** = it is a saucer shaped or wedge shaped lesion; loss of surface tooth structure due to a direct contact b/w teeth and external objects, e.g. tooth brush abrasion is most common; abrasives on powders, etc.; it is a **pathologic** process. It involves **only cementum**, as it is soft.
- **Erosion** = wedge shaped lesion; loss of tooth structure due to chemico-mechanical means in the absence of specific bacteria; it is one of the most predominant oral **pathologic changes,** e.g. by excessive soft drinks; hyperacidity; recurrent vomiting tendency; excessive intake of citrus juices; it involves **enamel** only.

DISCOLORATION OF TEETH It is of 2 types (Refer to pedosection also.)

- **Extrinsic** = is due to surface staining.
- **Intrinsic** = is internal and is due to changes in one or more tooth tissues.
- **Tetracycline** = it has 9 times more affinity for dentin than enamel; it forms chelates with calcium; can cross placenta; gets secreted in breast milk.
- **Fluorides**
- **Corrosion** products of amalgam enter in dentinal tubules; also the products of pulp necrosis, blood, etc.
- **Porphyria**

Bleaching

- 5 parts of 30% H_2O_2 + 1 part ethyl ether
  sodium perborate + 30% H_2O_2 to make paste
  heated at 110°–130°F for 1–3 min.

Indirect pulp capping

- Leaving some softened dentin at base of cavity to avoid pulp exposure.
- Softening of dentin preceeds bacterial invasion.
- Pulpitis does not occur until bacteria are within 0.5–1.0 mm of pulp.
- $Ca(OH)_2$ with alkaline pH is bacteriostatic and helps formation of calcific bridge of secondary dentin and arrests the caries.

Matcrials required

ZOE	Sterilises the underlying dentin Decreases PG synthesis Aids remineralization; hygroscopic
$Ca(OH)_2$	Alkaline pH Bacteriostatic Helps calcific barrier formation Zone of pulpal necrosis occurs, which gets mineralized with Ca^{++} ions from the pulp.

Materials required (*Contd.*)

Ledermix	Triamcinolone acetonide + demethyl chlortetracycline mixture Anti-inflammatory and bacteriostatic Also decreases pulp defenses.

CARIES (Also refer to section of oral pathology in Vol. I.)

Characteristics of caries

- **Caries** = it is the slowly progressing, irreversible decay of dental hard tissue, which is characterized by demineralization of inorganic part and disintegration of organic structure.
- Carious lesion tends to spread more rapidly in lateral direction along DEJ than along the dentinal tubules.
- **Bacteria responsible** for caries = Strept. mutans.
- Sugar responsible = sucrose.
- **First sign** of caries = is opacity.
- **Difference between opacity of caries and hypoplasia/ hypocalcification** = incipient caries lesion becomes translucent after wetting and again becomes opaque after drying. But, the developmental defects are not affected by wetting process.

Facts about caries

- **Miller's chemoparasitic theory** = dissolution of inorganic salts, i.e. HA crystals of the tooth occurs by acids produced.
- **Strept. mutans** = is main bacteria for initiation of caries, and **lactobacilli** is for P and F caries and **actrnomyces** in root caries.
- **Main sugar** implicated in caries = **sucrose.**
- **Rempant caries** = occurs on smooth facial surfaces of teeth; also seen in xerostomia after radiation therapy.
- **Initial caries** starts with *S mutans*; then lactobacilli aciduric bacteria predominate in the larger lesions.
- SnF_2 is the most effective in decreasing *S mutans*, levels in saliva, among the various Fluoride preparations available.

Caries disclosing dyes

- Used to find out the soundness of the dentin.
- **0.5% solution of basic fuchsin** in propylene glycol is used.
- Stained dentin has 1300 times more bacteria per mg of dentin than the unstained dentin.
- **Plaque disclosing agents** = 4% erythrosine.
- 5% Na–MFP is the abrasive in tooth powders.
- Saliva can be cultured on selective MSB medium to find out the count of *S mutans*. MSB contain bacitracin and sucrose broth.
- High caries Risk = if *S mutans* level is 10^6 CFU/ml (CFU = colony forming units).
- Best caries prevention is by = F + professional debridement + dietary counselling.
- Medium for lactobacilli uses pH = 5.
- If > 10^5 CFU/ml of lactobacilli = implies high caries.
- If < 10^4 CFU/ml of lactobacilli = low caries risk.
- **Xylitol is most effective sucrose substitute** in decreasing decay.
- 10^6 strept mutans bacteria/ml of saliva are required to start the caries.
- **Acidogenic theory** = acids produced from carbohydrates decalcifies inorganic part of teeth, and then the organic part is disintegrated creating cavities.
- **Proteolysis theory** = organic part of tooth is attacked first with certain lytic enzymes. This leaves the inorganic part without a matrix support, which gets washed away creating cavities.
- **Caries triad** = there must be 3 factors, i.e. host/tooth + parasite/ bacteria + medium/carbohydrate. A fourth factor has been added to it as time (Keyes triad).
- Caries susceptibility of a tooth is inversely proportional to its F, Ca and Sn contents.
- Caries susceptibility of a tooth is inversely proportional to salivary phosphate content.
- Higher organic content of saliva indicates more plaque accumulations.

- Higher alkaline saliva predisposes to less decay.
- Serous saliva/low viscosity causes more self-cleansing action.
- Higher quantities of saliva flow lead to less caries.
- Plaque adheres to tooth surface with a sticking polysaccharide know as **dextran**.
- Strept. mutans is the main cariogenic bacteria.
- Sucrose is the main carbohydrate causing caries.
- Anti-caries bacteria = veillonella.
- Genetic modification to prevent caries.
- **Fluorides** = decrease caries activity by decreasing solubility of tooth structure, decreasing surface energy of tooth surface, decreases plaque adhesion interferes in carbohydrate metabolism by bacteria.
- Increasing phosphate content in diet = decreases the solubility of inorganic substance of the tooth.
- Vitamin K = is anti-cariogenic.
- ***First component of enamel to be involved in caries is the interprismatic substance.*** Caries spreads in the form of a cone; the base of cone is towards DEJ in P and F caries and away from DEJ in smooth/convex surfaces.

Caries progress: Also refer to the sections of oral pathology and pedodontics.

- In P and F, the caries spreads along the divergence of enamel rods in the form of a CONE, the base of the cone is at DEJ.
- Spread of caries along DEJ is more RAPID than through enamel.
- Caries through dentin spreads as CONE, the base is also at DEJ.
- P and F caries = is seen as a small external clinical lesion, but internally more spread.
- Smooth surface lesions = base of cone is at outer enamel surface. Starts below plaque and below the contact areas.

First component of dentin involved is ***protoplasmic extensions within the dentinal tubules***, which are wider at DEJ and narrower at pulp. So caries cone in dentin has its base at DEJ.

Classification of caries–by Black–

Class	Features
I	P and F cavities at occlusal surfaces of M, PM, and pits on buccal/lingual surfaces of I/PM/M.
II	Cavities on proximal surfaces of PM/M. **Smooth surface** lesion.
III	Proximal surface of incisors/cuspids, but not involving incisal edges. **Smooth surface** lesion.
IV	On proximal surfaces of I/C, involving incisal edges. **Smooth surface** lesion.
V	In gingival 3rd of any tooth; mostly seen in older age group due to gingival recession.
VI	MOD cavity; and incisal edges and cusp tips of teeth.

Black's classification of caries = is a **therapeutic classification**; as it is based on Rx and restoration designs.

Class	Features
I. on all teeth	Begin in structural defects, e.g. P and F and grooves, e.g. occlusal surfaces of M and PM; the occlusal 2/3rd of buccal and lingual surfaces of molars; and the lingual surfaces of anteriors.
II. on posterior teeth	On proximal surfaces of M and PM.
III. on anterior teeth	On proximal surfaces of anteriors without involving incisal edge and angle.
IV. on anterior teeth	On proximal surfaces of anteriors and involving incisal edge and angle.
V. on all teeth	At gingival 3rd of facial/lingual surfaces of anterior and posterior teeth.
VI. on all teeth	On incisal edges and cuspal tips or on any highly self-cleansable areas.

Types of cavities: Classification of decay

Type	Features
Incipient/initial/	Is ***the first attack*** on a tooth surface.
Recurrent/secondary primary caries	Is seen ***under or around the margins*** or surrounding wall of an existing restoration.
Acute or rampant caries	Is a ***rapidly invading*** process, which involves several teeth. Lesions are soft and light coloured and mostly with severe pulpal reactions.
Chronic caries	Are of variable depth, longer standing; and tend to be fewer in number; dentin is hard and dark in colour.
Pit and fissure caries	Originates in P and F of teeth, e.g. on lingual surface of maxillary incisors; and buccal, lingual and occlusa surfaces of posterior teeth.
Smooth surface caries	Originates on all surfaces without P and F and grooves.
Forward decay	i.e. when caries cone in enamel is larger than in dentin or of same size, it is know as forward decay, as seen ***in Pit caries***.
Backward decay	When caries process in dentin is much faster than enamel, the lateral spread of caries may occur, which undermines the enamel. It may attack the enamel from the dentinal side. It is seen in ***smooth surface lesions***.
Senile caries	Are associated with ageing and are present almost on root surfaces.

Types of cavities: Classification of decay *(Contd.)*

Type	Features
Residual caries	Is that which is not removed during a restorative process, either by accident, neglect or intention.
Simple caries	Which involves ***only one surface*** of the tooth.
Compound caries	Which involves ***two surfaces*** of the tooth.
Complex caries	Which involves ***more than two surfaces*** of the tooth.

Features of carious lesions

- Opacity adjacent to Pit/fissure as evidence of undermining/ demineralization.
- Loss of normal translucency of enamel showing undermining.
- **Decalcification of enamel is first stage** of caries process.
- Decalcified enamel is white and opaque.
- White spot seen due to **subsurface demineralization**; the area is soft.

Smooth surface carious lesions = seen on proximal surfaces just below the contact area; have broad area of initiation. It is diagnosed by: –

- If MR (marginal ridge) is opaque due to undermining of enamel.
- R/G shows radiolucency due to break in surface continuity.
- Trans-illumination used for anterior teeth—loss of TRANS-LUCENCY is seen.
- Bite wing R/G are taken for posterior teeth.

Differences between acute and chronic caries

Acute caries	Chronic caries
The acids dissolving the tooth structure preceed the bacteria producing them i.r.t. pulp	The bacterial are preceding the acids produced by them or are at the same level pulpally.

Differences b/w acute and chronic caries (*Contd.*)

Acute caries	Chronic caries
Is of shorter duration	Longer duration
Soft and easily scooped out	Hard
Colour is straw yellow	Dark brown to black
Odourless	Foul smelling
In younger age	In older age
Little or no reparative reaction of pulp	+ve reaction
Deepest dentinal layer is considered sterile as it has only acids but no bacteria	Entire carious mass is infected

Number of line and point angles in different cavities

Cavity	Line angles	Point angles
I	8	4
II	11	6
III	6	3
IV	11	6
V	8	4
VI	14	8

Classification of prepared cavities: According to the depth of the cavity.

Class	Features
Class A depth	i.e. cavity with minimum depth. Remaining dentin is of maximum thickness possible.
B	Extends beyond the minimum depth required by mechanical and biological factors; a substantial thickness of dentins remains.
C	Extends into dentin such that only a thin, but intact wall of dentin remains.
D	Actual or subclinical exposure of pulp is observed.

Principles of cavity preparation: According to Black:

1. Outline form
2. Retention/resistance form
3. Convenience form
4. Removal of remaining carious dentin
5. Finishing of the enamel wall
6. Cleaning of cavity/toileting.

Steps in cavity preparation: From Marzouk:

- Outline form
- Resistance form
- Retention form
- Removal of carious dentin
- Convenience form
- Establishing the configuration and correlations of enamel walls
- Debridement
- Observing and practising the biologic forms

Outline form	Is the locations that the peripheries of cavity will occupy on tooth surface; for most intracoronal preparations: the depth of cavity should be to include DEJ and 0.5 mm in dentin. It is due to 3 reasons: • DEJ is very sensitive, where maximum inter-connections of dentinal tubules exist. • To give bulk to the restorations. • To take advantage of elasticity of dentin during insertion and function.
Retention form	**Principal means of retention are:** • Frictional retention. • Elastic deformation of dentin. • Inverted truncated cones or undercuts. • Dovetail **Auxillary means of retention:** • Grooves = cut in dentin. • Internal boxes = have definite walls and floors. • Posts = made from wrought/cast metals and placed in root canals. • Pins = made from cast/wrought metals. • Triangular area = placed in dentin. • Etching. • Cement/luting agents = **least effective** methods. • If occlusal loading helps to seat the restoration rather than displacing it, it is an ideal auxillary retention form.
Removal of	**0.2–0.5% basic fuschin dye** stains the dentin irreparable decay areas.
Debridement	• H_2O_2 • Water–air jet • Cavity cleaners = e.g. citric acid; ascorbic acid; acetic acid in a conc of 1–10%. • Smear layer is only removed by 10% EDTA • Chisel, etc.

- **Outline form** = is the form of area of the tooth surface to be included within the outline or enamel margins of finished cavity.
- **External outline form** = the external boundary or perimeter of the prepared cavity.
- **Internal outline form** = is the inner dimension and detail of the prepared cavity.
- **Retention form** = prevents the restoration from being displaced.
- **Resistance form** = enables the restoration to withstand the stresses of mastication.
- **Convenience form**–provides ease for placing the restorative materials, i.e. for instrumentation, condensation, adaptation and finishing.
- Enamel walls must be parallel to the general direction of enamel rods and be supported by an intact DEJ.
  - Heavy flow of thin saliva—helps in bathing the teeth and decreases caries. It has anti-caries effect due to immuno-globulins and fluorides.
  - A gingival sulcus depth of 1–2 mm buccally and lingually, and 2–3 mm inter-proximally is normal.
  - Normal physiologic changes in colour of tooth is deepening of colour and increased opacity due to loss of enamel, and thickening and sclerosis of dentin.

OCCLUSION

Central parts of TMJ are avascular and without sensory nerves. They are capable of functional stress bearing without injury or pain.

Supporting Cusps

- Lingual cusps of maxillary and buccal cusps of mandibular posteriors and cusps tips/incisal edges of anteriors.
- They contact in the **centric stops** of opposing teeth.
- In normal angle's class I occlusion = the centric stops on mandibular teeth are fossae and marginal ridges.
- Centric stops play a significant role as the physical determinants of occlusal stability.

- TMJ has **no receptors** that monitor forces on joint but may depend on inputs from teeth and muscles for monitoring loading.
- CR = is a position, where almost wholly rotary (hinge-like) open and closing jaw movements can be made upto approx 25 mm.
- Average movement/slide from CR to CO is approx 1 mm; it is in anterior direction; it is know as **freedom-in-centric**. CO is 1 mm anterior to CR.
- Optimal condylar position for maximum intercuspation is slightly anterior to the midmost uppermost position, i.e. on the anterior slope of articular eminence.
- RCP: seldom seen as a functional position in natural dentition; helps in relating the mandible to maxilla in a patient.

Position	**Features**
Premature contacts	areas for PC in CR are mesial inclines of maxillary teeth and the distal inclined of mandibular teeth (MU-DL).
Balancing interferences	on maxillary molars are mesial/distal cusps ridge along with the buccal incline of the lingual cusps.
Working side interferences	lingual inclines of buccal cusps of maxillary posterior teeth and buccal inclines of lingual cusps of mandibular molars.
Protrusive interferences	on Md Post tooth = mesial inclines of marginal ridges; mesial inclines of triangular ridges.
Protrusive interferences	On Mx molars/PM = distal inclines of triangular ridges; distal inclines of marginal ridges.

PERIODONTAL ASPECTS (Refer to perio section also.)

- Most vulnerable part of periodontium is the junction between gingival epithelium and the tooth.

- Epithelium which joins directly and adheres to the tooth surface is known as junctional epithelium; while the attachment itself is know as epithelial attachment.
- Epithelial attachment is weak and is supported and maintained by tonus of the firm, free and circular gingival collagen fibers, which hold the gingiva close to the tooth.
- JE and EA have cell turn over time of approx. 7–10 days.
- After injury, the EA is reestablished by regenerating epithelial cells within a week and during this time, the bacteria are eliminated by PMN cells.
- PD disease is most often initiated and maintained by PLAQUE.
- Depth of normal gingival sulcus is 1–2 mm buccally, lingually and 2–3 mm proximally.
- Probe stops approx. 0.5 mm short of CT attachment to the tooth under normal pressure.
- After Rx and PD diseases, 4–6 weeks time is required for gingival health to return to normal.
- Less the gingival shrinkage after the surgery—the better are the esthetic and functional results.

ELECTRO SURGERY (Also refer to section of oral surgery.)

- Can be used safely only for gingivoplasty of free gingiva.
- Hyperplastic tissues may be removed with it, but should be done before the preparation of a restoration.
- Margins of restoration should be placed SUPRA-GINGIVALLY.
- Subgingival margins cause inflammation of tissues.
- It should not extend more than 0.5–1.0 mm under free marginal gingival.
- **Contour** = over contouring is more damaging than under contouring. It interferes with plaque removal. It interferes with ***sealing-cuff effect*** of gingiva against the tooth.
- Contact areas or I/d soldering joints should be placed as far occlusally as possible and should be convex and easy to clear.

TYPES OF PONTICS (Refer to prostho section also.)

- **Sanitary pontics** = should be given in mandibular posterior area.

- **Ridge saddle pontics** = is in touch with the tissues—so makes plaque removal almost impossible.
- **Bullet pontics** = contact only at a point at the ridge.
- Antibiotics especially TETRACYCLINE may be required during maintenance plan for Rx of acute infection in a pocket.
- NaF and SnF_2 rinses help against sensitivity.
- APF should not be used for patients with porcelain crowns. It tends to stain the crowns.

SPLINTING (Also refer to perio for indications and details.)

- Used to maintain the PD support of teeth; it enhances the functional stability and esthetics. It also helps during healing phase.
- *Temporary/provisional splinting* = is required when continuous trauma interferes with comfortable function and to maintain teeth in favourable esthetic/functional position after ortho Rx.
- Ortho Rx can be done to intrude teeth with deep pockets.
- Intrusion does not eliminate the pocket, but makes them intra-bony due to new tooth position, which has better chance of reattachment after PD Rx.

PREVENTIVE MEASURES

- Acquired pellicle formation is the first stage of plaque formation due to absorption or precipitation of a protein layer on the tooth surface; it forms in less than 30 min, after through cleaning.
- Some cationic molecules about a nitrogen atom have preventive effect on plaque formation.
- Sucrose is the main sugar causing plaque and caries.
- Harmful effects of sucrose get increased by increasing thickness of plaque, because it then interferes with the ***buffer system of saliva*** and so low pH at tooth surface may lead to caries.
- Best prevention from caries and PD disease is by :
  - Regular professional tooth cleaning.
  - Fluoride application.
  - Tooth brushing instructions.

MECHANICAL MEANS OF PLAQUE CONTROL: (Also refer to pedo and perio sections for details and table.)

- Multi-tufted soft bristles brushes with a bristle diameter 0.007–0.008 inch and with will finished rounded tips.
- **Bass method** = at 45°, bristles pushed into gingival crevice, but it does not remove plaque over the free gingiva.
- **Circular scrub method** = better than Bass method; light pressure used; brush moved in 2–4 mm diameter with circular movements; more effective near the inter-dental areas.
- 5–8 circular scrub movements are to be made for each brushing position with some overlap as the brush is moved around the dental arch.
  - ***Disclosing solution*** = Bismarck brown.
  - Most effective cleaning of exposed I/D surfaces is provided by = **Charter's method**.

Floss (Classification of floss)

- Multi-tufted floss spreads out in a tape like fashion.
- More effective plaque removal occurs with unwaxed floss.
- For tight i/d contents = waxed floss is easier than unwaxed floss.
- Concave i/d surfaces that cannot be cleansed with floss are cleaned with special inter-proximal brushes.
  - Gingival massage helps in reducing gingival inflammation by removing plaque and crevicular toxins, rather than by stimulation of circulation and metabolism.
  - **Forced irrigation** = it should be used with caution in patient with active periodontitis especially with H/O rheumatic fever or diabetes, as it may lead to bactermia.

CHEMICAL MEANS OF PLAQUE CONTROL (Also refer to sections of pedo and oral pathology.)

- 0.2% **chlorhixidine gluconate,** but may cause taste change and staining of the teeth after prolonged use.
- Other cationic disinfections also have plaque inhibiting properties.
- Fluorides.

- SnF_2 and MFP decrease the incidence of caries.
- 2% NaF, 8% SnF_2, 1.23% APF can decrease decay by 40%.
- APF should not be used on ceramic crowns, as it tends to ERODE the surface of porcelain.
- NaF is easier to formulate than APF.
- Taste of SnF_2 is objectionable.
- 0.05% NaF = if used daily.
- 0.2% NaF = if used weekly.
- Maximum dose recommended in packs to be sold = ***264 mg of NaF***.

P AND F SEALANTS (Also refer to sections of pedo and dental materials.)

Prophylactic odontotomy is conservative preparation of non-carious fissures and filling them with Ag; by Hyatt 1923.

Enamel ›plasty—by Bodecker; enlarging the P and F to form wide, non-reten ive grooves to remove enamel faults.

Buonocore 1955—etching and bonding of resin helped 86% reduction of occlusal caries.

- Fluorides can decrease smooth surfaces caries but has little effect on P and F caries.
- A resin sealant coating is applied to enamel defect, which adheres to the demineralized ends of acid-etched enamel rods.
- Loss of this sealant can occur by abrasive wear, by bond failure or by premature contacts.
- So occlusal interferences should be removed esp if a fluid resin is used.
- P and F sealant should extend up the cuspal inclines adj. to the fissures to a sufficient distance to attain an undetectable junction with enamel.
- Most common materials used as P and F sealants = BIS–GMA, MMA, urethane diacrylate resins.
- Sealants can be pure or can have 15–20% wt. fillers of silanated glass particles.

- Filled resins have more viscosity/less flow and permit better control during placement, improved wear resistance.
- Sealants are **most effective in decreasing caries in young children** when applied shortly after permanent tooth eruption.
- So **sealant Rx in children and young adults is indicated** for non-carious teeth.
- Sealants are **C/I on primary molars**, on carious P and F, on inter-proximal lesions.
- It is best to seal non-carious P and F; however the bacteria present in sealed carious fissures loose their viability and potential to produce demineralization; because they get cut off from saliva and carbohydrates.
- **Sucrose** or other lightly refined carbohydrates in plaque are essential for caries.
- Ortho Rx creates a favourable dental alignment and may intrude periodontally involved teeth for a better bone support.
- Teeth active in mastication collect less plaque than non-functional teeth.
- Most common cause of gingival recession is FAULTY TOOTH BRUSHING.
- Recession also occurs in teeth with extreme facial or lingual inclination wrt the alveolar process.

INSTRUMENTS

Classification: Divided in 6 categories by black:

1. Cutting instruments: hand; rotatory
2. Condensing instruments
3. Plastic instruments
4. Finishing and polishing: hand; rotatory
5. Isolation instruments
6. Miscellaneous

INSTRUMENTS

- Hand cutting instruments
- Rotary cutting instruments
- Ultrasonic instruments

Hand cutting instruments

- Excavators = hatchet; hoe; spoon excavators; discoid and cleoids.
- Chisels = straight; monangle; binangle; triple angle.
- Special form of chisel = hatchets; GMT; angle formers; wedelstaedt chisel; offset hatchet; triangular chisels; hoe chisel.

Rotary instruments

- A rotary tool should be large in diameter, when used with low speeds.
- In ultra high speed, the diameter of tool should be decreased.
- Maximum cutting efficiency of a cutting tool of uniform width ranges b/w 5000–6000 surface feet/min.
- Heat production is directly proportional to = pressure; RPM; area of tooth in contact with the tool.
- Pulp gets permanently damaged if a temperature of 130°F is reached.
- **Vibration** = a rotation of approx 6,000 rpm sets up a fundamental vibrational wave of approx 100 cycles/sec. This is most annoying to the patient and dentist. But vibrations above 1300 cps are imperceptible to patients, which occur at ultra high speed.

Finishing and polishing instruments

- Burs
- Paper carried abrasives
- Brushes
- Rubber
- Cloth
- Felt

Restoring instruments

- Mixing instruments
- Plastic instruments
- Condensing instruments
- Burnishing instruments
- Carvers
- Files
- Knives
- Finishing and polishing instruments

HAND CUTTING INSTRUMENTS: 3 parts:

1. Handle/Shaft.
2. Shank—connects the shaft to blade.
3. Blade/Nib—also known as point/head. It is the functional end of instrument, bears cutting edge, etc.

INSTRUMENT FORMULA

3-unit formula

1. Width of blade = in tenths of a mm
2. Length of blade = in mm.
3. Angle of blade with axis of handle; in hundredths of a circle or centigrades.

4-Unit formula

- i.e. if cutting edge is at an angle other than 90° to blade length.
- It is placed at 2nd position in the formula.
- Describes the angle formed b/w cutting edge and central axis of the shaft; in centigrades.

Important points

- All hand-cutting instruments are Excavators differing in the shape of cutting edge.

- ♦ According to Angle/Angles in shank–4 types.

Straight	No angle
Monangle	One angle
Binangle	Two angles
Triple angle	Three angles

Contra angle = i.e. angling of shank to bring the cutting edge or working point into close proximity to the central axis of instrument.

- ♦ **Single plane instrument** = instrument with 2 or more angles in the shank in a single plane; it could be laid on the table top, e.g. hatchet.
- ♦ **Double plane instrument** = e.g. GMT; has a curved blade; curved blade has lateral scraping ability; All double plane instrument are *lateral cutting instrument*

TYPES OF HAND CUTTING INSTRUMENTS

Chisel
- One sided bevel.
- Cutting edge is ⊥ to plane of instrument.
- If cutting edge is distal to the shaft, it is know as CONTRA - BEVELED/REVERSE beveled chisel.
- Used with *push motion.*
- Monangle/Binangle chisels for MAXILLARY ARCH.

HOE
- Angle of blade is greater than 12.5°C
- Used with *pull motion.*

Hatchet
- CE/cutting edge is in the plane of instrument.
- R and L pair.
- Used for planning/cleaning Enamel and Dentin.
- May be bi-beveled placing the CE in the centre; used to refine line ∠ and point ∠.
- Generally used in MANDIBULAR ARCH.

Angle
- CE is at an ∠ to the BLADE.

Former
- ∠ of CE to the blade axis is 80–85°C.
- 4-unit formula = i.e. ∠ of CE to the shaft.
- Used to accentuate line and point ∠ in internal outline form in cavities.
- Used in *lateral scrapping motion*.
- Blade is beveled on sides and at ends to form 3 cutting edges.
- is a **modified chisel**.

Gingival margin trimmer—is a **modified hatchet**.

- CE is at an angle other than a right ∠ to the axis of blade (while in hatchet, CE is at 90° to blade axis).
- Blade of GMT is curved (while hatchet has straight blade).
- R and L pair.
- Used to bevel gingival cavosurface margin.
- Mesial GMT = 10–80–6–12.
- Distal GMT = 10–95–6–12 (Higher no. is always of Distal GMT).

Spoon excavators—modified hatchet; double plane.

- Rounded cutting edge.
- Action is *scooping/spooning nature.*
- Used for lateral scrapping.
- Paired.
- For removal of carious dentin.

Cleoid discoid instrument—modified double end chisel.

- Cutting edges = spoon shaped.
- Used for carving of amalgam and wax.

Abrasion

- Is the action of wearing away **by friction**.
- e.g. diamond, silicon carbide, aluminum oxide, silicon dioxide.

Air-brasive technique (By RB Black.)

- It is non-mechanical preparation of cavities.

- **30–50 micron aluminium oxide** particle under **110 psi pressure** of CO_2 stream are propelled at tooth surface and funneled through a tungsten carbide nozzle with a lumen of 0.018″.
- Precise, sharply defined cavities not possible with this technique.
- Used generally for smaller carious lesions.

Other important points:

- Mimp function of rotary instruments = action of cutting and abrading.
- Cutting instruments consist of = a six-bladed bur.
- Tungsten carbide burs = harder than SS burs.
  - At higher speeds (70,000 rpm) = lighter force increases cutting efficiency of diamond points.

ULTRASONIC METHOD

- Frequency used—15000–30000 cycles/sec.
- Al_2O_3 **particles** in water slurry is used.
  - **Atraumatic Restorative Techniques** (ART): here, no rotary instruments are used; gross caries removal is done with the help of excavators; the defect is filled with GI cements; it is mostly used in backward/developing countries.

Bur designs

Parts	Features
Bur tooth	It ends up in the cutting edge or blade. It has 2 surfaces: 1. tooth face = which is the side of the tooth on the leading edge. 2. back . flank = which is the side of the tooth on the trailing edge.
Rake angle	Angle which the face of the bur tooth makes with the radial line from the centre of the bur to the blade.

Bur designs (*Contd.*)

Parts	Features
	1. negative = if face is beyond or leading the radial line. 2. zero = if radial line and tooth face coincide with each other; also known as radial rake angle. 3. positive = if radial line leads the face ST rake angle is on the inside of the radial line.
Land	Plane surface immediately following the cutting edge.
Clearance	Angle b/w the back of tooth and the work. If back surface of tooth is curved—it is know as radial clearance.
Tooth angle	Is b/w face and back.
Flute or chip space	i.e. the space b/w adjacent teeth of the bur.

Important points about burs

- More positive the rake angle, greater is the bur's cutting efficiency.
- Radial rake angle bur cut more effectively than with negative rake angle.
- With negative rake angle = the cut chips move directly away from the blade edge and often fracture in small bits/dust.
- With positive rake angle, the chips are larger and tend to clog the chip space. The size of bur tooth is decreased and its tooth angle is decreased, so the bulk is decreased, which can get fractured during cutting.
- Larger clearance angle results in less rapid dulling of the bur.
- No. of teeth in a bur = 6–8.
- If no. of teeth is decreased = thickness of chip removed by each flute increases.
- If no. of teeth is less = the clogging tendency is decreased, but, because they remove more material, the bur wears faster and rougher.

- Bur with straight flutes produces less temperature than with spiral flutes.
- Fewer the no. of teeth, the greater is the tendency of vibrations.
- Burs can be latch type and friction grip types; burs revolve clockwise.
- Round burs = ¼; ½; 1, 2, ——— 10.
- Wheel burs = 14, 15.
- Inverted cones = 33 ¼; 33 ½; 34; 35 ——— 39.
- Plain cylindrical fissure burs = 55 ——— 59.
- Cross cut cylindrical fissure bur = 555 ——— 560.
- Plain tapered fissure bur = 169 ——— 172.
- Cross cut tapered fissure bur = 699 ——— 703.
- Round nose fissure burs = all burs can be round ended. The number 1 will be added to previous numbering, i.e. 155; 1555; 1169, etc.
- Pear shaped = 229 ——— 333; mainly used in **pedodontics.**
- End cutting burs = 900 ——— 904.
- **Run out** = is the eccentricity or maximum displacement of bur head from its axis of rotation. Average acceptable run out is 0.023 mm.
- **Load** = is the force exerted by the dentist on the tool head. For low speed, 1000 gm, i.e. 2 lbs; for high speed 2–4 oz is used.
- **Finishing burs** = should be at least 12 fluted.
- SS burs = for amalgam.
- Tungsten carbide burs = for composite resins.

Speeds used in dentistry

Ultra low speed	300–3000 rpm
Low speed	3000–6000 rpm
Medium high speed	20,000–45,000 rpm
High speed	45,000–100,000 rpm
Ultra high speed	> 100,000 rpm

Speed classification

Speed	Frequency
Conventional/low speed	< 10,000 rpm
Increased/high speed	10,000–1,50,000 rpm
Ultra speed	> 1,50,000 rpm

IMPORTANT POINTS

- Pulp is larger than it appears on R/G.
- Cutting instruments should be sharp, concentric and of proper shape and dimension for removal of caries.
- Removal of deep, pulp encroaching caries should be done by low rotational speeds and bulk removal of enamel and dentin by high speeds.

Instrumentation

- Position of pulpal floor of cavity should ideally be placed in = 0.5 mm into the dentin.
- Unsupported enamel should be removed.
- With spoon excavator, the forces of removal of dentin are directed LATERALLY.
- Slow speed is used for removal of carious dentin; use light forces while removing it.

Steel bur has more number of flutes than the carbide bur and so gives a smoother cutting action.

- Air water coolant = to dissipate heat.
- **Washed field technique** = i.e. high velocity evacuation of coolant.
- Fiber optic hand pieces = increases visualisation of the operative site.
- Ultra speed = is best for penetration through bulk of enamel and extensive removal of enamel.
- Low speeds = for caries removal and cavity refinements.

ROTARY PROCEDURES: For cavity preparation are:

1. **Penetration** = ultra speed; round bur is used.
2. **Extension** = ultra speed; straight/plain fissure bur.
3. **Excavation** = low speed; for caries removal; lighter touch; round bur used.
   - Round carbide bur is more sharp, with less cutting blades; more difficult to control in delicate procedures.
4. **Refinement** = with plain/non-cross cut fissure bur,
   - Excavation of caries lesion should be carried out at low rotational speeds, especially the deep caries encroaching the pulp.
   - Placement of retention areas and other refinements also require low speed. Should always be placed in the dentin without undermining the enamel.
   - Cross-cut burs should not be = used with ultra speed; as they become more of an abrading instrument than a milling instrument.

Noise emission is air turbines

- More noisy.
- Vibration frequencies are > 5000 cps.
- Speech range = 250–3000 cps.
- Intensity of > 85 decibels can lead to hearing diseases.
- Dental ball bearing air turbine noise is = 75–100 db.
- Air bearing hand piece = 60–70 db.
- Effective insulation of walls can increase noise absorption.
- Operate intermittently to reduce fatigue.

At ultra speed

1. At 3–5 lac rpm, only 2–4 oz light force are enough for cutting.
2. Tactile discrimination for the amount of tissue removed is absent.
3. Use small dimension burs for good control.

Instrument grasp methods

1. Pen grasp.
2. Inverted pen grasp.
3. Palm and thumb grasp.
4. Modified palm and thumb grasp.

Instrument grasps

Pen grasp grasp	Very accurate control most effective and universally used grasp.
Inverted pen	Used in upper teeth 3rd/4th finger rests on adjacent tooth of the same jaw.
Palm and thumb	Used on maxillary teeth esp of right side. Thumb rests at some distance from the point of operation.
Modified palm and thumb grasp	Greater freedom of movement and delicacy of control. Prevents instrument slippage. Hand is only about half-closed. End of thumb is used for the rest.

- **Pen grasp** = most frequently used; esp in **mandibular arch**; 2-handed control of both hand and rotary instrument is recommended.
- **Inverted pen grasp** = palm and finger tips are directed towards the operator. Used in maxillary arch on both L/R side. Dentist stands behind the patient at 11 O'clock .
- **Palm and thumb grasp** = Tip of thumb is the rest or pivot. Mostly used in **maxillary arch**.

Sterilization: (Refer to section of microbiology Vol. II)

- Is complete destruction of all microbial life including spores.
- Cutting edges of instrument must be protected during autoclaving by an oil emulsion coating.
- Autoclaving is the most reliable method; done at 121 C × 15 psi × 10 min.

Disinfection: It is the destruction of most of the pathogens from inanimate surfaces; can be done by:

1. 100°C water × 30 min.
2. 2% alkaline glutraldelyde for 10 min (for 10 hrs if instruments have been used in a TB patient or spores forming infection).
3. 1% NaOCl × 10 min.
4. 2% formaldehyde and 20–30 min.
5. Quaternary Ammonium compounds are not effective vs spores/virus and should not be used for disinfections.

For scrubbing the **chair/handles,** etc.

1. Detergents = to remove dried blood
2. 90% isopropyl alcohol or 70% ethyl alcohol = remove dried blood/saliva.
3. 5% iodophor in 70% isopropyl alcohol.
4. Air-water syringe line should be flushed for 3 min to decrease **Pseudomonas aeruginosa.**
   - Corrosion of instruments made of SS and Tungsten carbide can be prevented by using 2% sodium nitrite solution coating.
   - Autoclaving is done at 121 C × 15 psi × 10 min, i.e. (249.8°F) or at 258°F × 35 psi × 5 min
   - Ethylene oxide gas × 3 hrs applications; (total 24 hrs with aeration also).

BIOLOGICAL CONSIDERATIONS

Mechanical properties of teeth

- Compressive strength of enamel supported by vital dentin is = 36000–42000 psi.
- Compressive strength of vital dentin = 40000–50000 psi.
- Modulus of elasticity of enamel supported by vital dentin under compression = 70 lac psi.
- MOE of vital dentin = 19 lac psi.
- Tensile strength of dentin is about 10% less than its compressive strength.

- ♦ Tensile strength and compressive strength of enamel is same.
- Dentin is the secretory products of pulp.
- Enamel is hardest substance in the body due to its high mineral content, approx 95% inorganic and 5% organic + water.
- KHN of different dental tissues is

Enamel	–343
Dentin	– 68
C emcutum	– 40

- Enamel is 5–20 × more resistant to abrasion than dentin.
- Enamel rod = are made of many HA crystals, extend at right angles from dentin outward to the tooth surface.
- Rod sheath contains more ORAGANIC substance than the rod and so not as susceptible to demineralization by acids.
- Fluoride prevents caries by decreasing the enamel dissolution by making fluorapatite crystals, which are more resistant to acids produced. Fluoride facilitates redeposition of mineral as apatite, when acid attack has subsided.
- Walls of the cavity should be parallel to enamel rods direction leaving no unsupported enamel, which otherwise gets broken.
- Cavity preparation with an inter-cuspal distance of 1/4 to 1/3 results in sound enamel. If width is 1/2 the ICD, the cavity walls require increasingly greater divergence (inlay taper) to be parallel to enamel rods.
- For amalgam: the buccal/lingual/gingival walls of proximal box should be at right angles to the cavosurface for supported enamel rods.
- For gold: Bevel is used for proper adaptation of gold to the margins of the cavity.
- For class 5 cavity:
  1. Occlusal and gingival walls are diverging.
  2. Cavosurface angulation of occlusal walls must become more OBTUSE as the position of this margin approaches the occlusal surface of the tooth. It may be 120–130° to assure a sound enamel margin.
- Cuspal protection = minimum restoration required is gold only.

Biologic aspects of dental materials: Pulp injury may occur due to:

- Heat and dessication.
- Pressure generated during condensation of gold and silver
- Due to inherent irritational potential of materials, e.g. silicate cement; composite resin; so a protective base should be placed below them.
- Remaining dentin thickness is less.
- Presence or absence of reparative dentin below the cut dentin.

Acid etching

- Increases surface area by creating the micro-pores in the enamel surface **by 200 times** for bonding by creating micro-mechanical pores in the surface.
- 37–50% of buffered ortho-phosphoric acid for 1 minute. Latest researches say that etching time of 15–20 sec is enough.
- Rinse for at least 15 sec for washing; and air dry the surface for 60 sec. The air should be free of oil, etc.
- Etched Enamel surface appears as frosty/chalky white.
- Longer etching results in greater loss of enamel.
- A cavosurface bevel of enamel = gives more uniform etching.
- Etched pattern consists of 3 zones from surface inwards:

Pattern	**Depth**
Etched zone/enamel removed	10 micrometers
Qualitative porous zone	20 micrometers
Quantitative porous zone	20 micrometers

So composite resin tags can penetrate upto 50 microns into enamel to give retention.

- Provides higher surface energy to enhance WETTING.
- Demineralisation of rod ends occurs, in which resin flows to form RESIN TAGS.

- The bond is micro-mechanical/MECHANICAL.
- Salivary contamination deposits salivary mucoid material and remineralisation of etched enamel. So re-etching is to be done.
- Etched enamel returns to pre-etched state if exposed to oral atmosphere for 1 hrs.
- Complete remineralisation occurs within 45 days after etching.
- Acid etching of dentin = Removes smear layer, opens the dentinal tubules to the pulp, which act as pathway of micro-leakage to pulp.

Enamel

- 95% mineralized/inorganic component. Due to its uniformity, the pattern of acid etching is good; but the dentin contains both organic and inorganic components and so its etching pattern is not that good for good retention as of enamel. So dentin bonding agents are required.
- Demineralization—initially a **whitish lesion** with **decreased translucency**.
- Increased demineralization increases its OPACITY and friability, decreased hardness.

Dentin

- Carious dentin is soft and tends to be penetrated by explorer under light pressure.
- A clear **chatter sound** comes on normal dentin.
- KHN of sound/primary dentin = 61.
- KHN of reparative dentin = 40.
- **0.5% Basic Fuchsin** in propylene glycol for 10 sec = this stain affects that dentin, whose collegen fibers have been denatured irreversibly. Cross-linking of these fibers is reduced beyond REMINERALIZATION.

Dentin: refer to section of dental histology for details

DIFFERENT TYPES OF DENTIN: From lowest to highest permeability are:

- Calcific barrier dentin.

- Sclerosed dentin.
- Primary dentin.
- Secondary dentin.
- Tertiary/reparative dentin.
- Globular dentin.
- Granular dentin.
- Dead tract dentin.
- Forms the greatest bulk of the tooth.
- 70% inorganic + 30% organic.
- Made of collagen fibers and ground substances of muco-polysaccharide.
- KHN = 68, (enamel = 343), i.e. enamel is 5 times harder than dentin.
- Dentinal tubules = are of S shape curve.
- 30000–70000 /mm^2 of dentin = number of tubules per square mm of dentin.
- Only 100–150 micron thickness of dentin from the pulp contains free nerve endings. That is why the pain is felt during cavity preparation at that point.
- Pain in dentin is due to **tactile stimuli** like pressure; **probing**, etc. It is due to **rapid inflow** of the dentinal fluids from the dentinal tubules to the pulp.
- Pain due to osmotic stimuli like **sweets** is due to **rapid outflow** of the fluid form the dentinal tubules.
- Pain due to thermal stimuli is also due to **rapid outflow (cold stimuli)**; or **inflow (hot stimuli)** of dentinal fluid.
- **Pain transmission** = is through **hydrodynamic theory** of dentin sensitivity. Fluid in dentinal tubules moves under stimuli and stimulates the free nerve endings in pulp/dentin. No pain killer is effective in such conditions.
- Sensitive dentin indicates that the underlying tubules are open to the pulp.
- Fluid pressure is higher in pulp than in oral cavity.

- Air drying of freshly cut dentin causes evaporation of dentinal fluid causing fluid movement and sensitivity due to stimulation of pulpal nerves and pain.
- Bases applied in the cavity compensate for the lost dentin tissue. Bases/Varnish/Liner also compensate for setting shrinkage of restorative materials.
- Varnish/Base materials plug the dentinal tubules and prevent fluid movement in dentin, and thus prevent the hypersensitivity.
- Potassium nitrate containing tooth pastes also help in reducing the sensitivity.
- **Dentin bonding agents** = bonding to dentin is difficult due to its high organic and water content and presence of smear layer. DBA help to overcome these problems esp in class V and II cavities extending on dentin or cementum. DBA removes the smear layer, exposes the collagen and opens the dentinal tubules. Then DBA is applied, which has difunctional ends, the hydrophilic end attaches to dentin and the hydrophobic end bonds to the composite resin.

Important points

- 1 mm square of cut dentin exposes 30000–45000 dentinal tubules.
- Carbide burs are more cool–cutting than steel burs.
- Rotary abrasive instrument stones are not used on vital dentin as it may increase the temperature. So abrasive action should be confined to enamel and superficial 1 mm of dentin.
- **Effective depth** = is the thickness of dentin bridge b/w floor of cavity and roof of pulp chamber.
- If pulp temperature increases by 11 F—it may cause destructive reaction in pulp.
- Most deleterious speed is 3,000–30,000 rpm.
- In making pin holes, the speed should not exceed 3,000 rpm.
- Instrumentation pressure should not be more than 4 oz, when using high speed and 12 oz with low speed.
- When RPMs are increased, the size of cutting head should be decreased.

- Desiccation of vital dentin results in the **aspiration of nuclei of odontoblasts** into the tubules and may increase the permeability of vital dentin to the irritants.
- Cementum is thinnest over the cervical portion of the root and becomes thick towards the apex. It is the softest of all the hard tissues of tooth.

Factors affecting health of pulp and dentin

- Irritation stimuli lead to pulpal inflammation and then reparative dentin formation.
- *High speed cutting* with *copious water coolant* and a *light force* = results in MINIMAL HISTOLOGIC alteration of pulp.
- Cavity depth = dentin having remaining **thickness of 2 mm** or more acts as a good barrier vs the trauma of instrumentation.
- Pulpal response is more in larger and deeper cavity.
- Reparative dentin acts as an INSULATOR.
- Compressed air = prolonged use of dry air on a prepared cavity causes a DELAYED HEALING RESPONSE.
- 30 sec compressed air drying can cause pulpal inflammation and displacement of odontoblasts cells in the dentinal tubules. In most cases, this damage is REVERSIBLE.

DENTIN PRE-TREATMENT

Smear Layer: Amorphous layer of organic film and debris deposited on DENTIN during cutting is called smear layer.

- Acts as a cavity liner by sealing the dentinal tubules.
- But inhibits effective ion exchange and bonding of GI to tooth surfaces. So dentin should be pre-treated to remove it.
- Should be SELECTIVELY removed from dentin surface leaving the tubules filled.
- Open tubules may allow dentinal fluid to come on dentin surface, reducing proper bonding or/and irritant may go towards pulp.

Agents used

- Citric acid
  - (a) Poly-acrylic acid = Best; leaves tubules partially occluded
  - (b) EDTA
- Tannic acid
  - PAA/Poly-acrylic acid conditioning is done for 10–20 sec. But longer time can remove peritubular dentin and open the tubules.

Smear layer

- It is an uniform amorphous layer, which occludes the dentinal tubules.
- It prevents penetration of bacteria in the tubules, but does not prevent penetration of fluids through the dentin, e.g. bacterial products may cause pulpal inflammation.
- It greatly reduces dentin permeability and protects the dentin from hydrostatic forces.
- DILUTE EDTA is used to scrub the smear layer, but leaving the tubules blocked.
- **Potassium oxalate** can be used as a cavity liner. It removes smear layer and forms a calcium oxalate layer. It decreases dentin permeability and is resistant to ACID ATTACK.
- It can also provide ADEQUATE seal at the dentin interface and can be used to Rx dentin hypersensitivity.

Direct pulp capping (DPC)

- Its purpose is to preserve pulp vitality by using a medicament on exposure site, which provides an environment for the tooth to heal, e.g. $Ca(OH)_2$ is the best choice.
- A small, pin - point exposure **in young patient** has more chances of success due to VASCULARITY OF PULP AND SIZE OF exposure.
- Mechanically exposed teeth have greater chances of success than carious exposure, due to less pulpal inflammation and bacterial toxins.

Indirect pulp capping (IPC)

- Involves removal of all carious dentine except the deepest layer to prevent exposure.
- Placing calcium hydroxide dressing on some residual carious dentin, for the formation of reparative dentin.
- Helps in formation of reparative dentin by the pulp.
- It causes cell death of bacteria at high pH of 11–12, especially of those bacteria having pH optima below 7 as of most of aciduric organisms.
- It makes the remaining carious sterile of bacteria (with cannot withstand high pH).
- Best success in young patients due to large volume of pulpal tissues and good vascularity, which helps good healing.

BASIC Rx PROCEDURES

A. There are 4 **major zones of activity** around the operation field:

1. Operator's zone
2. Transfer zone
3. Assistant zone
4. Static zone.

B. **Positions**

- 12 O'clock = for U/L POSTERIOR segment.
  - Requires use of mouth mirror.
  - Requires severe bending of back and neck.
- 11 O'clock = most UNIVERSAL POSITION.

  Access to all areas except = most distal areas of mandibular right posterior teeth and cervical areas on right posterior teeth.
- 9 O'clock/7 O'clock = alternate position for mandibular right posterior teeth.

Transfer zone: Located near oral cavity, where instruments are transferred b/w operator and assistant. It is just in front of and slightly below the patient's mouth.

Assistant zone: At 3 O'clock position.

Static zone: Contains auxillary equipments.

Operator's position

- Operator seated well back on stool.
- Feet flat on floor.
- Legs relaxed and relatively together.
- **Thighs parallel** to the floor.
- Back straight and supported by back-rest.
- **16–18 inches** is the optimal eye to work distance.
- Usual operating position is b/w 10 to 12 O'clock wrt to the patient.
- Lower leg making a 90 degree angle with upper leg
- Straight line unobstructed of area of operations.

Patient's position

- In semi-supine or supine position.
- Operative field/oral cavity should be over the **operator's lap** at the height of operator's elbow.
- Operators **forearm should be parallel** to the floor.
- Pt's **ankles and chin should be at the same level**. If legs are higher than head, it may cause POSTURAL HYPOTENSION.
- For LA = supine position. But patient should be more upright for inferior alveolar block.

Dentist and patient seating positions

Quadrant	Dentist	Paticnt
Lower right	7–9 O'clock	2–4 O'clock
Lower front	Same	Same
Lower left	10–11 O'clock	3 O'clock
Upper and lower front	Same	Same
Upper arch with mirror	11–12 O'clock	3–5 O'clock
Upper right facial and left	7–10 O'clock	

Assistant's position: His head/stool should be 4–6″ higher than the operator to improve the vision. It is usually placed b/w 2 or 3 O'clock position. Assistant seated at a higher position than dr. so that his knees are at the level of pt's head and his feet rest on the foot rest of his stool.

Light position

- Operatory light should be placed at an arms length from the operator.
- Higher light position is used for mandibular arch.
- Lower light position is used for maxillary arch.
- Lower light position is used for indirect vision.
- Higher light position is used for direct vision.

ISOLATION

Various methods of attaining the isolation are:

1. Anti-Sialogogue drugs, e.g. atropinel; propantheline bromide.
2. An aesthetics.
3. Saliva ejectors and high vacuum evacuating devices.
4. Absorbents and cotton rolls.
5. Rubber dam.

Ideal isolation = by rubber dam.

An astringent retraction cord = decreases seepage from gingival crevice.

Adrenaline impregnated cord = **0.5 mg/inch adr**.

Rubber Dam: By SC Barnum (1860s).

♦ Parts of rubber dam:

Parts	Features
RD sheet	• rubber sheet of 5 × 5 or 6 × 6 inches size • 5 types = thin (0.006 inches); medium (0.008 inches); heavy (0.010 inches); extra heavy (0.012 inches); special duty (0.014 inches). • are of green or blue colour for colour contrast; • dull side of the sheet faces towards occlusal side to avoid light reflection.
RD holder	Mostly Young's holder is used.
RD clamp/	2 types = winged; wing less; smaller size retainers for premolars; larger size for molars; no. 212 clamp is used for retracting the RD sheet during class V restorations; its bow is placed towards distal side;
RD punch Clamp holding devices	

♦ Types = light, medium, heavy and extra heavy.

Hole punching

♦ 2 inches RD material peripheral to lower anteriors; lateral to U/L posteriors on each side.

♦ 1–1.5 inches peripheral to upper anteriors.

♦ Holes for anterior teeth follow a curve.

♦ Holes for premolars follow a straight line parallel to midline.

♦ Holes for molars follow a straight line, slightly inclined towards midline.

- For class V lesion, the hole is punched 2–3 mm away from normal arch line. And a clamp of 212 series is used.
- Isolation of anterior teeth = at least one tooth behind the one being operated to the opposite canine.
- Inter-septal rubber should have 4–5 mm width. It helps in gingival retraction and prevents the seepage due to its snug fit.
- Single tooth isolation is used for RCT.
- In RCT, light or medium RD sheet is used.
- Removal = done by clipping the inter-septal rubber.
    - Made of latex; indicated for **absolute dryness**.
    - **Dark coloured** = for good contrast; for decreasing light reflection.
    - 5″ wide = used with Young's frame.
    - 6″ wide = used with Enodon frame.
    - Mostly heavy weight is needed, as it also helps in **retraction of gingival** tissues.
    - RD clamp for securing on posterior tooth.
    - Enodon frame helps in formation of a RD pouch, in which water gets collected, which can be removed by saliva ejector.
    - Anti-sialogogues = atropine 5 mg given 1/2 hr before the appointment.

Factors/Imp points

- Involve at least one tooth posterior to the being operated extending to some position beyond the MIDLINE into the adjacent quadrant.
- More teeth isolated, the better is the access and easier isolation.
- Dental floss should be tied to the RD clamps = it helps in retrieval of the clamp, if it becomes dislodged toward pharynx.
- RD clamp is first placed in LIINGUAL CERVICAL position. A uniform **4-point contact** of the jaws of the clamp is ideal.
- Superior border of RD sheet should be JUST BELOW THE NARES, not obstructing BREATHING.

- Normal spacing from the border of one hole to the adjacent hole = 4 mm, except in Maxillary anterior region, where 5 mm space is required.
- While removing, the I/D rubber is cut for easy removal.

VARNISHES, BASES AND LINERS

Ideal requirements of a protective base:

- Well tolerated by the pulp (Blocompatible).
- Should promote reparative dentin formation.
- Should provide adequate pulp protection.
- Should have adequate physical properties to withstand forces.
- Anti-bacterial properties.
- Obtundent effect on pulp.
- Be compatible with restorative materials.
- Eg ZOE; $Ca(OH)_2$, glass-inomer, etc.

VARNISHES (Also refer to sections of pedo and dental materials.)

Varnishes are the film forming solutions.

- Made of natural gums, synthetic resins or rosins.
- e.g. copal resin dissolved is chloroform.
- These are the solution of resins in **volatile solvents**.
- Produce a resinous solute layer of a few micron thickness upon evaporation of organic solvent.
- Less soluble than cavity liners.
- Multiple layers (2–3) are better than single layer, it helps to seal the holes/defects due to formation of bubbles during evaporation of solvent.
- Should **not be used beneath composite resins,** because CR results in discontinuous varnish film.
- Provides no thermal insulation; but only helps to **prevent the microleakage.**
- Also helps to reduce the dentinal sensitivity.
- Decreases pulpal response.

- Decreases penetration of corrosion products in dentin and of acid from $ZnPO_4$ cement.
- Can be used even on CAVOSURFACE margins as it is **insoluble in the oral fluids**.
- Should be placed below Zn-PO_4 cement to prevent acidic attack on the pulp.
- Can be applied to enamel, dentin and cavo-surface margins.
- MMA (BIS–GMA monomers destroy varnish layers and should not be used.)

Liners (Intermediary bases) (Also refer to sections of pedo and dental materials.)

- These are the liquids in which $Ca(OH)_2$/ZnO are suspended in natural/synthetic resins.
- Minimize/prevent micro leakage.
- Also change physiologic environment by their peculiar chemical characteristics.
- It provides a chemical barrier; very thin layer is applied.
- Thin membrane is formed; it is **soluble in oral fluids**; so should not be placed on CAVO-SURFACE margins, it provides very little thermal insulation due to its thinness.
- Liners-Prevent micro-leakage; have some therapeutic effect on pulp. Does not have proper strength; are soluble in oral fluids.
- Sound dentin is the best barrier b/w pulp and restoration.
- Liner contains resin and ZnO/$Ca(OH)_2$ dissolved in volatile liquids.
- Varnish does not contain ZnO/$Ca(OH)_2$.
- Both are used in liquid form.

Cavity Liner suspensions

- Made of $Ca(OH)_2$, ZnO in resinous solutions; are used esp with composite resins.
- They form thicker films.
- Should not be placed on cavosurface margins, because of high solubility and so micro-leakage can occur.

- If placed on enamel, the opacity mars the esthetics, so must be restricted to dentin.
- $Ca(OH)_2$ in methyl-cellulose can also be used, but it does not adhere to dentin as compared to resin-containing liners.
- Can be used for pulp capping if $Ca(OH)_2$ is present in it.

Intermediary base

- Acts as a protective barrier.
- It has therapeutic effects also, e.g. $Ca(OH)_2$ in Direct Pulp Capping/IPC.
- It has low compressive strength and Mod of Elasticity (MOE).
- Provides a chemical protective barrier; if bulky, then provides thermal insulation.
- Thicker layer used—so better thermal insulators.
- e.g. $Ca(OH)_2$; modified ZOE, they retard penetration of acid.
- Eugenol–has topical anesthetic property; obtundent effect, decrease discomfort associated with dental caries and instrumentation; used to cover deeper dentin in class C deep caries.
- Eugenol is C/I with resin materials, as it hampers with the polymerization of resins.

ZOE

- Excellent sealing qualities.
- Bacteriostatic.
- **ZOE beneath composite resins is C/I,** because eugenol retards the polymerization of resin and dissolves the liner.
- A set matrix consists of unreacted ZnO particles held in a ZINC-EUGENOLATE material.
- Acts as a competitive inhibitor of ***Enz. PG synthetase*** at 10^{-5} to 10^{-4} mol/L range. Aspirin acts as anti-inflammatory effect by an irreversible inhibition of the same enzyme.
- It inhibits SENSORY N. ACTIVITY reversibly in 10^{-4} to 10^{-3} mol/L range.
- It is irreversibly NEUROTOXIC above 10^{-3} mol/L.

- A reversible VASODILATOR in 10^{-4} to 10^{-3} mol/L range.
- Reversibly inhibits RESPIRATION in mammalian cells in 10^{-4} to 10^{-3} mol/L range.
- Cells get killed by prolonged (12 hrs) exposure to 10^{-3} mol/L and by brief (minutes) to 10^{-2} mol/L. Cells survive prolonged exposure to 10^{-4} mol/L.
- Eugenol kills a range of intra oral organisms at 10^{-3} to 10^{-2} mol/L.

Mechanisms of ZOE (Also refer to sections of pedo and dental materials.)

- ZOE seals and excludes dietary substrate from bacteria, preventing decomposition.
- Kills microorganisms and halts spread of the lesion and bacterial toxins and so helps pulpal recovery.
- A conc. of 10^{-4} mol/L is there in the pulp adj. to intact dentin for at least 10 weeks—it decreases sensory nerve activity, increases blood flow and clearance of toxins; decreases PG synthesis and inflammation.
- Low thermal conductivity of ZOE and a good barrier to chemical diffusion will also decrease other insults to the pulp.

Calcium hydroxide (Also refer to sections of pedo and dental materials.)

- Used for direct and indirect pulp capping (DPC/IPC)
- Used for weeping canals in RCT.
- Used for Rx of internal resorption; apexification and apexogenesis; periapical resorption, etc.
- Is **acid etching resistant** liner beneath filled/unfilled CR.
- Helps in producing reparative dentin and so pulp to heal.
- BACTERICIDAL.
- May cause dystrophic calcification and obliteration of pulp chamber, which may be due to extensive and repeated irritation/micro-leakage and reparative dentin formation only.
- ZOE should not be used on exposed pulp or under CR.

Mechanism of action of calcium hydroxide

- $Ca(OH)_2$ in contact with pulp immediately causes severe inflammatory response. $Ca(OH)_2$ causes following reactions adjacent to the tissue it is placed:
  - LOCALISD NEOROSIS of pulp.
  - Inflammatory cells collect here.
  - Undifferentiated mesenchymal cells proliferate to form odontoblasts.
  - Reparative dentin forms in apprpox 1 month after the capping.
  - Causes formation of reparative dentin.
  - It is basic with pH = 11.
  - It causes a **superficial zone of coagulation necrosis**. New odontoblasts then develop through differentiation of undifferentiated mesenchymal cells in pulp and cause reparative dentin formation.

Cement Bases–e.g. Zinc phosphate/GI/Zinc poly-carboxylate/ Reinforced ZOE (Also refer to sections of pedo and dental materials.)

- Its main function is to **replace the dentin thickness lost** due to caries and cavity preparation.
  - **It provides** chemical/thermal insulation .
  - Have low thermal conductivity; high compressive strength and stiffness.
  - Replaces the lost bulk of dentin
  - Bases with compressive strength upto 200 psi are capable of supporting amalgam condensation.
- Provides bulk and strength; thermal insulation.
- $Zn(PO)_4$ cement has thermal conductivity similar to dentin and a high compressive strength.
- GI = has ability to bond to dentine and high compressive strength; a good sealing capacity. It chemically adheres to the dentin or enamel. No micro-leakage (Chemical adhesion).

- Bases are not required below CR, because the conductivity of CR is same as dentin. But $Ca(OH)_2$/GI may be used as liners to act as barrier to the monomer of resin and to micro-leakage.
- e.g. $ZnPO_4$/Reinforced ZOE/GI/Zinc-poly carboxylate cements.
- GI/Zn-PC = form chemical bond and get adhesion to dental tissues.
- Grooves may be placed for retention of cement bases into dentin by burs-grooves are directed LATERALLY from the pulp to avoid pulp exposures.

Strength requirement for cement bases

- Strongest cement, e.g. $ZnPO_4$/GI should be used to minimize tensile stresses and to bear the occlusal stresses.

$Ca(OH)_2$—used in 3 special circumstances.

- Direct pulp capping—as protective chemical barrier below the resins.
- Indirect pulp capping—as protective chemical barrier below the resins.
- For primary teeth esp if much loss of dentin is there.
- Thermal insulating property = can be used below silver-amalgam in class B depth cavities.
- Has no OBTUNDENT features.
- Compressive strength = 1500–4000 psi; not suitable under heavy occlusal pressure.
- Light cure $Ca(OH)_2$ material = has compressive strength = 12,000 psi.

$ZnPO_4$

- Varnish should be placed before $ZnPO_4$ to cover the dentin to prevent acid insult.

Reinforced ZOE

- Non–irritating to dentin
- No cavity varnish required.

Zn–PC

- No liner required below it.
- Adhesive to tooth.

GI cement = ABC

A. Adhesion to enamel/dentin.
   - Good support to restorative materials.

B. Biocompatible.
   - Under CR = for S and with technique.

C. Fluoride = anti-caries.

Mixing:

- Reaction b/w $ZnPO_4$ powder and liquid is **exothermic**. So use cool slab and wide area for mixing.
- Cool slab permits INCORPORATION of more powder and hence more strength.
- 70° F temperature is required for cooling slab.
- 6 increments spatulated for 15 sec each and so 90 sec are required for proper mixing.

Glass–Ionomer Cement

- Setting reaction is not exothermic.
- Reaction of PAA with alumino-silicate glass is fast = so cement must be placed, at proper time for proper adhesive bond.
- In water hardening cements – polyacid is dried, which is mixed with H_2O before mixing.
- Insertion of mix should be completed before the loss of gloss = to form a good adhesion to dentin.
- But in very deep cavity = the pulpal walls should be protected by using $Ca(OH)_2$.

Provisional restorations

- Maintains the position of the prepared tooth.
- ZOE acts as obtundent to the pulp.

- ZOE seals the cut dentin from oral fluids.
- After placing in the cavity = the hot water cotton pallet is wiped over the cement surface to HASTEN THE SETTING.

GI–CR laminate technique or scientist technique

It is used to fill the pits and fissures of a tooth to prevent the development of caries. Base of the fissures is sealed with GI cement as it is adhesive and releases the fluoride as anti-caries effect; the CR is placed on the GI after etching; as it is stronger and can withstand the heavy occlusal forces.

Gingival tissue M/M (Also refer to section on prostho.)

A. Mechanical method

- By extra heavy weight rubber dam = causes tissue retraction; prevent seepage of fluids.
- By placing cotton twills in gingival sulcus before starting the operative procedure.
- Fine cotton twills with ZOE cement are packed in sulcus. It puts GENTLE PRESSURE for some period of time for gingival displacement. It is most effective and conservative of all mechanical methods. But most time consuming (2–7 days).
- Tissues should be reflected laterally, but not compressed APICALLY.

B. Surgical removal

- Most effective = electro-surgery.
- Less bleeding.
- Cutting needle should not contact cementum and bone.

C. Chemical method

- Adrenaline impregnated cord = **0.5 mg/inch adr**.
- Should not be used in heart patients.
- Causes vasoconstriction and tissue shrinkage.

CHEMICAL TISSUE RETRACTION

- For impression of finish lines.
- But can damage the attachment of junctional epithelium.

- Cords = knitted/braided/loosely woven made of COTTON.
- May be plain/chemical.
- 2 types of drugs used = vasoconstrictor/astringents.
- **Vasoconstrictors** = Epinephrine; ***0.5 mg/inch of racemic epinephrine***; its causes shrinkage of tissues by constriction of blood vessels and thus decreasing local tissue contour.
- But C/I in HT/heart disease/DM/hyperthyroidism.
- **Astringent** = especially aluminium chloride, or ferric sulfate solutions. Its effect is shrinkage of tissues by decreasing flow of fluid and by coagulation and precipitation of thin surface films. Should not be used in excess, as can cause chemical burns due to low pH.
- Dry field is required for retraction, so anti-sialogogue drugs may be given.
- Chemical tissue peck should **not be left in sulcus for > 5 min**. It should be of WEDGE shape.

GINGIVAL RETRACTION

Method	Features
Physico-mechanical	• e.g. temporary restorations. • rolled cotton/synthetic cord. • heavy weight rubber dam sheet.
Chemical method	• **vasoconstrictor** = e.g. racemic Adr and N Adr. • **biologic fluid coagulants** = e.g. 100% alum; 15–25% aluminium chloride; 10% aluminum potassium sulfate; 15–25% tannic acid; they are very safe and no systemic effects. • **surface layer tissue coagulants** = 8% zinc chloride; silver nitrate; can produce local ulcerations, etc.

GINGIVAL RETRACTION (*Contd.*)

Method	Features
Electrosurgical means	• **cutting** = extremely precise; bloodless; with minimum tissue involvement and after effects. • **coagulations** = causes surface coagulation of tissues, their fluids; blood, etc. It occurs due to thermal energy; if overdone it leads to carbonization. • **fulgeration** = causes deeper tissue involvement; always accompanied by carbonization; greater energy is used. • **desiccation** = involve greater tissue depth and area; it is most unlimited uncontrolled, and unpredictable. • during electrosurgery, use light touches and rapid intermittent strokes. • never involve the crest of the free gingival, but only the internal walls of the sulcus. • probe type electrodes = J—or loop shaped. • **bipolar electrodes** are used for fulgerations and desiccation. • **unipolar electrodes** are used for cutting and coagulation.
Surgical methods	

SEPARATION OF TEETH

- Helps to detect a proximal carious lesion in direct visibility.
- Provides space for finishing, matrix band placement, etc.
- **Methods = active or immediate,** i.e. occurs within 30 sec.; **passive** or **slow,** which requires 24 hrs time.

- **Active** is done by wedge method **(Elliot** separator); or traction **(Ferrier** separator).
- Wedging method is preferred over traction, as wedging is less injurious to PD tissues; and applies less pressure than traction method.

  1. **Wedge method** = elliot separator; wood or plastic wedges.
  2. **Traction method** = ferrier double bow separator.
- **Passive separation or slow separation** = by rubber dam separator; separating ligature or brass wires; orthodontic separators; orthodontic appliances, etc. Orthodontic grass line ligature contracts under moisture and leads to separation.

WEDGE

It is defined as the wooden or plastic conical shaped device, which is inserted in the embrasure area in order to attain intimate adaptation of matrix band with the tooth and also to attain some sort of separation of teeth to provide room for the matrix band.

It is of 2 types = wooden or plastic; orange wood stick is the best.

Advantages of wedge

- It prevents the overhang of the filling.
- Helps in effective condensation of the material.
- Helps to attain anatomic contour of the restoration.
- Causes some separation of the teeth.
- Helps in intimate adaptation of the matrix band.
- Is placed below the gingival floor.
- Wooden, triangular in shape; base is placed apically towards the gingival papilla.
- Should be inserted from LINGUAL embrasure because it is wider.
- **Moistened wooden wedge** = better secured position and easier placement.
- **Hard wood wedge** = placed forcefully—separates the teeth due to PDL elasticity and compensates for the thickness of the matrix metal.

- Contact area with adjacent tooth should exhibit the resistance to the passage of dental floss. So the band should be slightly loosened (by 1/4–1/2 turn) after placing the wedge.
- Metal matrix band used is = 0.015″ thick.

Rules for placement

- It is placed from larger to narrower embrasure, i.e. from lingual to buccal.
- It is of triangular shape; the apex faces the occlusal surface and the base towards the gingival surface.
- Should fit snugly in the embrasure without hurting the gingival.
- Wooden wedges are preferred over plastic as they absorb the saliva and further improve the snugness and also easily placed.

MATRIX

It is defined as a thin contoured strip used to substitute the missing wall of a compound or complex cavity in order to attain proper condensation and to restore anatomical contour and contact areas.

Functions = Substitute for lost wall of cavity during restoration.

Ideal requirements of a matrix:

- Should be rigid.
- Arc form is helpful because, when it is tightened, the cervical part becomes constricted and upper part is widened, which conforms the anatomical contour of the tooth.
- Maximum edge strength is required in the cervical region during condensation, so wedge is placed to avoid overhang.
- Restores proper proximal contours. When a band is placed, it separates the teeth as per its thickness; and when band is removed after filling, the teeth come together to make proximal contacts.
- Circumferential band may produce a negative contour and open proximal contact. So the band - CONTOURING should be done to avoid it.
- **Thickness of the band material** = generally ranges from 0.0015 inch to 0.003 inches.

- In **anterior teeth** fillings; the matrix should be transparent to confirm proper adaptation. It also allows passage of light for light curing. Curved **Mylar matrix** strip is used mainly. It helps to make anterior inter-dental contacts.
- It should extend **1–2 mm below cervical edge** and above the incisal edge.
- Direction of pull of matrix strip is away from access opening of the prepared cavity.
- Matrix should be **pulled towards incisal to tighten the strip at cervical margin** and to minimize overextension of the filling material.
- Wedge helps in close cervical adaptation of material.
- Overfilling should be avoided, as filled CR is difficult to finish.
- Light cure allows more working time and incremental additions to build up proper contours.

Examples of MATRICES:

1. Toffelmire matrix = double banded for class I cavity and single banded for class II cavity. It is **in arc form**. The retainer can be placed either from lingual or buccal side; it is also know as **universal matrix band**; it is contra-angled.
2. Ivory no. 1 for **unilateral class II**; band is in curved form.
3. Ivory no. 8 for **bilateral class II cavity.**
4. **Ivory no. 9** = used for compound or complex cavities; MOD cavity; it is a straight metal strip.
5. **Auto-matrix** = is in the form of Cu-bands. Used for highly mutilated teeth or for taking impression of inlay cavities.
6. Black's matrix for Class II cavity.
7. Anatomical matrix = for mutilated and Class II cavity.
8. Roll-in-band matrix, i.e. auto-matrix.
9. S-shaped matrix band = for Class II with facial/lingual extensions; for cavity on the distal surfaces of cuspids.
10. Celluloid strips = for silicate cements; for Class III cavity.
11. Cellophane strips = for resins; for Class III cavity.

12. Mylar strips = for resin/silicates, etc.; for class III cavity.
13. Stock crown matrix = for Class IV cavity.
14. Aluminium foil = stock metallic matrix used for restoring incisal corner; it cannot be used for light cure restorations.
15. Window matrix = for Class V cavity.

Circumferential Retainers

- Completely encircle the tooth.
- e.g. Ivory no. 9 and Toffelmires.
- Straight and contra-angle Toffelmires.
- Used in MO/DO/MOD cavities.
- Retainers lie to buccal side, but Toffelmire contra-angle type lies on lingual side of the tooth.
- Are more stable than unilateral types (i.e. Ivory no. 1).
- Thickness of band material used = 0.0015″.

Medicaments

1. **Antisialogogues**:
   - Are anti-cholnergic agents.
   - Decrease saliva secretion.
   - e.g. Propanthelin bromide.
     - C/I in glaucoma/severe cardiac diseases.
2. **Antianxiety** drugs:
   - Control apprehensions (anxiety).
   - e.g. Benzodiazepines, e.g. Diazepam 10–15 mg, 1 hr before.
   - Barbiturate sedatives act at CNS, e.g. Pentobarbitol sodium; 50–100 mg 1 hr before the appointment.
3. **Antibiotics**
   - To avoid transient BACTEREMIA.
   - Penicillin–V 2.0 gm orally 1 hr before and 1.2 gm orally 6 hr after.
   - To penicillin–allergics—give Erythromycin.

Dentin hypersensitivity = it is an exaggerated response due to non-noxious sensory stimuli; it is due to dentinal fluid movement stimulating pulpal pain receptors. It has a tendency of spontaneous resolution due to deposition of insoluble inorganic precipitates on exposed dentinal tubules from saliva and due to formation of secondary dentin. Most common agent used for its Rx is potassium oxalate and 5% potassium nitrate.

Other methods of Rx of hypersensitivity

1. Cavity varnish.
2. Anti-inflammatory drugs.
3. Partially obturating the dentinal tubules by = burnishing of dentin; silver nitrate; zinc chloride; potassium ferricyanide; formalin, etc. They form insloluble precipitates or protein precipitates on dentin.
4. Calcium hydroxide.
5. Fluoride compounds.
6. Iontophoresis.
7. Dentin bonding agents.
8. GI cement.
9. Restorative resins.
10. Jacket crown in extreme cases.

Management of hypersensitive dentin

- By sealing the exposed dentinal tubules.
- Sensitivity is due to shifting of dentinal fluid by hydrodynamic forces and stimulation of mechano-receptors in pulp.
- 33% NaF/kaolin/glycerin paste creates smear layer in dentin.
- **Potassium oxalate** forms insoluble precipitates of Ca-oxalate, which occludes the dentinal tubules.
- K/Sr salts (KNO_3, etc.) = decrease nerve excitability.
- By **iontophoresis** also.
- Fluorides.

- Commercial pastes, e.g. sensodent K; sensodyne; thermoseal–RA, etc.

Anesthetics

- LA, with vasoconstrictor, which prolongs its duration of action and so a lesser volume of LA is required due to vasoconstriction of micro-circulation.

Astringents

- Cause constriction of tissues, and so arrest the secretions and hemorrhage.
- Aluminium compounds precipitate the protein in attaining their action.
- Vasoconstrictors constrict the blood vessels and controls tissue perfusion.
- Epinephrine or racemic epinephrine (is 15 times more active) = hemostatic due to vasoconstriction of capillaries.

Organic solvents/for degreasing

- Chloroform, acetone, alcohol but irritate tissue and dehydrate the dentin.
- Petroleum distillate, e.g. soltrol–130 has no above-said effects.

Acid neutralizers:

- Sodium bicarbonate in saturated solution is mostly used for neutralizing H_3PO_4 or polyacrylic acid.

DENTAL AMALGAM RESTORATIONS Also see Dental Materials in Vol. II P 210.

Classification of dental amalgam

According to the no. of alloyed metals	• Binary = Ag–Sn • Ternary = Ag–Sn–Cu • Quarternary = Ag–Sn–Cu, In • Unmixed • Admixed

Classification of dental amalgam (*Contd.*)

According to shape of particles	• Spherical = smooth surfaced • Irregular = lathe cut • Spheroidal
Powder's particle	• Micro cut • Fine cut • Coarse cut
According to Cu content	• Low Cu alloy = if Cu is < 4% • High Cu alloy = if Cu is > 10%
Generations	• First gen = Ag + Sn = 3:1 peritectically ratio • 2nd gen = Ag + Sn + 4% Cu + 1 % Zn • 3rd gen = Ag 71.9 % + Cu 28.1 %; it is Ag_3Cu eutectic alloy (spherical particles) added to the original alloy powder; mainly Ag_3Sn • 4th gen = upto 29 % Cu is alloyed to Ag and Sn to form a ternary alloy. Here, Sn is firmly bonded to Cu. • 5th gen = alloy of Ag, Cu, Sn, in to form a quaternary alloy; here none of Sn is available to react with Hg. • 6th gen = PD 10%, Ag 62%, Cu 28% eutectic alloy is lathe cut an is blended I 1st/ 2nd/ 3rd generation alloys in 1:2 ratio; has highest nobility.

- Reaction of Hg with silver amalgam is Physico-chemical in nature.
- Ag, Sn, Zn, and Au were the constituents of **BLACK's amalgam formula** (rather than Cu) initially. Latest is the high - Cu content in alloys as compared to Black's formula

- Zn = deoxidiser; scanvenger; decreases brittleness; increases deformability; resistance to oxidation; ultimate strength, but delayed expansion occurs in contact with moisture.
- Cu = increases strength, brittleness and proportional limit and hardness.
- Reaction = Ag Sn + Hg $\rightarrow$ Ag Hg + Sn Hg + Ag Sn + voids.

4 phases of amalgam mass

Phase	Properties
Gamma	remaining uncreated alloy **strongest, most predominant** phase esp Ag and Sn.
Gamma 1	next most predominant Strongest Ag–Hg phase.
Gamma 2	Sn–Hg phase; **weakest phase.**
Voids/air	Undesirable.

Different phases of amalgam

Phase	Composition	Properties
Gamma	Ag_3Sn	Strongest phase should occupy maximum space.
Gamma 1	Ag_2Hg_3	Noblest phase most resistant to corrosion should have maximum available space in bonding matrix.
Gamma 2	Sn_7Hg_8	Least resistant to corrosion; should occupy least space.
Hg	Hg	Weakest phase of the mass. Decreases strength and hardness. Increases flow and creep.
Voids	Air	Act as nidus for internal corrosion and stress conc.

- Conventional alloy = has Cu < 6% wt.
- Spherical particles are formed by ATOMIZING process.
- High-Cu content alloy = Cu-tin compound eliminates/decreases the WEAKEST and most corrodible phase of amalgam (gamma 2). Cu is upto 30 wt %.
- High Cu = less susceptible to corrosion.
- Compressive strength of amalgam = 5 × greater than tensile strength. So the thicker parts are stronger.

Strength

- Amalgam has a very weak tensile and a very high compressive strength.
- Amalgam looses 15% strength, when its temperature is increased from room to mouth temperature.
- 50% strength is lost if temperature is increased to 60°C.
- 50% compressive strength is lost, when Hg content is increased from 53 to 55 %.
- **Increase in strength** depends on:
  (a) reduction in particle size.
  (b) regularity and smoothness of particle shape and surface.
  (c) more trituration energy.
  (d) more condensation.
  (e) homogenization heat Rx of powder alloy.
  (f) minimum amount of Hg in the mix.
  (g) constituents on original alloy, which have good affinity to Hg, e.g. gamma phase.
  (h) spherical alloy attains strength quickly.
- Thermal conductivity is high, so base should be placed below silver.
- Galvanism and metallic taste can occur with different metal, but PASSIVITY soon takes place on the restorations surface.

Dimensional changes in amalgam: It occurs in 3 stages.

- **Stage 1** = is initial contraction occurs from the absorption of Hg in the inter-particular space of alloy powder.
- **Stage 2** = expansion, it is due to formation and growth of matrix crystals.
- **Stage 3** = limited delayed contraction due to the absorption of unreacted Hg.
- according to ADA–1 = –20 to + 20 micron/cm of D-change is acceptable.
- **Moisture contamination** = in Zn containing alloys, H_2 gas is produced. It occurs after 24–72 hrs and upto **2000 psi pressure** is created. Most obvious detrimental change is a **delayed expansion upto 400 micron/c.c**.

MAIN FEATURES OF CAVITY DESIGN FOR AMALGAM RESTORATION

- If grooves/fissures penetrate less than half the thickness of enamel —then it may be removed by ENAMELOPLASTY.
- **Enameloplasty** is the conversion of shallow fissure into a smooth based groove by removal of enamel; it becomes a part of the tooth surface.
- Unsupported enamel and opaque enamel should be removed.
- Buccal/lingual/cervical clearance of the adj. tooth should be 0.5 mm or less.
- Conservative cutting should be done. Latest in this methods is the ART, i.e. atraumatic restorative technique.
- While replacing any old restoration—keep in mind that cavity size is increased on an average by 0.6 mm each time a restoration is removed.

Reverse curve

- Used to conserve the tooth structure.
- Normally, it is a straight/convex curve where isthmus joins the Bucco-proximal flare.
- It preserves the triangular RIDGE of the affected cusp.

Internal outline form

- Pulpal floor is placed 0.5 mm in dentin; it gives 1.5–2.0 mm of bulk of amalgam for adequate strength.
- Axial walls are placed into dentin for placing RETENTIVE grooves without undermining the enamel.
- **Isthmus width** = 1/3rd of intercuspal distance.
  - 1/5th of BL dim of the tooth.
- Depth is = 0.6–0.7 mm from DEJ.
- Depth of axial wall is less at axio-gingival line angle than at pulpo-axial line angle, because thickness of enamel is LESS cervically.
- Proximal walls should meet the outer tooth surface at right angle to remove all unsupported enamel.
- **Less chances of tooth fracture** are there in cavities—with narrow isthmus and shallow pulpal floor than with wide isthmus and deep pulpal floor; on longer teeth than the smaller teeth; with rounded internal line angles as it help in better force distribution.

Effect of crossing the marginal ridge during cavity preparation:

By 1/4th of intercuspal distance	Decreases the strength of the tooth by 15 %.
By 1/3rd distance	Decreased by 30 %.
By 1/2 distance	Decreased by 40 %.

Effect of crossing the oblique ridge during cavity preparation:

If crossed by 1/4th	Strength decreased by 20 %.
If crossed by 1/3rd	Strength decreased by 35 %.
If crossed by 1/2	Strength decreased by 45 %.

Cement base

- To insulate the pulp against the thermal stimuli.
- Objective = to restore the lost dentin thickness with the cement.

RESISTANCE FORM

- To withstand the stresses of mastication.
- Pulpal and gingival walls should be perpendicular to long axis of the tooth.

RETENTION FORM

- Prevents the filling from being displaced.
- Proximal box = has truncated form or inversely tapered walls to resist occlusally directed tensile forces.
- Grooves are placed in dentin in the proximal box; should be parallel to the PULPAL TISSUES.
- **Dove-tail** = resist proximal displacement.

Removal of remaining carious dentin = should be done after staining with **0.5% basic fuchsin,** i.e. caries detection dye; use slow speed bur/sharp excavator.

Finishing

- Cavo-surface for amalgam should be = BUTT joint, i.e. at 90 degrees; it provides maximum bulk for strength.
- Leave no unsupported enamel.
- Cavo-surface should be parallel to enamel rods direction.
- Pulpal floor should be 0.5 mm beyond DEJ. It is done to pass the zone of maximum innervation of odontoblasts cells extensions. It helps to prevent the sensitivity.

ISTHMUS WIDTH

- Narrower the isthmus width of a cavity (1/4th the inter-cuspal distance) = enamel rods are more convergent towards the occlusal.
- Isthmus width = 1/3 ICD = E rods on the occlusal wall will be more nearly parallel.
- If isthmus width = 1/2 ICD = rods become divergent towards occlusal surface.
- Enamel rods = apically directed near CEJ, so gingival wall more near to CEJ should be reclined slightly apically.

Class V cavities

- Axial wall depth at occlusal wall is greater than at cervical, because enamel is thicker towards occlusal surface.
- A CURVED AXIAL wall is formed parallel to the pulpal contour to avoid over-cutting and encroachment of the pulp.
- Diverging walls are formed due to the direction of enamel rods and so retention grooves are placed in occlusal and cervical walls in the dentin.
- Retention grooves should not be placed in the mesial and distal walls of the cavity to avoid undermining the enamel at line angles.
- Occlusal stops should be on natural tooth surfaces and not on porcelain or porcelain–metal junction.

Class II cavity

- Dental caries starts just cervical to the contact area.
- Proximal margin of cavity should be cleared by 0.5 mm from the adjacent tooth and should be placed in self-cleansing area.
- Walls should be parallel with direction of enamel rods.
- Width of isthmus should be 1/4 to 1/5 of the inter-cuspal distance.
- Cavo-surface angle/ideal flare = 90 degrees/butt joint.
- Retention should be placed in SOUND tooth tissue.
- Gingival floor should incline apically if it is more near to the CEJ, to avoid unsupported enamel rods.
- Proximal box is triangular in shape, with its base at the gingival area, which is self retentive and exposes less area of the marginal ridge to the masticatory forces.
- Pulpo–AXIAL LINE angle should be ROUNDED/BEVELLED to avoid conc. of stresses in the amalgam.
- Retention should always be located in DENTIN, away from pulp; without undermining the enamel.

Tunnel approach = to inter-proximal caries via occlusal or buccal side; keeping marginal ridge intact; suitable for small lesions only.

Class 6 lesions, i.e. 2 class II lesions on the same tooth, which are to be restored with a single restoration, e.g. MOD cavity.

Class 3 lesions = on distal surfaces of canines = should be filled with AMALGAM for better load bear; not of esthetic concern.

- It is a smooth-surface lesion–like class II lesion.
- Starts just apical to contact area in anterior teeth.
- Lesion is entered from LINGUAL side for restoration.
- Proximal box with triangular shape and retention groove is formed.
- Lingual dovetail for retention is formed.

MERCURY TOXICITY

Mercury alloy ratio

- **Eames' technique** = 1:1 ratio so , 50% Hg in the final restoration.
- **High Hg technique** also know as **increasing dryness technique**; Hg is 52–53%.

METHODS TO PREVENT HGG TOXICITY

- Hg is volatile at room temperature; and is 14 times denser than the water.
- Greatest risk to Hg is by **inhalation**. During removal of old restorations OR during polishing of the restoration, a heat generation of 60°C leads to evaporation of Hg. So use adequate **water-cooling**.
- **Threshold limit volume** of Hg for producing Hg toxicity is = 50 micro-gm/cubic metre of the environment. Well ventilated operatory should be made.
- Waste amalgam **should be stored under old x-ray fixing solution or potassium permangnate** solution.
- Avoid spilling **Lead** from RG packets can be **used for absorbing small spillages** along with a paste of equal parts of $Ca(OH)_2$ and flowers of sulfur and water.
- Mercury suppressant powders are also available.
- Waste Hg/amlagam should be sealed in screw top bottles.
- Use **high volume aspiration** during removal of silver fillings.
- Use impervious containers, gloves, masks, etc.

- ♦ Hg may cause hypersensitivity/allergy/contact dermatitis (< 1%). Wash the skin with soap and water after contact.
- ♦ No significant effect on pregnant females, but avoid.
- ♦ Amalgam scrap should be stored in tight bottle and covered with **Sulfide-solutions**.
- ♦ ADA 1 = deals Ag–alloy.
- ♦ ADA 6 = deals with Hg–purity.

Mercury-alloy ratio (Also refer to section on DM in Vol. II, III roles of Hg.)

1. Hg is necessary reactant with alloy particles for developing suitable physical properties of restoration.
2. Hg helps trituration/wetting of alloy particles.
3. Hg influences the plasticity of amalgam and its adaptability to the cavity.
   - M/A are determined by wt-to-wt basis, (wt% of Hg).
   - In pre-weighted capsule, there is < 50% of the Hg.
   - Pre-weight capsule of M and A are best for dispensing.
   - Smaller particle size has more surface area and so trituration is more rapid and rapid setting occurs.
   - Lathe cut alloy particles are ROUGH/irregular; require more Hg.
   - Spherical alloy particles are smooth/regular; require less Hg.
   - Spheres provide MINIMUM SURFACE AREA per unit wt. so less Hg is required.
   - Plasticity of amalgam depends on M/A = higher the Hg more is plasticity. Higher residual Hg content in mix leads to poor properties.
   - Spherical particles exhibit GREATEST PALSTICITY > admixed > lathe cut type.

TRITURATION

- ♦ Wets all surfaces of alloy with Hg.
- ♦ Rubbing of alloy particles ABRADES AWAY the OXIDE FILM on them, which can be easily attacked by Hg.

- Trituration can be done by amalgamator; mortar and pestle; capsule and pestle.
- Mixing should produce a smooth, non-granular plastic mass of amalgam.

Mulling—helps to enhance the uniformity/plasticity of the mass.

Condensation

- Any delay in condensation decreases plasticity and increases residual Hg in final restoration.
- Helps to minimize Hg content as low as possible.
- Force of condensation should be perpendicular to walls of the cavity.
- Avoid voids in the filling; they weaken the mass.
- Mix should be condensed within = 3–3.5 min.
- At least 6 pounds force should be used.
- A minimum thickness of 1.5 mm of amalgam is required for proper strength.
- **Axio-pulpal line angle** has to be beveled **to avoid stress concentration** in class II cavity.
- Width of isthmus should be 1/4th–1/5th of inter-cuspal distance.
- Ideal length to width ratio of a cuspal wall surrounding a Class II cavity should be 1:1 or less in dimensions.
- Cavity varnish should be applied on all walls and floor to avoid micro-leakage and to seal the dentinal tubules.

During condensation—the excess Hg tends to migrate to the surfaces. Hg rich surface should be removed before placing additional increment. This surface Hg helps to bond the subsequent layer of amalgam to the previous one.

(a) Over-filing is done s.t. Hg-rich layer can be removed from final restoration contour and gains UNIFORMITY.

(b) Weakest phase of amalgam = gamma–2 = Sn–Hg

(c) **High Cu alloys** = Cu is 6–25%; are of 2 types = 1. Single composition, i.e. Ag, Sn, Cu these are most resistant to corrosion. 2. Dispersion mix of Ag, Sn, and Cu; Ag.

(d) **Micro-leakage** with amalgam decreases with time by corrosion products; can be decreased **by varnishes; by a bonding agent,** e.g. amalgam bond or **panavia**—21, which has a resin adhesive, which also bonds to set amalgam; and also **by fissure sealants** over the filled restorations.

Condensers—can be smooth/serrated.

- Force of condensation varies inversely with the area of the condenser face.
- If bigger restoration is to be done = then 2–3 fresh mixes should be used, to avoid loss of plasticity and for better condensation.
- Condensers of amalgam differ from those of gold-condensers.

Burnishing

- Helps further condensation and adaptation of amalgam at margins and surface of restoration.
- Helps in making surface strong.
- Adjustment of Marginal Ridges should be done prior to removal of the band.
- A premature contact on the filling should be removed to avoid fracture and Peri-Apical inflammation.

Polishing and Finishing

- Silex slurry with unwebbed rubber cup or soft cup.
- Tin oxide slurry and a soft cup brush used.
- Use low rotation speed with water spray and light intermittent forces to avoid heat production and so as to prevent leaching out of Hg.
- Silicone rubber points and cups.

Refilling (Replacement)

1. Mostly due to secondary caries, which are:
   - Mostly on proximal occlusal lesions, which are
   - Mostly on proximal surfaces of the tooth.

DIRECT ESTHETIC RESTORATIONS DIRECT TOOTH COLORED RESTORATIONS

- Silicate cement
- Unfilled resins
- Filled resins
- Composite resins
- GIC; alumino–silicate polyacrylate cements ASPA

For inter-dental lesions on 2 adjacent incisors = the larger lesion should be prepared first; but the smaller lesion should be filled first.

First translucent cement used = silicate cement by Fletcher.

Silicate cement = causes severe pulpal irritation, which is due to highly acidic H_3PO_4.

- Gel like matrix is formed to bond the unreacted powder particles.
- Gel matrix is **sensitive to early moisture contamination** and dehydration, which may cause severe CRAZING; increased solubility and opacity. So cavity varnish/coca butter/silicane grease is applied on the surface.
- **Fluoride released** = so decreases caries activity.
- High solubility and disintegration in oral fluids and so short clinical life.
- **Contraindicated in mouth breather** patients, otherwise crazing occurs.

Types of GI cements

Type	Features
I	Luting cements for crown/bridge orthodontic bands
II	Restorative cements = are of 2 types • esthetic • reinforced used also as fissure sealants.
III	Fast setting lining material
IV	Light cure and dual cure GI cements

Cermet = i.e. GI in which ion–leachable glass is fused with fine silver powder, held together by metal–salt matrix.

Resin-modified GI = in it, 5% resin (HEMA bis–GMA) is present; initial set of material is by formation of polymerization matrix; which is strengthened by acid–base reaction.

Compomer = i.e. GI with composite resins; composed of single hydrophobic resin filled with acid leachable glass particles.

Resin material

- Chemically activated.
- Lack colour stability.
- High degree of shrinkage during polymerization.
- High coefficient of thermal expansion and so poor marginal adaptation.
- Resilient and lack of abrasion resistance.
- INCREMENTAL METHOD of filling of resin = decreases initial shrinkage, by overcoming the shrinkage by successive increments.

TYPES OF COMPOSITE RESINS

Generation	Features
First	• Consists of macro-ceramics phases in the resin matrix. • Have **highest surface roughness.**
Second	• Have colloidal and micro-ceramic phases in a continuous rcsin phases. • Have **best surface texture.**
Third	• Is **hybrid composite,** i.e. have micro and macro ceramics as reinforcers in a suitable resin matrix in a **ratio of 3:1**.
Fourth	• Are **hybrid types.** • Contain **heat cured**, highly reinforced composite macro-particle with a reinforcing phase of micro-ceramics.

TYPES OF COMPOSITE RESINS *(Contd.)*

Generation	Features
Fifth	• **hybrid system.** • Continuous resin phase is reinforced with micro-ceramic and macro, spherical highly reinforced heat cured composite particles. • Improved workability. • Improved wettability; and chemical bonding of the particles.
Sixth	• Continuous phase is reinforced with a combination of micro-ceramics and agglomerates of sintered micro-ceramics. • Have **highest percentage of reinforcing particles.** • Exhibit **least shrinkage.**

Composite/filled resin system—By Bowen 1962.

- It has a polymeric, reactive phase (which is continuous) and an INERT phase of grand ceramic particle, is DISCONTINUOUS in nature.
- Ceramic decreases polymerization shrinkage and coefficient of thermal expansion.
- More stiff, durable.

Acid etched tip = i.e. for class IV lesions; the composite resin is the material of choice.

Posterior composites

- Hybrid material with more than 75% fillers should be used.
- Centric stops should be on sound tooth structures.
- Pre-wedging of teeth helps in creation of contact points. It helps in creation of the gap with wedge, which gets closed by bouncing back of the tooth after wedge removal.
- Incremental additions help to compensate for polymerization shrinkage.

Composite/filled resin: It has a 2-phase system

- Dispersed phase = ceramic particles as fillers.
- Continuous = polymer matrix.
- Silane coating on ceramic filler particles enhances bonding between 2-phases.
- Filler = 70–80% by wt.
  - Ductile resin matrix helps the STRESS TRANSFER b/w the particles.
  - e.g. BIS GMA or urethane diacrylates.
  - Setting reaction = free radical polymerization, which is initiated by BENZOYL PEROXIDE and is accelerated by TERTIARY AMINE.
  - Photo initiator = DIKETONE.
  - Visible LC = Blue light, 480–500 nm, for 20–30 sec.
  - Not soluble in oral fluids.
  - Silane bonding of particles decreases water sorption, and increases colour stability.
  - Filled resin are better able to withstand masticatory stresses.
  - Dimensional stability is more.
  - Shrinkage on polymerization is decreased to 1/4th as compared to unfilled resin.
  - Thermal coefficient of expansion is decreased by = 60%.
  - Low THERMAL conductivity and so insulates from thermal changes.
  - Loss marginal leakage.
  - Drawback = low resistance to ABRASION.
  - Functional Abrasion on contact area may occur, which is due to break down/hydrolysis of silane bond between filler particles and polymer.
  - Macrofilled resins (i.e. larger filler particles) rough surfaces texture and so more stainings.
  - Setting reaction of CR decreases in air or **with eugenol**.

- Pulpal irritation may occur in deep cavities due to penetration of low viscous resin or monomer in dentinal tubules.
- Cement base of liner should be placed as chemical barrier.
- **Dual cure composites** = first, light curing is done for 10 sec; and the final setting occurs chemically.

Microfilled resin

- Has mcirofine silica particles—55% by wt.
- Has smoother surface.
- Have better gingival response due to smoothness.
- Size of particles = 0.04 mm.
- Properties are not as desirable as for CR systems.
- Base resin is = BIS-GMA.
- Resin is impregnated with COLLOIDAL SILICA of sub-micron particle size.
- Its values for water sorption are higher than CR due to colloidal silica filler and so poor colour stability and marginal adaptation as compared to CR.

Hybrid/Blended resin

- Combination of micro filled particles.
- 1–5 μ size filler particles; radiopaque.
- Smoother surface finishing.

SHADE

- Vita shade guide is mostly used.
- Shade should be selected before rubber dam placement and before the eyes become fatigued.
- Operating **light should not be focused** while selecting the shade. Translucency and depth of chroma vary among the shades.
- Should be selected against **2 light sources**, one should be natural light.

Acid etching

- Preferential dissolution of inter-prismatic (inorganic part) enamel followed by top surfaces of prisms.
- Surface area is increased by approx **200 times**.
- Micro-irregularities develop with an average **depth of 25 microns**.
- It exposes proteinaceous organic matrix of enamel, which adds to retention of restoration (Primer).
- It **increases the surface energy** of enamel.
- Phosphoric acid adds a highly polar phosphate group to enamel surface, which increases the adhesive ability of enamel surface.
- A **micro-mechanical bonding** is achieved.
- ***Micro-leakage is zero***.
- 37% ortho phosphoric acid (30–50%).
- Low viscosity unfilled resin is used as the BONDING AGENT to gain retention (PRIMER).
- Etching causes
  - Removal of debris/pellicle from surfaces.
  - Increases surface energy of enamel, making it more reactive.
  - Ends of enamel rods are dissolved, which forms surface irregularities and increases the surface area for bonding.

Mechanical bonding occurs

- Primer (unfilled resin) goes into surface irregularities by CAPILLARY ACTION to form polymer tags.
- Re-mineralization of etched enamel occurs from saliva and after 24 hrs, it is not distinguishable form untreated enamel.
- Etched enamel is porous and has high surface energy. It has 3 zones from surface inwards:
  - Etched zone — 10 microns
  - Qualitative porous zone — 20 microns
  - Quantitative porous zone — 20 microns
  - So the resin tags are of approx — 50 microns long

Depth of micro-pores = approx 20–50 microns

- Acid etching is less effective on PRIMARY teeth = due to LESS (INORGANIC) PRISMATIC STRUCTURE.
- Acid etching is difficult on acid resistant fluorosed teeth also, so repeated etching may be required.
- Polymers = cross–linked BIS-GMA resin.
- Exposed dentin should be protected from acid.
- Acid applied for 60 sec. (latest = 15–30 sec).
- Washing = 30 sec.
- Drying = 15 sec.
- Apply BONDING agent immediately to avoid contamination of etches area.
- **Total etch concept** = enamel and dentin are etched.

Crystal growth bonding technique

It is the latest concept in which tooth surface is treated with a solution of polyacrylic acid containing SO_4^- i.e. sulphate ions. The liberated Ca ions will react with these sulfate ions forming $CaSO_4.2H_2O$. These crystals start growing outwards with irregular rough surface and are similar to etched enamel without loss of tooth structure. On it, primer and resin may be applied for restorations.

Class III cavity

- Dentin contains greater amount of ORGANIC material and has higher moisture. They interfere with wetting by resin bonding agent and formation of polymer tags.
- Acid etching of dentin opens the tubules, releases capillary fluid, contaminating the exposed surface during bonding.
- Cervical and gingival walls should converge towards the opening of the cavity for retention; lingual access is preferred; the walls should be parallel to the enamel rods.
- Retention grooves are placed in DENTIN, but should not encroach the pulp. Most prominent retention is formed in = CERVICAL WALL due to greater bulk of dentin.

- Mechanical bonding with acid etching is not a major retentive factor here because = E rods are etched in a LONGITUDINAL DIRECTION.

Class V cavity: Placed on gingival 3rd of the tooth.

- Due to enamel rod direction; the occlusal and gingival walls are parallel and the mesial and distal walls diverge outwards.
- Found more in old age due to gingival recession.
- Composite resin for esthetic purpose = use dentin bonding agents if cavity margin is not entirely on enamel.
- GIC is the material of choice.
- Wall direction should be parallel to enamel rods and the cavosurface margins should form right angles.
- Incisal enamel cavosurface margin should have a LONG BEVEL to improve retention by acid etching. It also helps in a BETTER COLOUR TRANSITION. The bevel of 1.0–1.5 mm is adequate.

Root caries = caused by **actinomyces viscosus**; GI cement is material of choice; occur after gingival recession; in older age group and due to decreased salivary flow, e.g. in irradiated patients;

Class IV cavity: i.e. caries of anterior teeth.

- Involves incisal edges also.
- Retention is mainly gained by placing CERVICAL RETENTION groove in dentin.
- Cavosurface margins should be BEVELLED to increase surface area.
- Incisal margin is not bevelled = because it will give a thin resin layer, which gets # ed under masticatory loads.
- 1–2 mm long bevel is given.
- A chamfer of 2 mm length in enamel, increases the surface area for bonding and improves plane of orientation of etched enamel rods.

PULPAL PROTECTION BELOW CR

- Placed on axial wall only.
- Liners/bases are used as thermal insulators below CR. But liners act as:
  - Barrier to irritating chemicals.
  - Help in attaining a healthy pulpal response.
  - GI liner in Class A, B, C depth cavities.
  - $Ca(OH)_2$ +GI liners in class C and D depth cavities.
  - Class D cavity = i.e. < 0.5 mm thick dentin remains. $Ca(OH)_2$ helps formation of secondary dentin.
  - GI cement bonds well to the dentin and prepares a seal vs etchant/monomer.
  - $Ca(OH)_2$ has **an air inhibited surface layer,** which can bond with resin, but not with dentin and so will not seal this interface (but GI can do).
  - But light-activated $Ca(OH)_2$ base is inert and will not interfere with resin polymerization.
  - Poly carboxylate cements = can bond with dentin as GI, but not with resin.
  - CR results in discontinuous film of the liner, making it ineffective.

Eugenol results in incomplete setting of resin materials

- Chemicals containing BENZENE RING, e.g. phenol, eugenol inhibit polymerization of resins.

LIGHT CURED RESINS

- No mixing required, so very less chances of air voids.
- Working time is under control = is greatest advantage.
- Better surface texture, strength, etc.
- Incremental filling is possible, which also decreases air, increased strength and compensates polymerization shrinkage.

- Chair light should be kept away from the material, as it may loose their flow properties.
- Composition–(Refer to section of dental materials).

HOW DOES THE BOND OCCUR

- Air inhibited, unpolymerized layer of a cured increment ACTS as a BONDING AGENT, which later cures when it is covered with the fresh resin and unites the 2 increments together.
- Conc. of light beam is greatest at the surface and so the polymerization is faster and more complete here.
- Smaller **increments of < 2.0 mm** should be used, for better curing.
- **Darker shades should be placed in THINNER increments** = because, they have more CHROMA and opaque and so have great difficulty in curing light rejection.
- Microfilled resins have smaller filler particles and less filler content = it does not cure to as great a depth as with longer filler particles.
- An unfilled resin boding agent is applied to etched enamel GI cement. Light cure it for 10–15 sec for optimum bond strength for resin tag formation.
- 450–500 nm, **blue light**, for 20–30 sec.
- Light source should not touch the resin, but should be away by 1 mm only.
- By finishing agents = the softer matrix is abraded at a relatively faster rate and the ceramic particles get projected on the surface, causing rough surface.
- Finishing discs of CR have Al_2O_3 particles on it.
- Abrasive strips = for I/d and gingival smoothening, has Al_2O_3 particles.
- Microfilled CR has better surface smooth finish.
- Etching for 60 sec washing for 30 sec.
- Etched surface appears FROSTY.

- Air inhibited surface of bonding agent becomes the bonding surface for Ist layer of the veneering resin.
- Darker/more chromatic layer should be placed first; should be 0.5 mm thick; should be thinned out as it approaches the incisal part of the tooth.
- A final increment of lighter shade is placed INCISALLY to make it translucent.
- Final curing is done for 60 sec to cure at all depths.
- Heavily filled hybrid material should be used in areas of FUNCTIONAL STRESSES.
- Hybrid resin veneer cementing surface should be ACID etched for 60 sec to clean it with debris and bonding agent should be applied.
- Porcelain veneer-internal surface should be etched with HF acid and a silane coupling agent is placed before final cementation to strengthen the polymer bond to porcelain.

GI cement

Powder = Ion-leachable calcium alumino-silicate glass and fluoride.

Liquid = Solution of polyacrylic and itaconic acids.

Initial setting reaction = Ca^{++} ions migrate in hydrated siliceous gel and form bridge between polycarboxylate ions (GEL MATRIX).

- **Final setting** = Aluminum salt bridges develop, cross linking occurs; F-complexes formed.
- **Anhydrous GI cement** = dehydrated polyacrylic acid is included in powder; its liquid is composed of distilled water and other additives.
- If dentin in < 0.5 mm thick, a protective layer of $Ca(OH)_2$ should be placed for formation of secondary dentin.
- High M.wt. of poly acrylic acid molecules - can't penetrate dentin tubules and so least pulpal irritant.
- GI gel is SENSITIVE to moisture, so should be protected during setting by varnish or LC unfilled bonding agent/Vaseline.

- Low resistance to abrasive wear = so should not be used in areas of functional stresses, e.g. contact areas, centric stops, etc.
- So GI should be limited to class 3, 5 cavities.
- Esthetic qualities and surface polish are inferior to CR. So GI is less preferred than CR in esthetic zones.
- It is the material of choice for class 3 caries extending on root surface.

Class V e.g. cervical abrasion.

- Usually found in patients with HIGH CARIES RISK.
- If on cementum also = GI is better for adhesion as it decreases micro-leakage.
- If lesion is surrounded by enamel = CR is better for surface finish.

DENTIN BONDING AGENTS (DBA)

- Dentin has high water and organic content.
- **Smear layer** = has amorphous layer of organic and inorganic debris; decreases dentin sensitivity and prevents loss of dentinal fluid; has more inorganic content as cp to dentin.
- They aim to modify and partially remove the smear layer by acidic primer, which exposes collagen and opens dentinal tubules; then a resin with bifunctional ends is placed, i.e. one end is hydrophilic which bonds with wet collagen and dentin and the hydrophobic end bonds with composite resin.
- Gets bond to dentin through CHEMICAL reaction.
- Bond is a WEAK POLAR BOND, which bonds the phosphate in Bis-GMA to Ca^{++} in tooth.
- Bond is also know as **SCOTCH BOND**.
- Bond strength to etched enamel = 3000 psi.
- Bond strength to dentin = 800–1000 psi.
- Better bond strength to dentin with either OXALATE pre-treatment or a GLUTERALDEHYDE base resin.

Generations of dentin bonding agents

I	Phosphate ester of BIS-GMA.
II	Chlor–phosphate ester of BIS-GMA.
III	GLUMA and 4-META.
IV	Moist dentin bonding; moist bonding technique; no air drying required.
V	Primer and adhesive agents combined; one-component system.
VI	Etching eliminated: No etch, no rinse, no cure technology.

GI with CR to restore cervical lesion

- GI is combined with micro-filled CR as 2-step procedure, using DBA.
- Dentin is conditioned with polyacrylic acid.
- GI lining is placed, i.e. GI is placed first as liner and then the CR is filled for bulk.
- Etching of GI and enamel is done for CR.
- It is also know as **SANDWICH TECHNIQUE**
- **Advantages**
  - GI provides chemical barriers to monomer of CR.
  - Provides seal at dentin.
  - Fluoride from GI is anti-caries.
  - CR gives improved esthetics smooth surface and greater durability

CR for posterior teeth

- Are hybrid CR, with greater strength and less dimensional changes.
- But have inadequate wear resistance.
- So it should be limited to those teeth where occlusal support is on sound enamel.

- Dentin should be protected from etchant to avoid pulpal irritation.
- Internal line angles **are more rounded** than for amalgam.
- Occlusal walls should have divergence toward occlusal.
- No BEVEL is placed on cavo-surface margin, as it provides a thin filling margin susceptible to fracture.
- Proximal box has convergence towards occlusal, with no cavo surface bevel.
- As cp to $Ca(OH)_2$, GIC bonds to dentin; prevents microleakage. It can also be acid etched for 20 sec to provide porous surface for mechanical bonding to CR.
- Filling is done in INCREMENTS, for proper curing of materials and to decrease total polymerization shrinkage and the internal stresses.
- Time of exposure of light beam should be increased to 40 sec when the distance from tip of light is more than 1.0 mm or the resin increment is > 2.0 mm thick.

Differences b/w light cure and chemical curing bonding

Light cured	Self/chemical cured
Less wastage of material	More
Filling/curing is done in increments	In one phase
Finishing is good	Poor
Strength is higher	Lesser
Controlled setting time	Starts setting with mixing of primer and adhesive
Working time is long	Less
No mixing is required mixed	2 components are to be
Colour stability is better	Poor
Wear resistance is better	Lesser
In orthodontic bonding, it gives adequate long time for adjusting the bracket position	This freedom is not allowed.

Fused porcelain: By Byram 1908.

- Better esthetics, durability, D-stability.
- But problem with proper marginal adaptation and so tinting agent is visible at cavo-surface margin. (BRITTLE).
- It can be prevented by acid itching and bonding with CR.

Porcelain veneer: The fitting surface is roughened with sand blasting, cleaned with alcohol and coated with silane–coupling agents, and then a dentin bonding agent is placed. The veneers are 0.5–0.7 mm thick.

All ceramic crowns: e.g. Empress, etc. are built on high strength alumina cores.

DIRECT GOLD RESTORATIONS

Are the only type of restoration which use pure gold, with the exception of electralloy.

2 types = precipitated gold; gold foils.

PRECIPITATED GOLD

- Gold is precipitated by atomization.
- Spherical particles are produced; of 5–75 microns size.
- 3 forms.

Form	Features
Powdered gold	• e.g. **goldent**; the precipitated gold particles are wrapped in cohesive gold foil to make balls of 1–4 mm diameter. Ratio of precipitated powder and cohesive gold foil is **19:1**.
Mat gold	• gold is precipitated through electrodeposition. • **mat foil** = mat gold strips wrapped in cohesive gold foil. • **electralloy** = is an alloy of **gold with calcium**. The calcium content is in 1% range.

Gold foils

- It is the oldest and most durable direct gold.
- Prepared by cold working/strain hardening of the ingot.
- Thickness range = 0.001–0.007 mm.
- 4 forms.

Form	Features
Plain gold foil	
Corrugated foils	Are more cohesive than plain foil.
Platinum gold foil	Used in areas of stress conc for improved mechanical properties.
Laminated gold foils	It has directional properties. It is much stronger and more resistant to stresses.

Pure cohesive gold foils restorations will be strongest; densest; hardest of all types of direct gold restorations, due to greater **cohesion** between foils.

Cohesive gold

- Surface is protected by chlorine or ammonia gases, which can be removed by degassing just before use.
- It can be done by **3 ways**.
- Heating by an open alcohol flame.
- Heating on a mica sheet over a flame.
- **Electric degassing**

Gold (Direct Filling)–(DFG)

Cohesion: i.e. force which bonds 2 similar molecules.

Forms of cohesive gold.

1. Fibrous gold foil = OLDEST
    - It is a wrought material.
    - Gold sheet formed are of **4″ size.**
    - Sizes vary from to 1/128.

2. **Mat gold**
   - Is a **crystalline deposit** deposited by **electrolytic process**. Extremely pure.
   - **Mat foil** = mat gold wrapped in a thin sheet of fibrous gold foil, which decreases its friability is know as mat foil.
3. **Encapsulated powdered gold**
   - Contain **organic annealing** indicator.
   - Better handling and little waste.
4. **Alloyed filling gold**
   - **Crystalline** structure.
   - **Ca^{++}** is the alloying agent.
   - Produces **Hardest surface** of all direct filling gold.

Type: Cohesive/Semi-cohesive/Non-cohesive

- Cohesive gold material has no surface contamination.
- The **ammonia compound** acts as adsorbent as **a protective covering** to prevent adsorption of non-volatile substances. It can be removed by heat for making it cohesive.
- **Annealing** = is the cleansing of gold by heating. Contaminants can be sulfides, oxides, etc.
- **Methods** = 1. **Bulk method**—foils placed on MICA Sheet on the open gas/flame, till the gold becomes DULL RED colour.
- DFG should never be annealed directly in open gas flame to prevent its contamination.

2. **Piece method** = most practical method; done on simple alcohol lamp; acetone–free alcohol should be used; it is known as DEGASSING; helps in selecting gold foil of desired size and avoids contamination of foil between annealing and use.

Storage of foils—with ***ammonia vapors***, which get adsorbed on surface and prevents contamination.

- Anneal all direct filling golds before use, to make it cohesive.

Condensation of pure gold

- Hand instrument condensation.
- Pneumatic condensation = i.e. by air pressure.
- Electronic condensation = at 2 ounces–15 lbs force; with 360 3600 cycles/min.
- Hand condensation and mallet.
  - Avoid voids/pits in the filling.
  - **Wedging principle** = condensation should begin at a central area and work towards the walls.
  - Gold foil should overlap each other.
  - Stepping of condenser point necessary over entire surface.
  - Gold is always worked from centre of restoration towards the margin (during finishing).
  - Silex + Tin oxide is used for polishing.
  - A tight proximal contact should be developed with adjacent teeth.
  - Hand pressure condensation-minimum pressure required is **15 psi**; sustained force is employed; condenser face is serrated and of **smaller diameter** than required for Ag-Hg; serration are CONICAL in shape to apply heavy localized, concentrated forces.
  - **Hand malleting** = helps in adapting denser cohesive golds into retention areas; 5 oz mallet is used.
  - **Mechanical method** = pneumatic; electro-mallet; lighter blows with high frequency are preferable.

Types of condensers

1. **Round** = used in retention grooves.
2. **Parallelogram** = used for BULK.
3. **Foot type** = used at cavo-surface.

Only fibrous gold foil is of fibrous/wrought nature, rest 3 are of crystalline nature.

Fibrous gold foil: Best suited for small pits and fissures and conservative cavities; on restricted surfaces.

- Gives excellent surface.
- Used to veneer other forms of cohesive gold.
- Used in cavities not having proper convenience form.

Mat foil: For BULK filling of **single surface** restorations, e.g. class I, V.

- Density greater than gold foil—so LESS TIME is required to fill the cavity.
- Not used on SURFACE, as pitting may occur due to its peculiar inadequate subsurface condensation.
- So restoration should be VENEERED with fibrous gold foil to maintain a good surface.
- Heavy hand force is required.

Encapsulated powdered gold

- Used both as a BULK filler and for surface restoration.
- Greater density than mat gold.
- Used **to fill all classes of cavities,** where cohesive gold may be indicated.
- Sustained hand pressure is required.

Alloyed filling gold

- Used **in all classes of cavities** especially, 1, 2, 3, 5.
- Heavy hand pressure is required for good surface.

Indications of DFG

1. Conservative cavities only.
2. No heavy biting stress areas.
3. Should be enclosed with in the cavity walls.

C/I: Should not be used if isolation is not proper; with larger cavities, etc.

CAVITY PREPARATIONS

1. Angular undercut placed in dentin walls of conservative class I cavities = permits easy placement for fibrous gold foil.
2. If more dense gold is to be used = the less angular or a rounded groove should be placed.
3. Fibrous gold foils are WEDGED in the angular retention grooves = wedging helped by ELASTICITY OF DENTIN.
   - Bevel = short cavo-surface bevel is required for condensing fibrous/wrought gold foil, as it provides adequate margin strength in thinner cross section.
   - Bevel is protective, as it removes unsupported enamel.
   - It should be at 45 degrees and 0.5 mm in length.
   - Bevel should not be placed for crystalline gold as it will get fragmented in thinner layers under masticatory pressure.

Filling

1. Thin layer of varnish applied, should not block the retention grooves; should be on DENTIN only.
   - Condensation is started in retention points for fibrous gold.
   - Condenser is stepped in an overlapping manner.
   - Periphery is built slightly ahead of central area of the cavity.

Veneered gold foil restoration = i.e. combined use of alloyed filing gold/mat gold and gold foil on the surface. It is used if SIZE of cavity is LARGE. Heavy pressure is used. Walls of cavity are covered ahead of floor/axial walls, till cavity is 95% filled.

Then = a veneer of **fibrous gold** is started at cavo-surface bevel, till whole surface is veneered.

- Burnishing should be done from metal towards the enamel; it helps in work-hardening.
- Silex and tin oxide paste in rubber cup is used for polishing.
- Gold is a malleable material and is always burnished TOWARDS the margins of restorations.

Class III cavity

- For mx incisors = lingual approach to make class 3.
- For md incisors = labial approach to make class 3.

Class II cavity

- Alloyed filling gold/encapsulated powdered gold preferred.
- Should be limited to conservative defects
- Proximal box prepared with triangularity slightly more than used for amalgam cavity.
- A 35° short bevel on gingival margin.
- Internal line/point angles should be well defined.

Matrix

- A Cu-band heated to redness and quenched in alcohol to soften it is used.
- Quenching in water allows formation of oxides, which may contaminate the gold.

CAST GOLD RESTORATIONS

- Pure gold is used only occasionally for inlays in LOW-STRESS BEARING AREAS.
- Types = I, II, III, IV gold alloys.
- From Type I to IV alloys.
    - Hardness increases.
    - PL and strength increase.
    - Elongation decrease.

Type I gold

- Soft gold alloys
- For low stress bearing areas, e.g. small Cl I, 3, 5 cavities.
- Direct method of INLAY preparation is used.

Type II

- Medium hard alloys
- Used for majority of castings, e.g. crowns for single tooth.
- Supports occlusal stresses without deformations.
- INDIRECT method casting is used.

Type III alloy

- HARD alloys
- Greater Tensile strength Required, e.g. FPDs, i.e. for abutment crowns.
- Has lesser elongation.

Type IV

- Extra hard alloy.
- For RPD castings.

CAVITY DESIGN

1. Cavity wall should DIVERGE towards the occlusal. (As cp to silver amalgam and DFG, in which cavity walls should converge.)
2. **Line of draw** = is the axis of taper. Taper permits unobstructed removal of wax pattern. Axis of taper for class 1, 2 cavity = Parallel to long axis (LA) of tooth. Axis of taper for class 5 cavity = Perpendicular to LA of tooth.
3. **Cone angle taper** = 10–16 degrees; it is the relation of all prepared walls of the cavity.
4. Longer preparation require taper in higher range; short preparation in lower range.

INLAY CAVITY

- Divergent walls.
- Rounded line angles.
- No undercuts.

- For onlays = a minimum of 1.5 mm reduction of cusps is necessary.
- For porcelain = silane coupling agent is used on the fitting surface.
- Do not use eugenol with composite resin.

TYPES OF BEVELS

- **Partial bevel** = involves part of enamel wall, not more than 2/3rd of its dimensions.
- **Short bevel** = includes entire enamel wall but not dentin.
- **Long bevel** = include entire enamel wall and upto one half of dentinal wall.
- **Full bevel** = includes all of the enamel and dentin walls. But its use should be avoided as it decreases internal resistance and retention.
- **Counter bevel** = it is used when capping the cusps to protect and support them.
- **Hollow ground/concave bevel** = it allows more space.

Bevels

Helps in adaptation of margins; as gold is ductile and malleable.

1. **Butt joint**
   - 90 degrees
   - Most difficult to adapt
2. **Lap joint**
   - 35 degrees metal margin
   - Easy to adapt
3. **Sliding lap joint**
   - 25° margin
   - Margin should be burnished beyond its P.L. for adaptation.
4. Axio-pulpal line angle is rounded to avoid stress and concentration in this area.
5. Flare of proximal walls should form axio-proximal angle of 100–110 degrees.

6. Occlusal dovetail.
7. Pin holes/post holes = to prevent ROTATIONAL displacement.
8.. CERVICAL MARGIN bevel—is important feature. For indirect wax pattern–smaller; for direct wax pattern - bevel should be of greater bulk and of greater MD width across the cervical floor. It should be 1/4th–1/3rd the MD width of cervical floor; it helps easy manipulation of wax, and manipulation of gold margins.
   - Also pulpal floor is SLANTED to the lingual side and so cervical floor will not be parallel to the pulpal floor.

Cuspal protection

- ♦ 1.5 mm reduction is done for adequate thickness.

Class 3 = Class 3 inlay is best used on the **distal surface of canines**.

Class IV cavity

- ♦ is a 2–surface cavity involving incisal and proximal surfaces.
- ♦ Retentive pin hole in cervical and incisal areas are placed (approx 1 mm deep).

Class 5

- ♦ Trapezoidal smooth flowing shape.
- ♦ Walls should be prepared parallel to enamel rods.
- ♦ Axial wall must be curved parallel to pulp chamber.
- ♦ Walls are made divergent so that they are parallel to enamel rods.

Cervical finish lines may be:

FINISH LINES

Type	Features
Chamfer	• **Most commonly** used. • 0.5 mm is the maximal depth. • Assures bulk and definite margins. • But limited burnishability.

FINISH LINES (*Contd.*)

Type	Features
Knife edge/ feather edge	• **Least tooth structure involvement.** • Should be used only if alloy is very castable–burnishable type, e.g. gold alloy type II. • Its **disadvantage** is = possibility of indefinite termination for the casting; over contoning.
Beveled shoulder	• **Involves most tooth structure** indicated if **maximum bulk** of cast is needed marginally. • It maximally reduces marginal problems of internal spacing. • Ideal design for subgingivally located margins.
Hollow ground	• Is **exaggerated chamfer** tooth involvement is greater than chamfer and less than the beveled shoulder. • Is **superior to chamfer.**
Shoulder	• Finish line **at 90 degrees** to axial wall. • Used for **porcelain** for maximum bulk. • No burnishing is possible or required.

Die (Also refer to section of prostho.)

- ♦ Electroformed metal die is better than stone dies as there is minimum danger of abrasion and overfinishing.
- ♦ Dies for long and thin preparation especially on anterior teeth are best formed of metal, as it is least prone to fracture.
- ♦ Epoxy/resin materials exhibit polymerisation shrinkage.

SILVER ELECTROFORMING of rubber/Impression

- ♦ Helps to form metal dies.
- ♦ But polysulfide RBM can't be copper plated due to lack of throwing power of $CuSO_4$.
- ♦ Silicone impressions can be copper plated easily.

- Ag = plating of dies is also done, esp. of prepared teeth only.
- Alkaline silver cyanide (Ag-CN) solution and pure silver anode are used.
- Current = 10 ma; (low current can lead to formation of gas bubbles and powdery deposits of silver.
- Electroplating is done for > 12 hrs.

ELASTIC IMPRESSION MATERIALS

- Ist elastic material was = Agar.
- Agar is a reversible gel; due to a physical phenomenon of temperature change.
- Alginates = irreversible gel, a chemical reaction occurs.
- First rubber base impression material was-polysulfide and then silicone and then polyether.

Polysulfide

- Useful for impression of deeper subgingival areas.
- Hydrophilic.
- Dimensionally stable if dies are to be formed even 1 hr after the impression.
- More difficult to mix.
- Least costly.
- But long WT and ST; less cross linked.

Condensation silicones

- Medium WT/ST.
- Mix easily.
- **Hydrophobic**; require dry field.
- More shrinkage due to loss of Bye-products.

Addition silicones

- Newest.
- ***Least amount of shrinkage***—no formation of Bye-products.
- MOST ACCURATE.

- If delay in die formation is there—these are the best impression materials.
- Highly cross-linked.
- High hardness-low flexibility.

Polyether

- Short WT/ST.
- Low flexibility, tear strength and flow.
- So LESS VERSATILE than others.

AGAR: Reversible; due to physical change.

- Impression **must be poured soon after** removal from mouth.
- Only stone dies can be made.
- Agar has high water content, so it is dimensionally instable.
- Conditioning and storage:
  - In liquefying bath for 15 min.
  - In storage bath = 150 degrees F.
  - Tempering bath = 115 ± 5 F for 5 min.

Cooling is done under running tap water for at least 4 min. It is a poor thermal conductor and gelation occurs from outside to inside.

SPRUING

- Hollow sprues better than solid sprue, because they carry less heat and so less distortion of wax pattern; also give firm attachment to the pattern.
- Should be attached in the bulky part of pattern in an area least disturbing the contours/margins.
- Slight **funneling** is done at attachment point to decrease heat build up.
- Should be attached at approx **45 degrees** to occlusal plane; while a casting which has to gain its major portion of compensation by hygroscopic setting expansion HSE, should be placed symmetrically in the investment.
- A Y-shaped sprue is made for MOD casting.

- Sprue length above the sprue former should be **6–8 mm** only.
- Most frequently used sprue diameters are 12, 14, 16 gauge.

INVESTING

- Internal stresses in the wax pattern get released and lead to distortion = so should be invested quickly.
- Linear contraction is 0.4% in wax.
- Casting shrinkage occurs on cooling.
- Expansion in investment compensates this by 3 procedures.
  - NSE = due to crystalline growth of gypsum binder
  - TE = when investment is heated to remove wax
  - HSE = when investment sets in contact with H_2O.
- HSE and TE provide larger amount of expansion.
- HSE is also know as **low heat casting technique.**
- TE is know as **thermal technique.**
- HSE = investment is placed in 100 F water bath for 35 min.

CASTING

- Investment is placed in preheated oven at 900 ± 25 F for 1 hr for wax removal.
- Sprue hole should be down for 1/2 hr and then for 30–45 min with hole upright. So O_2 comes in contact with wax for **complete oxidation of residual wax**.
- Metal is heated by, natural gas and compressed air flame.
- Blue flame is used, it is a reducing zone.
- Metal is heated to light red colour with good fluidity.
- After casting, **quench** the casting; it helps in **breakage of investment**.
- **Pickling** = done to remove surface oxides.
- Saturated Sod. Bicarbonate solution is used to remove residual acid.
- Previously cast gold can be re-used after adding some new gold to **replenish the ZINC** content.

- Internal surface of casting is etched by **air-abrasive tech** under low pressure.

SOLDERING (Also refer to the section on dental materials Vol. II).

- Done to make proximal contact area.
- Free-hand soldering is simple/efficient.
- Anti-flux = carbon pencil; graphite.
- Flux = Borax and Boric acid.
- Type II casting gold, 650 fine, 18 K solder is used to make the contact and other contours.
- If during seating—a heavy consistency of cement mix is placed ON CASTING and tooth, then a saturated solution of $NaHCO_3$ is applied for disintegration of cement and its removal.
- **Proximal contacts are first adjusted before seating.**
- Cervical margin of seated inlay is the **first to be adapted**.

Direct wax pattern—for class II cavity.

- Type I wax is used.
- Matrix adapted = 0.002″ matrix band.
- Wax heated in water at 122 F for 5 min.
- Heavy finger pressure maintained for 3 min.
- 20 gauge hollow sprue placed just inside the Marginal Ridge on occlusal surface for removal of wax pattern.
- Hollow 14 or 16 gauge sprue attached to proximal surface, slightly to LINGUAL SIDE of contact area; should form 45 degree angle with the occlusal plane after investing.
- Type I soft gold is most often used for class 2 casting.
- For class 3 wax pattern = 0.0015″ mylar matrix is selected.
- Soft type I gold alloy is good for class 3, 5 inlays, because of low functional stresses encountered.

PORCELAIN FUSED TO METAL (PFM) RESTORATIONS

- Dicor crown = **cast** ceramic crown.
- Cerestore crown = **injection molded** crown.

- Colour/shade = is produced by the REFRACTION, INTERFERENCE, ABSORPTION.
- **Refraction**-occurs when light passes from one medium to another, in which its velocity is different.
- **Interference** = is by thin transparent films on a surface st light waves travel at different rates.
- **Absorption** = colours of object is the reflection of wavelength (colours) not absorbed.
- UV light produces chemical changes; damages the retina (retional determent) and the infrared is a source of heat.
- **Hue** = describes colour, i.e. red, yellow, blue.
- **Chroma** = describes intensity of colour; it is the strength/ saturation of colour.
- **Value** = describes brightness/dullness of colour. It is determined by amount of gray/white present.
- **Opaque** = blocking the passage of light.
- **Transparent** = permitting the passage of light.
- **Translucent** = permitting the passage of light, but diffusing it.
- For shade selection = both artificial and natural lights should be used.
- PFM crown = it has a cast substructure, of special alloy to which porcelain is fused.
- Feldspathic percelain = feldspar (81%), quartz = (15%), kaolin (4%) and metallic oxides (< 1%). But it is TRANSLUCENT.
- **Aluminium porcelain jacket crown** = its CORE has 50% high strength alumina + 50% porcelain. It was developed by John McLean. It is OPAQUE.
- Mostly, the failure of porcelain jacket crowns is due to propagation of micro-cracks, which occur during cooling. This propagation is interrupted by HIGH-STRENGTH ALUMINA CORE.

BONDED ALUMINA CORE

- Stress concentration is high around microcracks on the inner surface of ceramic.

- Metal can relieve stress concentration around the crack, and thus prevents its propagation under loading.
- Aluminous porcelain is bonded to pure Pt foil by first coating the foil with 0.2–2.0 mm of TIN before firing on the porcelain. Then porcelain is CHEMICALLY-BONDED to the metal coping.

CERESTORE CROWN

- It is a ceramic restoration, which uses a ***shrink free alumina ceramic core***, with an ***aluminous porcelain veneer***.
- High strength alumina core, so the crown is **better for posterior teeth**.
- Made by **injection molding technique** and so has an EXCELLENT MARGINAL FIT.
- ***No metal substructure.***
- Has translucency.

DICOR CROWN

It is a truly castable–ceramic restoration.

It is used for posterior teeth.

- ***No metal substructure*** or underlying core.
- Its shade is not durable, because it is applied to the SURFACE of restoration.

Acrylic jacket crown

- Mainly used for PROVISIONAL RESTORATION
- Used for YOUNG patients with large pulpal chambers; and so extensive crown cutting cannot be done for ceramic.
- Colour stability of heat cured is better than the self cured acrylic.

ABUTMENT PREPARATION

- For anterior tooth = the shoulder is extended to lingual line angle of the tooth—for esthetic season.
- For posterior tooth = the shoulder is just beyond the buccal line angle.

- Width of shoulder = 1.5 mm till I/D area and it narrows as it extends toward the lingual for anterior teeth.
- Incisal/occlusal reduction = 2–2.5 mm.
- Lingual surface reduction = 0.5–1.0 mm.
- **Bevel** is placed on labial shoulder = it provides metal collar, which is the most resistant to distortion during the stages of porcelain firing = where esthetics is not of much concern.
- If esthetics is required = than SLOPING SHOULDER provides space for both metal and porcelain.
- A BUTT-JOINT = is best for an ALL-PORCELAIN margin. Strength of porcelain depends on its bulk, and the butt joint provides most bulk in the restoration.
- A 10° convergent taper towards INCISAL.

Die fabrication

- Metal die is preferred for fabrication of PFM crown—as it resists the abrasion.
- Electroformed dies can be formed on rubber base impressions.
- Fabrication of cerestore restoration requires use of **special epoxy die**, for the development of alumina core.
- A ***canine–guided occlusion*** favors the use of porcelain occlusal surface, as there is no facial contact on porcelain in lateral movements.

PIN RETAINED RESTORATIONS

- To enhance retention during filling of extensively decayed tooth.
- Help in transmitting occlusal stresses to the surrounding tissues and so fracture of filling is reduced.
- Pins decrease the TENSILE STRENGTH values of amalgam.

Types of pins

1. Cemented = helpful for non vital teeth.
2. Self-threading pins = also known as TMS pins; best.
3. Friction lock type retained by RESILIENCY OF DENTIN

Most commonly used pin = self threading type.

Features	Cemented pins	Frictional grip/ friction lock	Threaded
Pin channels	Larger in diameter	Slightly narrower	**Narrower**
Stresses	Little/ no stress	**Maximum**	Intermediate
Retention	**Least**	Intermediate 2–3 times	Most 5–6 times
Crazing	Nil/little	**Maximum**	Intermediate
Retention to restorative materials	More retentive	**Least retentive** to amalgam and resin; **least used pin**	More retentive
Distance from DEJ	0.5–1.0 mm	**>2.5 mm**	1.5 mm

Basic rules

1. Should be placed in dentin only due to its elasticity. 1–1.5 mm from DEJ.
2. Dentinal engagement : pin protrusion in cavity = ideal is 2:1; for best retention.
3. A minimum of 2 mm distance should be there between 2 pins for better retention.
4. Cemented pin is the only technique to be used for RCT teeth and/or to be located very close to DEJ. 0.5–1.0 mm.
5. Threaded pin technique is used for vital teeth. Pin is located at least 1.5 mm from DEJ.
6. Staple post = i.e. post in 2 adjacent root canals is continuous.

GUIDELINES

1. Pins should be placed as close as possible to **the line angle of the tooth**, which is the area of greatest bulk of dentin.

2. Pin holes should be in the dentin, **at least 0.5 mm from DEJ and** no closer than 1.5 mm to external surface of the cavity.
3. If more than one pin is to be placed-the optimum inter-pin distance is 5 mm.
4. Pins should be placed s.t. their axes are not parallel. It helps to increase the retention.
5. Direction of pin holes should be parallel to the external contour of the tooth.
6. Should be placed at least **0.5 mm from the axial wall** of tooth. It allows adequate condensation of restorative material. Smaller size of the condensers are used.
7. Minimum no. of pins should be used to avoid crazing; to maintain inter-pin distance; in general one pin is used for replacing one cusp and marginal ridge.
8. For molars = 1 pin/missing cusp.
9. For premolars = 2 pins/missing cusp.
10. Pin depth of **2 mm into dentin** provides sufficient retention.
11. Optimum length of pin extending **into amalgam is 2 mm**. If more, it can lead to fracture of amalgam
12. Holes are drilled at the speed of 300–500 rpm. It is done in one thrust for uniformity of the hole.

CEMENTED PINS

- Pin holes should be 0.001–0.002 inches wider than the size of the pin.
- Twist drill = 0.021 or 0.0027″ diameter.
- Holes are placed at 3–4 mm depth, at dissimilar angles.
- GI or reinforced ZOE used for cementation, as they have more favorable pulpal response.
- **Least TRAUMATIC to dentin**, as placed in oversized holes.
- Preferred for NON-VITAL TEETH, because no crazing or internal stresses produced.
- RETENTION is LEAS, because cement may be soluble. Micro-leakage is more.

Friction lock type pins

- Size of the pin hole is 0.001 inches smaller than the size of the pin.
- They are retained by friction.
- Introduce maximum stresses in the dentin.
- Give maximum discomfort to the patient.
- Retention is 2–3 times more than the cemented pins.

Self-threading pins—(also known as TMS = thread made system)

- Best and **most widely used.**
- Mechanical retention due to visco-elastic property of dentin.
- Pin - hole = is 0.0015-0.004″ smaller than the pin size.
- Pin–hole size is SMALLER than diameter of PIN.
- No cement used.
- Best retention (5–8 × more than the cemented pin).
- Lesser depth of pin-holes is required.
- Least micro–leakage.
- Disadvantage-rauma to dentin, may lead to CRAZING AND CRACKING AND fracture.
- Less discomfort to the patient.
- **Pin hole perforation**—pulpal perforation is treated by $Ca(OH)_2$ intermediary base into the pin hole.
- Periodontal perforation—is sealed by AMALGAM.

Types of the Pins: pins are of 3 types:

Pin type	Diameter
Minikin	0.019 inch
Minim	0.024 inch
Minuta	0.015 inch

Amalgapin

- Here pins are not used, but 2–3 mm deep holes are made, in which amalgam is condensed for retention.
- But amalgapin chambers are more wide than pin holes and so more conservative.

Post for restoration of devital teeth

- RCTed teeth are BRITTLE and DRY.
- Get fractured with time, so should be restored.
- Instrumentation of RC leads to weakening of tooth and fracture
- Only 9% loss of free water in a pulpless tooth occurs as cp to vital tooth and there is no change in BOUND water.
- Devital teeth will fracture if they are not restored with CUSPAL COVERAGE.
- Post and core may be placed. The CORE replaces the lost crown structure, the post is used for retention for a core.

Characteristics of a POST

- Minimal length of post should be equal to the clinical crown.
- Apical RC seal should be 5–6 mm (apical 3rd) to prevent microleakage.
- Parallel-sided posts have better retention than TAPERED post, but less than threaded post.
- Internal tooth structure should be preserved to provide maximum resistance to fracture.
- A safe ended GATES-GLIDDEN or peeso reamer is used for preparing the dowel space.
- An external cavo-surface bevel is placed to provide a degree of resistance to prevent tooth fracture.
- Anti-rotation lock/keyway placed to prevent rotation.
- On max. first PM-lingual canal is used for POST—as it is STRAIGHTER.
- In max. molars-PALATAL canal is used-as it is largest and widest.
- On mandibular molar-DISTAL canal is used.

- A vent is placed along the length of post for escape of cement during cementation.
- A generally accepted rule for restoring RCTed posterior tooth = MOD protected cusp gold inlay is used as a minimum restoration.
- Types of post and cores: (1) prefabricated/custom made; (2) parallel sided/tapered; (3) threaded/smooth/serrated.
- Parallel sided have better retention; but tapered are less likely to cause apical 3rd perforations of root canal.

Important points

- For achieving proper proximal contact, the best material is = cast gold.
- For thin margins restoration and cusp restoration, the best material is = gold foil because it is malleable and ductile.
- Saliva is cultured upon MSB medium or on 20% sucrose + sulphasomidine at a pH of 5.0.
- Xylitol is the most effective of the sucrose substitutes in reducing decay.
- Maximum fluoride is deposited in = cementum.
- Acid etching cannot be done on cementum, because acid dissolves it uniformly rather than creating the micropores; cementum has only 45–50% of inorganic part.
- **Cusp protection** is required if the occlusal margin of the lesion is more than halfway to the cusp tip.
- **Supporting cusps** require more BULK or thickness of protection than balancing cusp, due to more occlusal load.
- Up to 2 mm should be removed from working cusp, but only 0.5 mm from non-working cusp for bulk of metal.
- Internal line angles should be rounded for better stress distribution in the tooth and the material.
- Occlusal taper should be approx 5 degrees.
- Retention grooves are placed in the dentin, away from the pulp.
- MTA is the latest material being used as a setrograde filling material after epicoectomy.

2

MCQs in Operative Dentistry

1. The optimum fluoride concentration in community drinking water is:

A. 0.1 ppm
B. 0.12 ppm
C. 1.0 ppm
D. 10.0 ppm

2. Which of the following is not an essential factor needed for the initiation of a carious lesion?

A. Susceptible host (tooth)
B. Microflora with cariogenic potential (plaque)
C. Saliva
D. Suitable substrate (dietary carbohydrates)

3. The principal feature of a sealant that is required for success is:

A. High viscosity
B. Adequate retention
C. An added colorant to make the appearance slightly different from the occlusal enamel
D. High strength

4. The outline form of a Class V composite preparation resembles that of a Class V amalgam preparation except for what important feature listed below?

A. No retentive grooves are necessary
B. The internal line angles are much more rounded
C. Pulp protection is not required
D. None of the above

5. **Which of the following is formed very rapidly in response to irritants?**
   A. Primary dentin
   B. Secondary dentin
   C. Reparative dentin
   D. Sclerotic dentin

6. **The gypsum bonded investments are used with**
   A. Type 1 gold allows
   B. Type II gold alloys
   C. Type III gold alloys
   D. All of the above

7. **Caries that is often found in older patients and attacks the cementum and radicular (root) dentin is called?**
   A. Residual caries
   B. Secondary (recurrent) caries
   C. Root surface (senile) caries
   D. None of the above

8. **For an efficient four handed dental delivery system, the position of the chairside assistant should be:**
   A. Lower than the dentist
   B. At the same height as the dentist
   C. Higher than the dentist
   D. None of the above

9. **The number one indication for the use of direct filling gold is:**
   A. The large Class II lesion
   B. The small initial Class III lesion
   C. The small Class II lesion
   D. The large Class III lesion

10. **How is high mercury content generally manifested in the clinical amalgam restoration?**
    A. By tissue irritation adjacent to the restoration
    B. By severe marginal breakdown
    C. By delayed expansion
    D. By increased thermal shock resulting from hot and cold foods.

11. **Rapid cooling by immersion in water, of a dental casting from the high temperature at which it has been shaped is referred to as:**
    A. Annealing
    B. Tempering
    C. Quenching
    D. None of the above

12. **High copper and low mercury content of an amalgam restoration will tend to**
    A. Increase creep
    B. Decrease creep
    C. Will not effect creep
    D. Can either decrease or increase

13. **The amount of mercury remaining in dental amalgam after condensation directly affects which of the following?**
    A. The porosity of the restoration
    B. The compressive strength of the restoration
    C. The corrosion resistance of the restoration
    D. The surface finish of the restoration
    E. All of the above

14. **Which cement below, when set, has the potential to inhibit the development of recurrent caries at its margin as a result of fluoride release from its surface?**
    A. Zinc polycarboxylate cement
    B. Zinc oxide-eugenol
    C. Zinc phosphate cement
    D. Glass ionomer cement

15. **All of the following are radiographic signs of trauma from occlusion except**
    A. Hypercementosis
    B. Root resorption
    C. Periodontal pockets
    D. Alternation of the lamina dura
    E. Widening of the periodontal ligament space

16. Frequently, the surface of a gold casting is dark due to the formation of a surface oxide film. This surface film is removed by:

A. Quenching
B. Age Hardening
C. Pickling
D. Fusion

17. A short, painful response to cold suggests:

A. Pulpal necrosis
B. Irreversible pulpitis
C. Pulpal hyperemia
D. Acute apical periodontitis

18. A properly acid-etched enamel surface appears:

A. Somewhat yellow in color
B. Identical to unetched enamel
C. Dull white and chalky
D. Slightly gray with a shine

19. The total energy absorbed to the point of fracture is referred to as:

A. Resilience
B. Brittleness
C. Toughness
D. Modulus of elasticity

20. The attraction of unlike molecules is referred to as:

A. Adhesion
B. Cohesion
C. Attraction
D. None of the above

21. Which cement system listed below was the first system developed with a potential for adhesion to tooth structure?

A. Zinc phosphate cement
B. Zinc polycarboxylate cement
C. Zinc oxide-eugenol
D. Calcium hydroxide cement

22. A lesser number of blades on a bur result in
A. More efficient cutting and a smoother surface
B. Less efficient cutting and a rougher surface
C. More efficient cutting but a rougher surface
D. Less efficient cutting but a smoother surface

23. Filled resins *(Composite resin)*
A. Are harder and stronger than unfilled resins
B. Have a lower coefficient of thermal expansion than unfilled resins
C. Are more resistant to abrasion than unfilled resins
D. All of the above

24. Which of the following instruments is designed to most effectively plane the enamel of the facial and lingual walls of a class II amalgam preparation?
A. A gingival margin trimmer
B. A straight chisel
C. An enamel hatchet
D. Spoon excavator

25. Today the most popular way to polymerize matrix monomers is:
A. Self-cured
B. Chemically cured
C. Ultraviolet light-cured
D. Visible light-cured

26. Which of the following are indications for the use of pins
A. A class II amalgam preparation where one or more cusps have been lost or where the outline form otherwise far exceeds that which is considered normal.
B. A very large class III amalgam preparation
C. A class V amalgam preparation which far exceeds minimal dimensions especially in the gingivo-incisal area
D. A preparation for an amalgam buildup over which a cast restoration will be fabricated
E. All of the above

27. All of the following are major parts of a hand - cutting instrument *except*

A. Handle
B. Shank
C. Nib
D. Blade

28. Which of the following statements in reference to amalgam is false?

A. Increased trituration time will **increase** compressive strength and **decrease** setting expansion
B. A decrease in particle size will decrease compressive strength and increase setting expansion
C. Increased condensation pressure will increase compressive strength and decrease setting expansion
D. All are false.

29. Essential properties of a Class V cavity prepared for direct filling gold include:

A. Sharp internal line angles
B. Small retentive undercuts placed in the axio-occlusal and axio-gingival line angles
C. Mesial and distal walls that flair and meet the cavosurface at a 90^0 angle
D. An axial wall that is convex and follows the external contour of the tooth, 5 mm into dentin
E. All of the above

30. The selection of a base to be used under a permanent restoration is governed by

A. The design of the cavity
B. The type of permanent restorative material used
C. The proximity of the pulp in relation to the cavity wall
D. All of the above

31. What is the proper amount of time to wait until an amalgam restoration can be finished and polished ?

A. 2 hours
B. 12 hours
C. 24-48 hours
D. Makes no difference

32. Which cavity lining agent below does not provide thermal protection ?

A. Calcium hydroxide
B. Zinc oxide eugenol
C. Copalite
D. All of the above

33. When attempting to isolate an operating field in the oral cavity, which method listed below would be the best to use ?

A. Mouth prop
B. Cotton roll isolation with saliva ejectors
C. Rubber dam
D. All of the above

34. Starting from the lowest to the highest rate, arrange the following materials based on their coefficient of thermal expansion:

- Unfilled resin, 5
- Composite resins, 4
- Amalgam, 3
- Direct gold , 2
- Tooth, 1

A. 3, 4, 5, 2, 1
B. 3, 2 , 1, 5, 4,
C. 5, 4, 3, 2, 1
D. 1, 2, 3, 4, 5

35. Composite filler particles function to do all of the following *except*

A. Increase the coefficient of thermal expansion
B. Increase the tensile strength and compressive strength
C. Reduce the polymerization shrinkage
D. Increase the hardness
E. Improve the wear resistance

36. Which of the statements are true concerning posterior composite restorations

A. Posterior composite restoration are frequently indicated in the treatment of occlusal lesions which allow conservative preparations

B. Posterior composite restoration are contraindicated in patient with heavy occlusion *(bruxims)*
C. Posterior composite restorations are contraindicated in a patient with a carries active mouth
D. Posterior composite restorations may be indicated for the restorations of class II cavities in premolar teeth where the appearances is very important, the cavity margins are in the enamel, and the occlusal contacts are on the enamel
E. All of the above statements are true

37. The one characteristic that is common to all Class II gold inlay preparations is
A. The uniform depth of the pulpal floor
B. The lack of undercuts
C. The placement of a base
D. All of the above

38. Which of the following methods of investing is more dependable in the prevention of surface nodules on a casting?
A. Hand investing
B. Vacuum investing
C. Both produce similar result
D. Hand – cum – vacuum casting

39. The most important design characteristic of a bur blade is :
A. The clearance face
B. The rake face
C. The edge angle
D. The clearance angle
E. The rake angle

40. Silver's major effect in a gold casting alloy is :
A. Corrosion resistance
B. To increase the hardness
C. To offset the color contributions of copper
D. To elevate the melting range

41. The success of pulp capping is recognized by :
A. The symptoms of pulpitis
B. The lack of a vital response after several weeks or months

C. The formation of a complete barrier of dentin at the site of pulpal exposure
D. The patient being able to bite down hard on the tooth.

42. Which tooth below requires special attention when preparing the occlusal aspect for a restoration?
A. Maxillary first bicuspid
B. Mandibular first bicuspid
C. Maxillary second bicuspid
D. Mandibular second bicuspid

43. When is the matrix band removed from the tooth?
A. Prior the final caving of the restoration
B. As soon as the amalgam has been condensed into the prep
C. After the final carving of the restoration
D. None of the above

44. The retention of a pin:
A. Decrease as the diameter of the pin increases
B. Increases as the diameter of the pin increases
C. Increases as the diameter of the pin decreases
D. The retention of a pin has nothing to do with the diameter of the pin

45. When mixing zinc phosphate cement, a cool slab is used to :
A. Accelerate the setting time
B. Create more free zinc oxide in the cement
C. Increase the powder-liquid ratio
D. Increase expansion of the set cement

46. Which preparations listed below has a proximal cavosurface margin that form a 90 angle with the external surface?
A. A conservative class II amalgam
B. A conservative class II inlay
C. Neither of the above
D. Both of the above

47. All of the following statements concerning direct gold are true except:
A. It is most nearly permanent of all restorative materials
B. It provides good adaptation to the cavity walls

C. Its coefficient of thermal expansion is close to that of tooth structure
D. It has a low tensile strength *(edge strength)*
E. It will not corrode

48. Bases are materials that function:
A. As barriers against pulpally irritating agents
B. To provide thermal insulation below a restoration
C. To provide adequate resistance to the compressive forces of mastication
D. All of the above

49. Which class III lesions listed below should not be filled with composite resin
A. Mesial-lingual of canines
B. Distal-lingual of laterals
C. Mesial-lingual of centrals
D. Distal-lingual of canines

50. Zone II of carious dentin is also referred to as :
A. Normal dentin
B. Sub-transparent dentin
C. Transparent dentin
D. Turbid dentin
E. Infected dentin

51. Which rubber dam frame listed below provides more retraction of the tissues
A. Woodbury
B. Young's
C. Both are the same
D. None of the above

52. The main advantage of using an 8% solution of stannous fluoride instead of a 2% solution of sodium fluoride for a topical fluoride treatment is :
A. It will not stain
B. It has a better taste
C. It is stable when kept in a polyethylene container
D. A single treatment may be given

53. The pH of acidulated phosphate fluoride gels is in which of the following ranges?
A. 1 to 4
B. 4 to 7
C. 7 to 10
D. 10 to 12

54. A dental patient may experience a sharp pain when two restorations constructed of dissimilar materials in opposing arches make contact in the wet environment of the oral cavity This clinical phenomenon is commonly known as:
A. Current explosion
B. Voltage flow
C. Electrolyte explosion
D. Galvanic shock

55. Small hybrid size filler particles in composite resins :
A. Result in a composite resin that has better finishing characteristics but a lesser resistance to wear
B. Result in a composite resin that has greater resistance to wear but doesn't finish well
C. Result in a composite resin that has better finishing characteristics and a greater resistance to wear
D. Result in a composite resin that has a lesser resistance to wear and also doesn't finish well

56. Which of the following are advantages of the visible light curing systems compared to the old ultraviolet light curing system ?
A. A greater depth of resin can be cured by visible light
B. The resin can be polymerized through enamel, which is particularly advantageous in class III restorations
C. The intensity of visible light remains relatively constant until the bulb fails completely
D. All of the above

57. A diagonal cut across the cavosurface margin that is flat in one dimension only and curved in other dimensions is called a:
A. Plane
B. Bevel

C. Chamfer
D. Butt

58. Which grasp used with hand instruments allows for the greatest intricacy or delicacy of touch ?
A. The modified pen grasp
B. The inverted pen grasp
C. The palm and thumb grasp
D. The modified palm and thumb grasp

59. All of the following statements concerning the use of base metal casting alloys compared to using noble metal casting alloys for cast restorations are true *except*
A. Base metal alloys are harder to cast and finish
B. Base metal alloys are less dense
C. Base metal alloys are stronger
D. Base metal alloys are more resistant to corrosion

60. Favorable factors for direct pulp capping include:
A. The visual evidence of uninflamed *(pink)* pulp tissue
B. The absence of copious hemorrhage through the exposure
C. No previous symptoms of pulpitis
D. A small non-carious exposure (a mechanical pulp exposure)
E. A clean cavity uncontaminated with saliva
F. All of the above

61. Which of the following cavosurface margins is the only one that is beveled when preparing class II amalgam preparation?
A. The occlusal cavosurface margin
B. The facial cavosurface margin of the proximal box
C. The lingual cavosurface margin of the proximal box
D. The gingival cavosurface margin of the proximal box

62. The outline form of the classical class V amalgam preparation is :
A. Square
B. Deformed trapezoid
C. Triangle
D. Rectangle

63. A short, painful response to cold suggests:
A. Pulpal necrosis
B. Irreversible pulpits
C. Pulpal hyperemia
D. Acute apical periodontitis

64. Which cement listed below is the oldest of the luting cements and thus is the one that has the longest "track record" and serves as the standard to which newer systems can be compared?
A. Glass ionomer cement
B. Zinc polycarboxylate cement
C. Zinc phosphate cement
D. Zinc oxide eugenol

65. The greatest stress to which a material can be subjected such that it will return to his original dimensions when the forces are released is referred to as the.
A. Proportional limit
B. Elastic limit
C. Yield strength
D. Tensile strength

66. Which cement (luting agent) below is also used as a permanent restorative agent ?
A. Zinc polycarboxylate
B. Zinc phosphate
C. Glass ionomer
D. Zinc oxide-eugenol

67. Unfilled resin *(acrylic)* temporaries fabricated for inlays and on lays should have which of the following properties?
A. Restore and maintain proximal contacts
B. Restore and maintain tooth occlusion
C. Restore and maintain tooth contours
D. The margins should be closed and flush with the tooth
E. All of the above

68. All of the following are contraindications to the placement of sealants except

A. Patient behavior does not allow for the maintenance of the dry field necessary for successful application
B. There is a carious lesion on the occlusal surface
C. Children whose teeth have a deep pits and fissures
D. There is a carious lesion on the smooth surface that necessitates preparation of the occlusal surface
E. Tooth has been previously restored
F. Tooth is not fully erupted and a dry field can not be maintained

69. Which of the following instruments is designed for the removal of caries and refinement of the internal parts of a preparations?

A. A hoe
B. A file
C. An excavator
D. A scaler

70. When comparing the physical properties of filled resins to unfilled resin, all of the following are true *except*

A. Filled resins are harder
B. Unfilled resins have a lower coefficient of thermal expansion
C. Filled resins have a higher compressive strength
D. Unfilled resins have a lower modulus of elasticity
E. Filled resin have higher tensile strength

71. The most frequently used pins are :

A. Cemented pins
B. Frictions- locked pins
C. Self-threaded pins
D. All of the above

72. The edge angle of a bur blade is:

A. The angle made between the line connecting the edge of the blade to the axis of the bur and the rake face.
B. The angle formed between the rake face and the clearance face

C. The angle formed between the clearance face and a tangent to the path of rotation.
D. None of the above

73. Which of the following characteristics of amalgam would explain why cold sensitivity is the most common problem encountered after placing a dental amalgam restoration?
A. Its coefficient of thermal expansion
B. Its biocompatibility
C. Its thermal insulation properties
D. Its high edge strength

74. Annealing is the process of heating and cooling a metal to make it:
A. Weaker and more brittle
B. Tougher and less brittle
C. More tarnish resistant
D. Easier to cast and finish

75. If a zinc phosphate cement base is used restoring a tooth, when should the varnish be applied?
A. Prior to placement of the base
B. After placement of the base
C. Makes no difference when the varnish is applied
D. Varnish should not be used in conjunction with zinc phosphate cement

76. Which circumference of the matrix band is always place toward the occlusal surface of the tooth?
A. Smaller
B. Larger
C. Both openings of the band have the same circumference
D. Does not matter

77. Cavity liners are used to:
A. Help retain the restorative material
B. Protect the pulp
C. Add strength to the restorative material
D. Decrease the setting expansion of amalgam

78. The two most frequently quoted disadvantages of using the rubber dam are :

A. Time consumption
B. Patient objection
C. Cost
D. Staff allergies to material

79. Which of the following statements concerning sealants are true:

A. Sealants are highly effectively in preventing pit and fissure caries
B. When sealants are applied correctly, there is a decreased development of new carious lesions and a decreased progression of pre-existing lesions
C. A close correlation exists between the retention of sealants and their effectiveness
D. The effectiveness of sealants appears to be equal whether applied by dentist, dental hygienists or dental assistant, provided that they have received appropriate training
E. Acid-etch resin sealants are classified into three types, based on the method by which they are cured
F. All of the above statements are true

80. All of the following facts concerning fluoride are true *except.*

A. Most fluoride is absorbed in the small intestine and excreted through the kidneys
B. Fluorosis may result from excessive fluoride consumed during the mineralization stage of tooth development and can occur in permanent and deciduous teeth
C. Fluoride passes the placental barrier slowly
D. Fluoride is deposited in calcified tissues *(i.e. bones)*
E. At 1.0 ppm, fluoride is tasteless, colorless and odorless
F. The US Public health Service sets the optimal fluoride level at 1.2 to 2.5 ppm for public water
G. The cariostatic effect of fluoride is produced during the calcification stage of tooth development
H. The uptake of fluoride by the teeth depends on the amount of fluoride ingested (not delivered) and the length of time of exposure.

81. The squeezing of material by external forces is called?
A. Compression
B. Tension
C. Shear
D. Brittleness

82. The most susceptible area of a tooth for the retention of dental plaque is :
A. The cusp tips
B. The proximal surfaces
C. The developmental pits and fissures
D. The buccal and lingual surfaces

83. Pit and fissure caries does not spread laterally to a extent until the
A. Pulp is reached
B. Dentinoenamel junction *(DEJ)* is reached
C. Cementoenamel junction (CEJ) is reached
D. Marginal ridge is reached

84. Enamel is etched with
A. Boric acid
B. Phosphoric acid
C. Acetic acid
D. Nitric acid

85. Crystalline gold is also known as :
A. Mat gold
B. Gold foil
C. Powdered gold
D. Electraloy

86. The softest dental inlay wax is :
A. Type A
B. Type B
C. Type C
D. None of the above

87. With respect to onlay preparations, "shoeing" of a functional cusp is :
A. Sometimes indicated

B. Always indicated
C. Never indicated
D. None of the above

88. The most conservative way to lighten vital teeth is:
A. Bleaching
B. Direct composites
C. Laboratory- fabricated porcelain veneers
D. Full coverage crowns

89. Surrounding the wax pattern with a material which can accurately duplicate its shape and anatomical feature is referred to as :
A. Investing
B. Burnout
C. Casting
D. Picking

90. The outline form a cavity preparation is defined as:
A. That form the cavity takes to resist the forces of mastication
B. That from the cavity takes to resist dislodgement or displacement of the restoration
C. The shape or form of the cavity on the surface of the tooth
D. All of the above

91. A 15-year old female has lived in a non-fluoridated area all of her life. Which of the following is most likely to occur in this female when she moves to a community where the drinking water naturally contains 6 ppm of fluoride ?
A. A 50% reduction in dental caries
B. Moderate dental fluorosis
C. An increase in the amount of fluoride stored in her bones
D. Gastrointestinal problems

92. After the initial setting period, which of the following cements is the least soluble?
A. Zinc phosphate cement
B. Zinc polycarboxylate cement
C. Glass ionomer cement
D. Zinc eugenol cement

93. Which property of filled resins is primarily to blame for the failure of class II composite restoration?

A. Low flexural strength
B. Low compressive strength
C. Low Tensile strength
D. Low wear resistance

94. Head and neck cancer patients can benefit by using which of the following fluoride types for home-care custom tray use?

A. Stannous fluoride only
B. Acidulated phosphate fluoride only
C. Sodium fluoride and stannous fluoride
D. Sodium fluoride and acidulated phosphate fluoride

95. A necrotic pulp may

A. Have no painful symptoms
B. Not respond to the electric pulp tester at any current level
C. Respond to heat
D. Not respond to acid
E. All of the above

96. If a casting fails to completely seat in a cavity, one should first check for :

A. Undercuts in the tooth preparation
B. Residual temporary cement or other debris in the cavity
C. Premature internal contact
D. Excessively light proximal contacts

97. The mesial and distal walls of a class I amalgam preparation should diverge slightly towards the occlusal surface to :

A. Provide convenience form
B. Provide resistance from
C. Afford support for the mesial and distal marginal ridges
D. Make condensing of the amalgam easier

98. All of the following are disadvantages of cast gold restorations *except*

A. Esthetic
B. Cost
C. Time-consuming

D. Difficulty of technique
E. Gold has a low thermal conductivity
F. The need to use cement, which is the weakest point in the cast gold restoration

99. Match the following four types of ZOE material with their indications for use.

Types of ZOE Materials	Indications for use	Matching
Type I ZOE	Cavity liner	4
Type II ZOE	Temporary cement	1
Type III ZOE	Permanent cement	2
Type IV ZOE	Temporary filling or base	3

100. Which line angle listed below is rounded when preparing a class II amalgam preparation

A. Axiobuccal
B. Axiolingual
C. Axiopulpal
D. None of the above

101. All of the following statements are true regarding glass ionomer restorations *except*

A. Glass ionomer is often the ideal material of choice for restoring root surface carries in patients with high caries activity
B. The best surface finish for a glass ionomer restorations is that obtained against surface matrix
C. Glass ionomer adheres to mineralized tooth issue
D. Glass ionomers are somewhat esthetic and polish much better than composites

102. Pulpal pain, either spontaneous or elicited by an irritant, that lingers more than 10 seconds suggest:

A. Pulpal necrosis
B. Pulpal hyperemia
C. Irreversible pulpits
D. Acute apical periodontitis

103. All of the following statements concerning fluoride are true *except*
   A. The substantial reduction in dental decay that have occurred in the young population in the United States are due, for the most part, to the use of systemic and topical fluorides
   B. Fluoride reduces caries by increasing the enamel hardness
   C. Fluoride converts hydroxyapatite into fluorapatite by the substitution of the OH ion for the fluoride ion
   D. The fluoride ion decreases the solubility of the hydroxy-apatite crystal and at the same time increases the size of the crystal itself.

104. All of the following are components of sodium fluoride paste that can be used to treat sensitivity except.
   A. Sodium fluoride
   B. Kaolin
   C. Glycerin
   D. Eugenol

105. Which of the following is defined as "that form the cavity preparation takes to aid the operator in preparing, or finishing the restoration"?
   A. Retention form
   B. Resistance form
   C. Convenience form
   D. Outline form

106. There is abundant evidençe that the initiation of dental caries requires a high proportion of:
   A. Staphylococcus aureus within saliva
   B. Streptococcus mutans within dental plaque
   C. Streptococcus mutans within food
   D. Staphylococcus aureus within dental plaque

107. Acute caries is characterized by all of the following except:
   A. Most frequently found in children
   B. Often multiple, soft in children
   C. Slowly progressing
   D. Little or no staining

108. Which component of a dentin bonding system listed below functions primarily to remove the smear layer of the dentin?

A. Etchant
B. Conditioner
C. Primer
D. Adhesive

109. The best angle to attach the sprue pin to the proximal wall of a wax pattern is:

A. 20°
B. 45°
C. 90°
D. The angle makes no difference

110. Which of the following are indications for a cast gold onlay?

A. Restoration of large lesions: involving more than one-third intercuspal dimension, extensive loss of supporting structure where at least half of the clinical cusps. Loss of cusp (s) with at least 1 mm of dentin supporting remaining cusps
B. Restoration of ideal occlusion in cases of drifting, hypo- and hyper eruption, etc.
C. Restoration of optimum contour and proximal contact
D. Restoration of brittle teeth (endodontically treated)
E. Restoration of a tooth as an abutment for removable prosthesis, creating ideal guiding planes, rest seals and undercuts
F. Restoration of teeth to meet patient preference for gold
G. All of the above

111. All of the following are advantages or indications for a Class II gold inlay except

A. The desire for permanency
B. A low caries index
C. Less expensive
D. Moderate size lesions with conservative outlines

112. All of the following drugs may be useful in controlling salivary secretions to help in obtaining a dry field except:

A. Atropine
B. Methantheline

C. Diazepam
D. Belladonna derivatives
E. Propantheline bromide

113. Which of the following factors tends to reduce the setting expansion of amalgam.
A. Increasing the amount of mercury in the mix
B. Increasing the silver content of alloy
C. Increasing the trituration time
D. Increasing the zinc content of the alloy

114. Which of the following is the strongest phase of the set amalgam?
A. Gamma
B. Gamma-one
C. Gamma-two
D. They are all the same strength

115. Why is it important to restore proper proximal contact when restoring teeth?
A. To minimize periodontal pocket formation
B. To maintain the proper height of the interproximal papillae
C. To maintain the mesiodistal dimension of the tooth
D. To minimize food impaction
E. All of the above

116. All of the following are true concerning a Class V amalgam preparation except:
A. The outline form is determined primarily by the location of the free gingival margin
B. The mesial, distal, gingival, and incisal walls of the cavity preparation diverge outward
C. The retention form is provided by the gingival retention groove placed along the incisoaxial line angle
D. A cervical clamp is usually necessary to retract gingival tissues

117. The most ductile and malleable metal is:
A. Silver
B. Gold
C. Copper
D. Platinum

118. In zinc oxide-eugenol (ZOE) cements, the powder is zinc oxide and the liquid is:

A. Phosphate acid
B. Eugenol
C. Zinc polyacrylic acid
D. Saline solution

119. Which restorative material listed below has the lowest thermal conductivity and diffusivity?

A. Amalgam
B. Gold
C. Unfilled resin
D. Filled resin

120. A patient is evaluated about eight months after her sealants were applied. She has lost two out of the four sealants.that were placed. Which of the following could be blamed for thes : sealants being lost?

A. The etchant was not rinsed thoroughly off the tooth surface
B. A dry field was not maintained and the tooth surface was contaminated by saliva after etching
C. A contaminated air supply to air/water syringe
D. The tooth wasn't thoroughly dried prior to application of sealants
E. All of the above.

121. A cavosurface bevel is used when preparing a tooth for a cast gold inlay or onlay. What is the principal reason for its use?

A. To allow room for the cement
B. To improve the marginal adaptation
C. To compensate for shrinkage of the casting gold allow
D. To provide resistance form to the preparation

122. Cavities developing on the proximal surfaces of anterior teeth not involving the incisal edge are classified as:

A. Class I
B. Class II
C. Class III
D. Class IV

E. Class V
F. Class VI

123. Match up the fluoride concentration with the appropriate type of professionally applied topical fluoride.

Topical Fluoride	Concentration	Matching
Sodium fluoride (NaF)	8.0%,	3
Acidulated phosphate fluoride (APF)	2.0%,	1
Stannous fluoride (SnF_2)	1.23%,	2

124. How many milligrams of fluoride are contained in an 8.2 ounce tube of toothpaste?
A. 130 mg
B. 232 mg
C. 350 mg
D. 400 mg

125. High-gold alloys used for cast restorations are:
A. Greater than 20% gold or other noble metals
B. Greater than 30% gold or other noble metals
C. Greater than 50% gold or other noble metals
D. Greater than 75% gold or other noble metals

126. Which cavities below can involve any teeth, anterior or posterior?
A. Class I
B. Class II
C. Class III
D. Class IV
E. Class V
F. Class VI

127. The position of the gingival margin of a Class II amalgam restoration is dictated primarily by:
A. Aesthetics
B. The location of the gingival margin
C. The extent of the carious lesion
D. The thickness of the enamel

128. Delayed expansion of amalgam restorations is associated with which two factors listed below?

A. Insufficient trituration and condensation
B. High residual mercury
C. The contamination of the amalgam by moisture during trituration and condensation
D. The failure to use a cavity varnish

129. Triangularly shaped spaces located between the proximal surfaces of adjacent teeth are called?

A. Contact area
B. Heights of contour
C. Embrasures
D. Contact points

130. High copper dental amalgam alloys involve what ranges of copper in their composition?

A. 1 to 4%
B. 5 to 8%
C. 10 to 30%
D. 50 to 60%

131. The minimal reduction of working cusps for protection from the forces of mastication should be?

A. 2.5 to 3 mm for both amalgam and cast gold restorations
B. 1.5 to 2.0 mm for both amalgam and cast gold restorations
C. 2 mm for amalgam and 1 mm for cast gold restorations
D. 2.5 to 3 mm for amalgam and 1.5 mm for cast gold restorations

132. All of the following are true concerning dental caries except:

A. Dental caries is an infectious microbiological disease of the teeth that results in localized dissolution and destruction of the calcified tissues
B. The evidence for the role of bacteria in the genesis of dental caries is overwhelming
C. Streptococcus sanguis is considered to be a principal etiological agent in dental caries
D. Organisms which cause caries are called “cariogenic”

E. Lactic acid produced by acidogenic bacteria is the main cause of enamel decalcification

133. Pins should be inserted into:

A. Enamel only
B. Dentin only
C. Enamel and dentin (DEJ)
D. Any of the above

134. Chisels are used primarily to cut:

A. Cementum
B. Dentin
C. Enamel
D. Amalgam

Answer Key to MCQs in Operative Dentistry

1	C	2	C	3	B	4	B
5	C	6	D	7	C	8	C
9	B	10	B	11	C	12	B
13	E	14	D	15	C	16	C
17	C	18	C	19	C	20	A
21	B	22	C	23	D	24	C
25	D	26	E	27	C	28	B
29	E	30	D	31	C	32	C
33	C	34	C	35	A	36	E
37	B	38	B	39	E	40	C
41	C	42	B	43	A	44	B
45	C	46	A	47	D	48	D
49	D	50	B	51	A	52	D
53	A	54	D	55	C	56	D
57	B	58	A	59	D	60	F
61	D	62	B	63	C	64	C
65	B	66	C	67	E	68	C
69	C	70	B	71	C	72	B
73	C	74	B	75	A	76	B
77	B	78	A, B	79	F	80	F
81	A	82	C	83	B	84	B
85	A	86	C	87	C	88	A
89	A	90	C	91	C	92	C
93	D	94	C	95	E	96	B
97	C	98	E	99	—	100	C
101	D	102	C	103	B	104	D
105	C	106	B	107	C	108	B
109	B	110	G	111	C	112	C
113	C	114	A	115	E	116	A
117	B	118	B	119	C	120	E
121	B	122	C	123	—	124	B
125	D	126	A, E, F	127	C	128	C
129	C	130	C	131	D	132	C
133	B	134	C				

3

Endodontics

Most common complaint of the patient that leads to dental treatment = pain

A delta fibres = sharp, piercing, lancinating pain, usually **responds to cold**, easy to localise, not referred

C delta fibres = dull, boring, gnawing and excruciating pain, respond **abnormally to heat**, not easy localisable, referred

Acute reversible pulpitis / hyperemia = more responsive to cold than heat,

Irreversible pulpitis = pain caused by heat, relieved by cold

Disease	Vitality of associated Tooth	E.PT
Acute periodontal abscess	Vital	
Periapical osteofibrosis	Vital	
Response to cold	Vital	
Acute apical periodontitis	Vital/non vital	
Odontogenic cyst	Vital	
Fissural cyst	Vital	
Central giant cell granuloma	Vital	
Cementoblastoma	Vital	
Cementoma	Vital	

Ossifying fibroma	Vital	
Radicular cysts	Non vital	Commom in max. ant. area
Granuloma	Non vital	Negative
Phoenix abscess	Non vital	
Chronic alveolar abscess/ gum boil	Non vital	
Condensing osteitis		Common in mand first molar area

Mobility of teeth

First degree: noticeable movement of tooth in its socket.

Second degree: movement of tooth within 1 mm range.

Third degree: movement of tooth more than 1 mm range. Or tooth is depressible in the socket.

DIAGNOSIS

A lesion on r/g is not seen until the cortical bone has been reached

Loss of cancellous bone is undetectable until at least 6.6 % of mineral content of cortical bone in the direct path of x-ray beam has been lost.

Pulp vitality depends on intrapulpal blood circulation.

A **false positive** electric pulp testing test indicates: moist, gangrenous pulp, or partially necrotic pulp in multirooted teeth.

In full coverage restoration electric pulp testing is not done, so test is by CO_2 snow, frigident spray (– 50° C), or diflorodicholoro methane.

Recently traumatised teeth, open apex in young teeth, = misleading electric pulp testing.

A false negative test is more misleading than false positive electric pulp test.

Electric pulp testing is better than thermal testing.

In **liquifaction necrosis** = a minimum response to maximum current of electric pulp testing.

Thermal test

Response to **cold** = vital pulp, can be easily localised.

Heat test = preferred temp. is 65.5° C

16°–55° C is well tolerated by pulp.

Anaesthic test = localisation of specific tooth by intraligamentary inj, is the last resort.

Test cavity = drilling is done at slow speed without coolant, if pain / sensitivity occurs => vital pulp.

Acute alveolar abscess = is phoenix abscess. **conduction anaesthesia** is used to block its pain.

Acute periodontal abscess: aka parietal abscess.

Trepanation = artificial opening thro cortical plate

Root fracture = more closer to the apex, better the prognosis.

Pulp is not responsive to pulp vitality tests for 6–8 weeks = **stunned pulp**, wait and watch.

Avulsion: tooth should be kept in the socket > milk > saliva > water, because milk preserves the vitality of PDL longer than saliva.

Extraoral time for an avulsed tooth should be < 30 min for best progresses.

Most effective antibiotic in RCT is = penicillin

least effective antibiotic in RCT is = tetracycline.

Normal **intrapulpal pressure**: 10 mm Hg

If intrapulpal pressure is upto 13 mm Hg = reversible changes in pulp.

If intrapulpal pressure is up to 35 mm Hg = irreversible changes in pulp.

All stimuli from pulp are = pain

Pain due to decreased atmospheric pressure = **barodontolgia**

C fibres	A delta fibres
80 %	20 %
Unmyelinated	Myelinated
0.3 – 1.2 micron diameter	2–5 micron diameter
0.4 – 2 m/sec. Conduction velocity	6–30 m/sec. Conduction velocity
Slow, distributed thro out pulp	Fast, present in odontoblastic and sub-odontoblastic zone, associated with dentinal pain
Conduct throbbing and aching pain	Sharp and piercing pain
Excitation due to injury or chemicals leads to pain	Excitation is associated with dentinal sensitivity and is difficult to explain.

Referred pain = pain of pulpitis of different teeth is referred to :

Mandibular molar	Preauricular area and in the ear
Mandibular 3rd molar	Angle of mouth
Max Ist molar and canine	Infra orbital region
Max 2nd molar	Preauricular region
Max incisors	Supraorbital region
Mand incisors	Mand frenum
Pain of dental origin is always IPSILATERAL; never crosses the midline. Also pain of non-dental origin in mand angle area is due to = myocardial infarction and sub acute thyroiditis.	

Impulses travel through **plexus of Rashkow** to trigeminal nerve (II, III div.)

Efferent motor pathway in pulp = are sympathetic fibres from **cervical ganglion**.

Parasympathetic fibres thro 5th nerve = involved with **dentinogenesis**.

Hydrodynamic theory is the most acceptable theory for pain transmission.

Cementum = 20–50 micron thick at CEJ, 20–150 micron at apical third.

Average deviation of apical foramen = 0.2–0.5 mm from center of root apex.

Average width of PDL = 0.15–0.38 mm

CAUSES OF PULP DAMAGE

CHEMICAL INSULT

Poor recuperative ability of pulp is due to = **high plasminogen activity**.

Dehydration of pulp by air stream may cause aspiration of odontoblast nuclei, e.g. by alcohol, hydrophilic restorative materials, etc.

Silicate cement is one of the most common cause of pulp death in incisors.

Sodium fluoride for 5 min is not dangerous to avoid secondary caries, but 8 % stannous fluoride for more than 30 sec is C/I.

BACTERIA

Most common cause of pulp injury = bacterial

Anachoresis = attraction / fixation of blood-borne bacteria in areas of inflammation causing pulpitis.

Gnotobiotic = germ-free

Lactobacilli acidogenic are common in carious dentin, but seldom in pulp.

Commonest bacteria of mouth = streptococci

Commonest bacteria of root canal = streptococci

Most common bacteria in RC = alpha-hemolytic streptococci (*S. viridans*)

0.1 % agar in TSA facilitates growth of anaerobes.

Most common bacteria in infected vital pulp = streptococci, staphylococci.

Most common bacteria in chronic alveolar abscess = alpha – hemolytic streptococci and obligate anaerobes.

Chronic hyperplastic pulpitis = pulp polyp, seen in teeth of children and young adults

Internal resorption = mostly seen in maxillary anterior teeth.

Its treatment is removal of cause. If perforated then seal with $Ca(OH)_2$

External resorption = Its treatment is removal of cause. RCT and dressing with $Ca(OH)_2$.

Three types of resorption =

1. Surface = in it, cementum gets deposited
2. Inflammatory = replaced by granulomatous tissues
3. Replacement = leads to ankylosis.

Discoloration of tooth is the first indication that the pulp is dead.

Abscess = pus takes the path of least resistance.

Sinus tract is generally on labial/ buccal mucosa

Labial alveolar plate = upper jaw

Palatal plate = upper lateral incisor, palatal root of upper molar

In vestibule along buccal alveolar plate = lower jaw

May be on lingual alveolar wall = lower molars

Sinus tract opens near symphysis = lower anteriors

Sinus tract opens near inferior mandibular border = lower posteriors

Bay cyst = the lesion in which the cyst lumen communicated with apical foramen.

Only disorder which is chronic periradicular disease in the area of condensation is = **condensing osteitis**

Pulpotomy = done in children and young adults, surgical removal of coronal pulp. Preserves the vitality of radicular pulp. Helps complete **apexogenesis.** Under $Ca(OH)_2$, odontoblasts form reparative dentin to bridge the gap.

CHEMICALS USED IN ENDODONTICS

- **Formoacresol** does not help to form reparative dentin, but just fixes the tissues, acts antibacterial. Coagulation necrosis occurs. Used with recently exposed primary teeth only for pulpotomy.
- **Glutraldehyde** does not go beyond apex due to high cross–linking, so it is better than formoacresol.
- **Functions of $Ca(OH)_2$:**

1. Root resorption treatment
2. Healing of pulp
3. Apexogenesis, closure of root apex.
4. Formation of tertiary dentin due to high pH.
5. Antimicrobial properties.
6. It should be in contact with tissues to be effective. Excess material is removed by multinucleated giant cells.
7. In deci roots canals, it causes internal root resorption.
8. Pulpotomy with it is C/I in irreversible pulpitis and in deciduous teeth.
9. **Mechanism of action** = It causes coagulative necrosis in adjacent pulp tissues and inflammation of contagious tissues. The anion of its maintains local alkaline pH which is necessary for the bone and dentin formation below the area of coagulation necrosis. Cells of pulp differentiate into odontoblasts and form dentin matrix. Calcium required comes from the blood.

- ZOE also heals the pulp, but does not cause formation of dentin bridge,
- H_2O_2 for washing and irrigation of RC.

- 5.2 % NaOCl for irrigation of RC; completely dissolves the pulp in 20 min–2 hrs. liberates 5% chlorine; antiseptic, destroys bacteria;
- 5.2 % NaOCl should be used as a last solution to irrigate rather than H_2O_2, because otherwise nascent oxygen liberated in PA area from H_2O_2 may cause pain.
- 15 % EDTA = is a chelating agent; helps to open calcified RCs by softening the dentin.
- Normal saline = for irrigation of RCs.
- Metronidazole solution = for irrigation of RCs for anaerobes.
- ZOE paste = for obturation
- Chloroform = for dissolving the gutta percha during removal of GP form the RCs.
- 30% H_2O_2 = for bleaching

DIFFERENT PROCEDURES

PULP CAPPING: to maintain the vitality of the exposed pulp; it is done by placing $Ca(OH)_2$. Done for a pinpoint, recent pulp exposure only.

Direct pulp capping, i.e. pulp is exposed

Indirect pulp capping, i.e. on a thin layer of slightly soft dentin

PULPOTOMY or partial pulpectomy: removal of inflamed coronal pulp, to preserve the vitality of root pulp, to continue normal development of the root, i.e. APEXOGENESIS.

Done mainly on vital teeth; if exposure is larger.

$Ca(OH)_2$ pulpotomy is used in permanent teeth; but not in primary teeth where it causes internal root resorption.

Formoacresol pulpotomy / vital pulpotomy: done only on primary teeth, it causes the fixation of pulp tissues by combining with cellular proteins. It diffuses through the pulp and may be through apical foramen in PA tissues. But it does not promote pulp healing.

Glutaraldehyde is considered better because of its large molecular size and does not diffuse through the pulp tissues.

Devitalisation pulpotomy = is a 2-stage procedure. Here, paraformaldehyde is used to fix entire coronal and radicular pulp tissue. Formaldehyde gas liberated permeates through the coronal and radicular pulp, fixing the tissues.

<u>Non- vital pulpotomy</u> = in primary teeth, 2-stage procedure is used first, necrotic coronal pulp is removed and then infected radicular pulp as treated with a strong antiseptic solution, e.g. Beechwood creosote, CMCP, etc.

Apexification: to induce the development of apex in immature, pulpless tooth to form a bridge AGAINST WHICH OBTURATION IS TO BE DONE, root length does not increase.

Difference between apexification and apexogenesis = apexogenesis is the natural formation and completion of the apex in presence of vital radicular pulp; while the apexification is to create a dentinal bridge across the open root-ends, against which obturation can be done. Root length may not be achieved in it.

Pulpectomy / RCT = is complete removal of the pulp tissues.

B-cells = humoral immunity, produce antibodies.

T-cells = cell mediated immunity esp by effector T-cells.

Extravasation Igs in the inflammed tissues of pulp and plasma cells = IgG

Some endodontic flare up is mediated by = IgE reactions.

Selection of cases

If PA radiolucency is < 10 mm, then RCT

If PA radiolucency is > 10 mm, then SURGERY

If more than 1/3 rd root is involved = surgery.

RCT treated tooth can erupt normally and can be moved orthodontically normally, because a viable PDL is required for OTM.

STERILIZATION OF INSTRUMENTS

- **Burs** = heated on the flame of ethyl alcohol + formalin (3 :1), it destroys spore-formers also.
- **Quaternary ammonium compounds** = effective against vegetative bacteria
- **Ethyl alcohol and isopropyl alcohol** = effective against vegetative bacteria and TB
- **Alcohol – formalin solution** = effective against vegetative bacteria and TB and spores.
- **Orthophenyl alcohol and benzyl- p-chlorophenol** = effective against vegetative bacteria, TB, fungi, virus but not spores.
- **Hot salt sterilizer** = 425 – 475 F° × 5 sec, i.e. 218–246° C (for files, broaches) and for 10 sec (for absorbent points, cotton pellets)
- Pure NaCl should not be used, it should be mixed with **1% sod silicoaluminate**, $MgCO_3$ or Na_2CO_3= to avoid fusion of salt in heat.
- Hot salt steriliser is better than glass bead
- Hottest part of salt bath is along its outer rim.
- Smallest temp. is in centre of surface layer of salt.
- Beads of glass should be < 1 mm in diameter.
- Temp in glass bead steriliser = 218–246° C for 5 or 10 sec as above.
- **Laser beam** for 3 sec = kills bacteria and spores
- **Alcohol – formalin solution** = for tips of cotton pliers, blades of scissors, etc.
- **Flaming** = for 2 sec for cotton pliers, cement spatulas.
- **Autoclaving** = 120° C × 15 min × 15 lbs.
- **Dry heat oven** = 320° F × 2 hrs / 340° F × 1 hr / 380° F × 30 min.
- **Gutta percha** = 5.2 % NaOCl × 1 min., then rinse with H_2O_2
- **Silver cones** = on flame / hot salt steriliser × 5 sec

ANATOMY OF ROOT CANAL

Types of root canals

1. Type I = RC have one canal and one apical foramen.
2. Type II = two separate canals leaving the pulp chamber, but merging at apex to form single apex.
3. Type III = two separate canals opening through two separate apical foramina.
4. Type IV = one RC opening with two apical foramina.

- **Accessory canals** =apical 3rd and furcation of root
- Mesial root of mandibular first molar = 2 canals
- Distal root of mandibular first molar = occasionally has 2 canals
- Mesiobuccal root of maxillary first molar = sometimes has 2 canals
- **Apical constriction area** = 0.5 – 1.0 mm from apex.
- Apical foramen opens slightly eccentrically = 0.4 – 0.7 mm from apex.
- R.C. Obturation should end 0.5 mm from anatomic apex as seen on R/G
- A root apex completes 2–3 years after eruption of tooth.
- Abscess of max canine perforates in buccal vestibule below the insertion **of levator labii superioris.**
- If perforation is above LLS = abscess drains in canine space and causes cellulitis.
- **Dentinal map** = anatomic dark lines in the pulpal floor

ANOMALIES

- Hereditary opalescent dentin = **RC very small, obliterated**.
- Hyperparathyroidism = pulp calcification, loss of lamina dura.
- Hypopituitarism = retarded eruption, open root apices.
- Dentinal dysplasia = **obliterated pulp chambers**, defective root formation, RC obliterated sometimes.
- Taurodontism = short tooth, **very larger pulp chambers**

- Neanderthal man = **very larger pulp chambers**
- Dens in dente = invagination within crown /root of lingual surface, lined by enamel. Mostly max lateral incisors.
- Dens evaginatus = talon's cusp, mostly on premolars.
- Palatal dev groove = on max central and lateral incisors,
- 0.5–1.0 % **zinc acetate** added to ZOE cement accelerates its setting and prevents its deformation
- **Cavit** = ZnO–polyvinyl material should not be used in the vital teeth.
- **Tooth discoloration** = due to infiltration of blood in dentinal tubules. It can be avoided by irrigation with 5.2 % NaOCl.
- **Calcified root canals** = **EDTA** for 24 hrs in the RC, it softens the dentin.
- After pulp removal, **hemorrhage** should be controlled by 5.2 % NaOCl.
- Cleaning of barbed broaches = in 5.2% NaOCl × 30 min.
- 2.6–5.2 % NaOCl. completely dissolves pulp in 20 min–2 hrs.
- Alternate irrigation with 5.2% NaOCl and H_2O_2 is done, last solution should be 5.2% NaOCl. To remove H_2O_2, otherwise nascent O_2 can cause pain.

INSTRUMENTS

- Instruments (10–100) = increase in size by 5 units upto 60 and by 10 units upto 100.
- **Instruments no.** is = diameter at the tip in 1/100 th mm
- Length of flute part = 16 mm
- Diameter at D2 = 0.32 mm greater than at D1
- Constant increase in diameter from D1 to D2 = by 0.02 mm/ mm (0.32/ 16 = 0.02)
- Tip angle of instrument = 75° ± 15°.

Instrument are in 21, 25, 28, 30 mm sizes,

Mostly 25 mm are used; 40 mm for endodontic implants; 28–30 mm for canines.

- Color coding = PGP BYR BGB (6, 8, 10, 15, 20, 25, 30, 35, 40)

SMALL INSTRUMENTS ARE FORMED BY **SQUARE BLANK**

Larger INSTRUMENTS ARE FORMED BY **triangular BLANK**

Reamers	**k-files**
Pushing, rotatory motion	Pulling, rasping motion
Less flutes	More
Triangular	Square blank
Resist fracture less	More
Larger	Small, fragile instruments
Cut 2.5 × more efficiently	Less

k-flex file	**H file**	**Unifiles**
More flexibility,	Spiral flutes	Made form two spiral
More cutting efficiency than k-files	Higher cutting	Less efficient
Rhomboidal/diamond	Low flexibility	Double helix design blank design
Alternate high and low flutes	Used for finishing coronal 3rd	High fracture resistance
Fragile, fracture easily	Less fractured	

RECAPITULATION, i.e. return to smaller instruments to prevent packing of debris from RC

Diagnostic/ exploratory instruments are no. 10 – 20 k-files

<u>Actual length of canal</u> = 1.2 mm less than R/G

Working length of the file should be 2 mm less than the root length to prevent injury to periapical tissues.

Apical foramen is 0.3 mm short of actual root tip.

DCJ is 0.4–0.7 mm away from the root apex.

Instruments should stop 0.5–1.0 mm short of RC length.

Ideally, RC should be at least enlarged to no. 25 –30 size in apical third area and to 40 or more in coronal/ mid part of RC.

Step back method aka flare / telescopic method – better method.

H- file 1–2 sizes larger than last file should be used to finish the coronal third of RC.

Gates Glidden drill = for cleaning/shaping cervical 3 rd of RC

Peeso reamer = for preparing post space.

Ultrasonic = 0.001 – 0.004 " movement of file at 20,000–25,000/ sec.

Sonic = 1500–6500 rpm

Gutta percha = can be softened by chloroform, xylol

EDTA = helps in softening the dentin by forming Ca – chelates for easy removal. 15% EDTA has pH = 7.3

DISINFECTION OF RC

Eugenol = anodyne, antiseptic,

Phenol = carbolic acid, necrosis of tissues

1% *p*-chlorophenol = antimicrobial,

camphorated *p*-chlorophenol = antibacterial

formocresol = strong disinfectant, causes necrosis, and fixation of tissues, causes CMI thro T-cells.

2% glutraldehyde = strong disinfectant, fixative, but no CMI

$Ca(OH)_2$ = antiseptic, increases pH of circumpulpal dentin

NaOCl = disinfectant action of halogens is inversely proportional to their atomic number, so chlorine has maximum effect.

OBTURATION

No obturation is done if there is persistent sinus/fistula.

Best material = gutta percha; it has ZnO as in maximum/main component.

Different techniques are = lateral condensation; vertical condensation; sectional condensation; compaction

Tug back = important process; it is the snug fitting of the master cone of GP, resisting removal. It is placed within 1 mm of the apex.

Compaction = ka McSpadden technique, the RC should be enlarged to > 45 no. size by **step-back technique**

Vertical condensation tech. is used with **step-back technique** of RC preparation

Vertical condensation is better than compaction technique, but has a risk of vertical root fracture.

Sectional tech = GP cones of 3 – 4 mm size are used to pack, but voids may form.

Silver cone = used in fine tortuous canals. C/I if post and core is required.

Eucapercha has replaced chloropercha b'coz chloroform is carcinogenic; shrinks after setting = poor seal

Thermoplasticized GP technique = used with injection technique; disadvantage is lack of precision near apex.

Hydron is hydrophilic; polymer of HEMA; but more leakage from RC.; used with injection technique.

Diaket = is polyvinyl resin; but has a tendency towards fibrous encapsulation.

Long term use of Corticosteroids = interferes with fibroblastic activity and retards the healing.

Pulpless teeth have approx 9 % less moisture than a vital tooth.

In retrograde filling = 2 mm of RC is filled;

Transplantation is not as successful as replantation; however, both lead to root resorption and loss of tooth.

BLEACHING

- Normal color of primary teeth = bluish white
- Normal color of permanent teeth = greyish yellow
- Decomposition of pulp tissue = more common cause of discoloration
- Congenital porphyria = red/purple
- Hereditary opalescent dentin = violaceous
- Fluorosis = mottled brown
- Erythroblastosis fetalis = grayish brown
- Jaundice = brown
- Nasmyth's membrane = green
- Silver amalgam = slate gray to dark gray
- Copper amalgam = bluish black to black
- Gold = dark brown

BLEACHING AGENTS

Superoxol = 30 % H_2O_2 by wt and 100 % by vol. In pure distilled water

Walking bleach = superoxol + sodium perborate .

Sodium perborate liberates nascent oxygen.

Vital tooth bleaching = for mottled enamel; by a solution containing 36% HCl and 30% H_2O_2 for bleaching.

- Tetracycline stains are irreversible because they form complexes in dentin.

TRAUMA

- Most common fractured teeth : max anteriors
- Most prone to trauma = children 8–12 years of age.
- Incidence of fracture = 5 %, male > females
- Fracture of crown is diagonal, frequently involving mesial corner
- Fracture of root is horizontal

- Fracture of root near apical third = prognosis is better
- Vertical fracture = prognosis is poorest
- Avulsion = do not curette the socket, RCT should be done within 7–14 days,
- If extraoral time is < 30 min, PDL will survive.
- In endo–perio cases = endo treatment is done before perio treatment
- Radisectomy = endo treatment is done before root removal
- Trephination = is making a perforation in cortical bone.

Ellis' classification of tooth trauma

Class 1	Crown fracture, with little/ no dentin
Class 2	Extensive fracture of crown, involving enamel; dentin but no pulp
Class 3	Exposing the dental pulp
Class 4	Tooth becomes non-vital, with/without loss of crown structure
Class 5	Teeth lost as a result of trauma
Class 6	Fracture of root, with / without loss of crown structure
Class 7	Displacement of tooth, without fracture of crown or root
Class 8	Fracture of crown en-masse and its replacement
Class 9	Trauma to deciduous teeth

ENDODONTIC IMPLANTS

Apical foramen is widened to no. 60–90 size

40 mm long reamer is required.

RC must be enlarged to at least to 60 size.

RC should be irrigated with LA solution, because NaOCl irritates the PA tissues

MTA

- It is used for sealing off the pathways of communication b.w root canal system and external surface of the tooth.
- It is a powder which has fine hydrophilic particles which sets in presence of moisture. Hydration of the powder results in the formation of a colloidal gel with a pH 12.5 which solidifies to a hard structure.
- MTA is a mixture of tricalcium silicate, tricalcium aluminate ; tricalcium oxide and silicate oxide; it also cntains small amount of other mineral oxides which modify its physical and chemical properties.
- Bismuth oxide is added to provide radiopacity.
- Calcium and phosphorus are the main ions in MTA.
- Setting time is approx 4 hrs. compressive strength is 70 Mpa at 21 days; whichy si compartble to IRM and super – EBA,, but less than amalgam (311 Mpa).
- Other materials used for root canal sealting are : amalgam; ZOE based cements; eg super – EBA; and IRM; GIC; and compostite resins.
- MTA- leads to direct bone apposition; is biocompatible;
- **It has an inductive effect on cementoblasts**.
- It may facilitate regenration of PDL.
- It has been used as capping material in mechanically exposed pulp; root end induction and rerpair of root perforations, barrier during internal bleaching of RCTed tooth.
- It is prepared immedialtely before use by mixing with sterile water; P: L ratio is 3 : 1.
- It stimulates dentin bridge formation adjacent to dental pulp ie dentinogenesis; it can be due to alkalinity etc
- It helps to form apical plug ie apexification in teeth with immature apices and it causes lesser inflammation
- Biocompatible, good sealing, prevents microleakage
- But gets dissolved in presence of acidic environment, so it should not come in contact with oral cavity for an extended period of time.

- Its pH is 12.5 ie approx equal to calcium hydroxide; which gives it **antimicrobial** properties.
- Its radiopacity is slightly > dentin.
- Presence of moisture is essential for setting.
- Helps in Rx of perforation; furcation involvement and PD regeneration etc.

Mtwo instrument for RCT

- Are NiTi ROTARY instruments and used with pulling out movements;
- Used at 300 rpm
- Tip is non-cutting
- **Cross section** of M – two is **ITALICS – S,** with 2 cutting blades.
- **4 instrument sizes** are available – from # 10 to # 25; these are basic instruments.
- Taper is from 0.04 to 0.06
- # 10 has 0.04 taper; It is the first instrument to be placed in the root canal.
- # 15 has 0.05 taper; # 20 & # 25 have 0.06 taper;
- **Colored ring** on handle identifies the size.
- No. of grooved rings on handle identifies taper ie one ring is 0.04 taper; 2 rings is 0.05 taper; 3 ring is 0.06 taper; & 4 rings is 0.07 taper;
- lengths available are 21 mm, 25 mm; 31 mm.
- Conventional cutting part is 16 mm long.
- Extended cutting part is 21 mm for cutting in coronal part.
- Helical angle HA increases from apex toward crown
- HA is more open / greater for the bigger sizes; less flutes for the instrument length and vice versa
- Flutes are deeper from apex towards coronal area increasing the capacity to remove debris coronally. It is also called as **PITCH PROGRESSION**.

- RETREATMENT FILE: are 2 types of files ie # 15 with 0.05 taper; and # 25 with 0.05 taper. They have active tip as compared to RC preparing files; to easily enter the obturated material.
- Crown down technique is used; here it is specifically called as **simultaneous technique** because full length of root canal is approached at the same time.
- It can be safely used in curved root canals.

CALCIUM HYDROXIDE:

- Introduced by Herman in 1920
- PH is 12.5, alkaline; antimicrobial;
- Tissue dissolving ability; inhibition of tooth resorption; induces repair by hard tissue formation
- Mechanism of action: it released hydroxyl ions in aqueous environment which are highly oxidant free radicals showing extreme reactivity they kill bacteria by damaging cytoplasmic membrane; protein denaturation and damage to DNA.

DENTINAL HYPERSENSITIVITY:

Methods to check dentinal hypersensitivity:

- Tactile: by using dental explorer; electronic probe; pressure probe device; etc
- Thermal: by bursting room temperature air for one second; between 65 to 70 degree Fahrenheit and at a pressure of 60 psi.
- Osmotic; by using sweet stimuli.
- Electrical:

Management of hypersensitivity:

- Potassium nitrate: 5 or 10 %; it reduces dentinal sensory nerve activity due to the depolarizing activity of the K – ions.
- Strontium chloride: strontium gets deposited in der in in place of calcium resulting in recrystallisation of strontium apatite complex.
- Sodium fluoride: it increases the resistance of dentin to acid decalcification. Also the precipitated fluoride compounds

mechanically block the exposed dentinal tubules and thus blocking transmission of stimuli.

- Sodium monofluorophosphate:
- Stannous fluoride: it helps creating a calcific barrier blocking the tubular openings on the dentin surface.
- Fluoride iontophoresis: iontophoresis is the process of influencing i0onic motion by an electrical current. It uses sodium fluoride.
- Oxalates: oxalate ions react with calcium ions in dentinal fluid to form insoluble calcium oxalates crystals which block the dentinal tubules apertures.
- Resins and adhesives
- Lasers: Nd: YAG laser is used with fluoride varnish. Also $CO2$ laser with stannous fluoride gel is effective.
- Combination agents: ie a combination of 5 % $KNO3$ and Fluoride
- Restorative materials
- Tooth mousse.

4

Oral Surgery

Electrosurgery = it involves the use of electric current in performing various surgical procedures.

Principal = passing of an alternating current thro the body using 2 electrodes. The large electrode is dispersive and small is active.

- Effects of the current = dehydration; warming of the area; coagulation; tissue destruction.

Types of electrosurgery

Electro-fulguration/ electro-dessication	High frequency High voltage Low amperage	One electrode used
Electro-coagulation	High frequency Low voltage Low amperage	2 electrodes
Electro-cutting	High frequency	2 electrodes
Electrocautery	Low voltage High amperage	One electrode

Principles of surgery

1. Asepsis/sterilization
2. Atraumatic procedure
3. Infection control
4. Hemostasis

- Increased susceptibility to infections occurs in:
  - D. Mellitus
  - Leukemia
  - Pt. on corticosteroid treatment
  - Uremia, etc.
  - Quinidine can cause thrombocytopenia

Response of the patient to an operation is divided in **4 phases of convalescence:**

1. Acute injury; **catabolic state**; for 2–5 days; negative N_2 balance; increased production of catecholamines and corticosteroids.
2. Patient's appetite increases; diuresis begins.
3. **Anabolic phase**—increased appetite; gains strength; positive N_2-balance; for 2–3 weeks; lean muscle mass is restored.
4. Gain in fat.
   - For approx 2 days after operation, there is Na and H_2O retention and so less Na and H_2O should be given I/V.
   - Increased production of corticosteroid occurs after injury especially free 17-hydroxy-corticosteroids esp CORTISOL.
   - If patient was on a prolonged steroid therapy, his adrenal-pituitary axis gets suppressed and so he is not able to respond to trauma. These patients require **replacement therapy** with steroids to avoid PROFOUND shock, etc. during extractions/surgery, etc.

STERILIZATION (Also refer to the section of microbiology for details.)

- Moist heat is most reliable and least expensive method.
- Sterilization = means the total destruction of microbes, virus and spores.
- Bactericide = destroys the bacteria.
- Bacteriostatic = inhibits the bacterial growth.
- Autoclaving = 121°C × 15 psi × 15 min or 134°C × 30 psi × 3 min.
- 3 min FLASH CYCLE is best for unwrapped instruments.

Dry heat	120°C
Boiling water	100°C
Autoclaving	12°C
Oil bath	175°C
Gas	10.8°C
Irradiations	
Filteration	

Antisepsis and disinfection

- Alcohol 70%
- Hexachlorophene 3%
- $Iodine_2$ and its compounds 2–5%
- Aq. Quat. Ammonium compounds
- H_2O_2 3%
- Sodium hypochlorite
- Phenols
- Formaldehyde and glutraldehyde
- Chlorhexidine 20%
- Cetrimide 0.5%

Boiling water sterilization

- Cannot remove spores.
- At 100°C × 30 min.

DRY HEAT STERILIZATION/HOT AIR OVEN

- For disinfection of dental hand-pieces, oils, powders, papers, clothes, etc.
- Slow method
- 121°C × 6 hrs.
- 60°C × 2 hrs.

- Dry heat will not attack glass and will not rust instruments.
- Less expensive.

Chemical or cold sterilization: SLOW = 18–24 hrs required.

- Most widely used for DISINFECTION.

1. 70–90% solution by wt. of ***ISOPROPYL ALCOHOL***
   - Poorly effective vs all micro organism.
   - NOT AT ALL effective vs spore formers.
   - Expensive.
   - Does not work in p.o. body fluids.
   - Can rust the instruments.
2. ***Benzalkonium chloride*** (a quaternary ammonium compound.)
   - Used for general sanitation and house-keeping.
3. ***2% glutraldehyde*** = best; bactericidal.
4. ***2–5 % Hexachlorophene.***
   - Bacteriostatic
5. ***8% formaldehyde***
   - ***20% formalin***
   - ***I_2 and iodophores***
   - ***Chlorinated bis-phenols***

GAS STERILIZATION

- For heat-sensitive and water-sensitive instruments.
- **Ethylene oxide** gas is used = bactericidal.
- Use ethylene oxide at room temperature and a 30% HUMIDITY for 12 hrs.
- Used for dental hand-pieces, etc.
- Gas is expensive.
- Gas > 3% of room air can be EXPLOSIVE.
- Items should be aerated after sterilization for 24 hrs.
- Used for INDUSTRIAL use.

CHEMICAL VAPOUR STERILIZATION–(CHEMICLAVE)

- Formaldehyde + Alcohol + water vapors.
- 132°C (270°F) × 20–40 psi × 20–25 min.

Adv. SHORT cycle; No rusting of instruments; No aeration required; But high cost.

For industrial sterilization

- ***Ionizing radiations.***
- **Gamma** and accelerated beta rays.
- **e.g.** for the mass sterilization of syringes, etc.

RADIATION SOURCES

1. Electron accelerators
2. Radio-isotopes
   - Co 60 and Cerium 137 = give gamma–rays

Important points

- Oils and grease should be removed before sterilisation.
- Instruments should be completely immersed in water to prevent RUSTING.
- Hypodermic needles and syringes should be sterilized by AUTOCLAVING.
- Instruments should be stored in AUTOCLAVED MUSLIN or paper packs.

Conversion data

1. To change F to C = subtract 32 from F and divide by 1.8. (F = Fahrenheit; C = celsius).
2. To change C to F = multiply C by 1.8 and add 32.
3. 1" = 2.54 cm.
4. 1 oz = 28.35 gm.
5. 1lb = 453.5 gm.
6. 1kg = 2.2 lbs.
7. 1 gallon = 3.78 liters.

For **hand-scrubbing**

- Soaps containing HEXA CHLORO PHENE or Iodophors are used.
- 10 minutes scrubbing is required.

Other principles

- Surgeon's back and the gown **below the level of waist** is UNSTERILE.
- ONLY the interior of glove should be touched with hands. Exterior of the glove is considered STERILE.
- Surgeons and nurse/assistant **should pass BACK-TO-BACK** in the OT.
- In OT—the **level of surgical table** is the line of demarcation for asepsis.
- In dental clinics—**level of ARM–REST** of the dental chair is line of demarcation of asepsis.
- Gloved hands may be scrubbed between patients, using a 2 min. scrub with HEXACHLOROPHENE SOAPS.
- O_2 cylinder = black cylinder with white collars.
- N_2O cylinder = blue cylinder.

INCISIONS

1. Pen-grasp method.
2. Table knife method.
   - Skin is more difficult to incise than mucosa.
   - Incision on skin should be placed into the creases of skin relaxation. It helps in wide exposure as they are the cleavage lines of superficial tissue planes.

- Cleavage Dissection = here, the tissue layers are exposed by accurate clipping of tissues with a sharp scissors or scalpel; it produces a LESS BLIND TRAUMA than blunt dissection.
- If incision is placed in LINE OF TENSION = sutures will be under maximum stress and so more SCAR.
- Gentle handling of tissues; aseptic conditions.

- Incision should be clean, atraumatic, perpendicular to skin.
- During suturing on skin—a slight EVERSION of skin edges is preferred.
- Avoid infections.

Principles of skin incisions

- Incision can be placed in a relatively hidden area.
- Incision can follow LANGER'S lines. These lines are the direction of collagen fibers, i.e. lines of tension in the collagen fibers of dermis. Incision parallel to them does not gape and a thin scar is formed after suturing.
- Incision should not be placed in a direction so that muscles may pull the edges of wound and widen the scar.
- Best place of incision is skin crease, these are the areas where muscle pull is absent.
- Incision in growing children tend to heal with a broad scar, it is due to stretch of scar due to somatic growth.
- Always mark the incision on skin with pen, etc. before incision.
- Skin is incised at right angles to the surface except within the eyebrow, where the cut should be angled along the line of the eyebrow hairs.
- Skin edges of neck and facial wounds should not be grasped with dissecting forceps, etc. or they will get crushed and damaged.
- Stitch should enter not more than 2 mm from the wound edges and pass to a depth of 4 mm, embracing a greater width of s/c tissues.
- There should be no dead spaces.
- Cut edges at the surface should be slightly raised in order to produce a final scar, which is flat and level with the rest of the surface.

SUTURE TECHNIQUES–classification

1. Interrupted sutures.
2. Continuous sutures.

3. Continuous locked or blanket sutures.
4. Sub-cuticular sutures.
5. Continuous mattress or horizontal sutures.
6. Vertical mattress sutures.
7. Square knot sutures.
8. Halsted interrupted mattress sutures.

Bandages

1. Stockinette bandage.
2. Barton's bandage.
3. Towel bandage.
4. Barrel bandage.
5. 4-tailed bandage.

Poor wound healing—why?

- Diabetes.
- Poor nutritional status especially Vitamin C deficiency.
- Protein deficiency.
- Poor amino acid metabolism.

Suture materials—classification

(a) absorbable/non-absorbable.

(b) braided/non-braided.

(c) monofilament/multifilament.

(d) metallic/non-metallic.

1. Absorbable

e.g. Catgut = made from serosa of sheep intestine; chromic gut.

- Must be wet to be manageable.
- Absorbed by metabolic activity.
- Highly tissue reactive.

- Polyglycolic acid sutures—easy to handle; less tissue reactive; less expensive.
- Polyglactin 910 and collagen.

(a) **Natural fibre** (enzymatic absorption)

- **monofilament**—catgut/collagen.
- **multifilament**—none.

(b) **Synthetic fibre** (hydrolytic absorption)

- **Monofilament**—glycolide/caprolactone (monoacryl).
- – Glycolide/dioxanone/trimethylene carbonate (biosyn).
- – Polydioxanone (PDS).
- – Polyglycolide/trimethylene carbonate (maxon).
- **Multifilament**—glycolide/lactide (vicryl, polysorb, dexon).

2. Non-absorbable material

(a) Natural fibers = silk, cotton, linen.

(b) Synthetic fibers = Dacron, nyclon, polyester, polypropylene.

- Have superior tensile strength
- **Minimum capillary action**
- Less inflammatory reaction
- But difficult to handle and **hard to tie**.

(a) **Natural fibre**

- **monofilament**–none
- **multifilament**–cotton; silk

(b) **Synthetic**

- **monofilament**
- – Polyamide (nylon)
- – Polybutester (novafil)
- – Polypropylene (prolene, surgipro, surgilene)
- – Polytetra fluoroethylene (PTFE)
- – Steel
- **multifilament** = polyamide (nylon); polyester (e.g. dacron); steel

Ideal properties

1. It should have adequate strength.
2. It should be sterilizable.
3. It should evoke little tissue reaction.
4. It should have a contrasting colour.
5. It should have good handling and knot tying characteristics.

Sutures are sized such that **No. 3 is the largest and 7–0 is the smallest** in general use. The more zeros in the number, the smaller the diameter of the strand. 3–0 and 4–0 are used intraorally.

A. Absorbable sutures

1. Gut
2. Collagen
3. Polyglycolic acid and polyglactin 910.

GUT: It is derived from sheep's intestinal submucosa or bovine intestinal serosa. It is of 2 types:

- **Plain gut** = this is stiff and has **insecure knot handling** characteristics.
- **Chromic gut** = this is plain gut, which has been **tanned with a solution of chromium salts** prior to being spun, ground and polished.

Gut suture is **absorbed by proteolytic degradation** and phagocytosis. This is accompanied by considerable inflammation and tissue reaction.

COLLAGEN: Is obtained by grinding the native collagen of deep flexor tendons of cattle.

POLYGLYCOLIC ACID and POLYGLACTIN 910: They are resorbed by hydrolysis. They are synthetic polymers, and produce very little tissue reaction. When braided, they are the **strongest of the absorbable materials**.

B. Non-absorbable materials

1. Silk
2. Nylon
3. Cotton and linen

4. Metal
5. Dacron polyester, teflon coated polyethylene, polypropylene.

SILK

- **Most popular suture material** for intraoral use.
- Excellent handling characteristics.
- Produces a moderate tissue reaction.
- It is inexpensive.
- Does not irritate the adjacent mucous membrane.
- If retained for a long time, produces a **rail-track scar.**
- Its complications are suture abscess, inclusion cyst (the epithelium invades down into the connective tissue).
- Remove silk in 5–10 days.

NYLON

- Can be obtained in braided or monofilament forms.
- Because of its stiffness, a **large knot is required.**
- It has a tendency to tear through the non-keratinized tissue, therefore **nylon is not frequently used intraorally.**

COTTON and LINEN

- Cotton suture is made from non-continuous natural fibers of cotton, which are combined into yarns and then twisted into piles.

METAL

- Stainless steel or tantalum sutures, either monofilament or braided.

Multifilament sutures = source of infections as cp to mono-filament sutures due to capillary actions; monofilament sutures get loose more often.

Suture needles - 1/2–5/8″ length; types are:

1/2 circle round edge

1/2 circle cutting edge

Swaged needle

Eyed/non-eyed needles

- Lateral cutting edge helps easy suturing thro' Ligamentous tissues.
- 18" length of suture material.
- Wire is strongest of all suture materials.
- Wire mesh = used to fill in the bony defects and lost bone contours. TANTALUM mesh is best, but expensive.
- Sutures should be placed at > 5 mm intervals; helps in proper seepage of exudate.
- Chromic gut resorbs more slowly than the plain gut.
- Interrupted sutures are preferable to continuous sutures on skin.
- Slightly EVERT the line of skin incision during closure. It permits some sub-dermal contractures without separation in the line of incision.

Consistency of swellings/growth

Soft	In lipoma
Firm	Fibroma
Cartilage hard	Pleomorphic adenoma
Bony hard	Osteoma
Rock hard	Malignant lymphatic nodes
Rubbery hard	Affected nodes in Hodgkin's disease

Edges of ulcers

Undermined	Tuberculous
Punched-out	Gummatous ulcer
Rolled	Rodent ulcer
Rolled, raised and everted	Malignant ulcer

Different cells

PMN cells	Increase in **acute infections** and after trauma; trauma; blood loss and cardiac infarction, etc.
Lymphocytes	Increased in pertusis, **glandular fever** and lymphocytic leukemia.
Monocytes	Increases in **protozoal infections;** in monocytic leukemia; in glandular fever.
Eosinophils	Increased in **parasitic disease;** intestinal worm infestations; **allergies,** e.g. asthma, urticaria.
Punctate basophilia	In **lead poisoning**.

Eye signs seen in toxic goiter

Von-Graefe's sign	Lid lag sign.
Joffroy's sign	Absence of wrinkling of forehead, when head is bent down and patient looks up.
Moebius's sign **Exophalthmos** **Anxious looks**	Difficulty in convergence.

Sub mandibular approach

- Cut placed 2 cm below the inferior borders of mandible; in the line of skin tension; it avoids cutting of the mandibular br of 7th N.
- Incision should rest on solid bone/firm base.
- Major facial vessels lie deep to superficial ms of expression and PLATYSMA.
- Md Br of 7th N lies just deep to platysma, directly over the facial A; superficial to anterior border of masseter.
- STYLOMANDIBULAR lig separates parotid and submandibular glands.

Surgical approach to TMJ

- Danger of damage to 7th N.
- Blair = inverted-L or reverse question-mark incision.
- Wakely = T-incision; horizontal bar of T is placed over the zygomatic arch.
- Lampert's ENDAURAL approach.

Hypertensionion

Essential HT = increased BP for which definite etiology is unknown.

Mild or moderate HT =	systolic BP	< 200 mm Hg
	Diastolic BP	< 110 mm Hg
Severe HT =	SBP	> 200 mm Hg
	DBP	> 110 mm Hg

Avoid Na-containing I/V solutions.

Cyclosporine-A = may cause gingival hyperplasia.

Vitamin K deficiency–2, 7, 9, 10 clotting factors depressed.

B.P.	mild	if	DBP 90–104 mm Hg
	moderate		105–114 mm Hg
	severe		> 115–125 mm Hg
	malignant		> 125 mm Hg

Adrenal insufficiency

S/s—Weakness; wt loss; fatigue and hyper-pigmentation of skin and mucosa.

Secondary adrenal insufficiency

- Due to chronic therapeutic steroid administration.
- S/s of patient are moon facies, buffalo hump and thin translucent skin.

Thyrotoxicosis: Only thyroid disease, in which an acute crisis may occur. It is due to raised circulating levels of T_3 and T_4 hormones.

S/s of excessive thyroid H

- Fine brittle hair
- Hyper-pigmentation of skin
- Increased sweating
- ↑ BMR; ↑ HR
- **Wt. Loss**
- Palpitation
- Exophthalmos

Thyroid gland **should not be palpated** as it can also trigger crisis.

Atropine and Adr should be avoided in these cases.

PREGNANCY

- Elective procedures should be avoided in 1st and 3rd trimesters.
- Best time for elective procedures–2nd trimester.
- Position of the patient during the Rx.
- Maximum time of procedure allowed.
- How much LA can be given.
- What are the C/I during pregnancy.

Dental medicines to be avoided in pregnancy

- Aspirin and other NSAIDS
- Carbamazepine
- Chloral hydrate
- Corticosteroids
- Diazepam, etc.
- Diphenhydramine hydrochloride
- Morphine
- Nitrous oxide
- Pentazocine HCl
- Phenobarbital
- Promethazine HCl
- Propoxyphene

- Tetracyclines
- If N_2O gas is to be used, at least 50% O_2 should be used with it.
- N_2O should not be used during first trimester.
- Drugs least likely to cause fetal harm are: lidocaine/bupiva caine/acetaminophen/codeine/penicillin/erythromycin.
- Aspirin should not be given in late 3rd trimester = due to its ANTICOAGULANT property.
- Pt. should not be in SUPINE position, to avoid compression of IVC (inferior vena cava).
- Should be placed slightly to one side during surgery.

Drugs to be avoided in LACTATION

- Ampicillin
- Aspirin
- Atropine
- Barbiturate
- Chloral hydrate
- Corticosteroids
- Diazepam
- Metronidazole
- Penicillin
- Propoxyphene
- Tetracycline

Safer drugs in lactation

- Accetaminophen
- Antihistamines
- Cephlaxin
- Codeine
- Erythromycin
- Fluoride
- Meperidine

- Oxacillin
- Pentazocine

ASA classification of physical status

ASA I	A normal healthy patient.
II	A patient with mild systemic dis, or significant health risk factor.
III	A patient with severe systemic dis. which is not incapacitating.
IV	A patient with severe systemic dis, which is a constant threat to life.
V	A moribund patient, who is not expected to survive without operation.
VI	A declared brain-dead patient, whose organs are being removed for donor purposes.

Instruments (details/classification)

- Most commonly used scalpel blade for intra-oral surgery = No. 15 blade.
- **Hemostat** = for controlling bleeding from incised Vs and As.
- **Halsted's mosquito/Artery forceps** = used as hemostats.
- **Adson forceps** = to grasp the soft tissues, to stabilize the flaps during suturing.
- **Allies tissue forceps** = has locking handles and teeth to grip the soft tissues firmly, during removal of soft tissues/fibrous/granulation tissues.
- **Russian tissue forceps** = large, round-ended, tissue forceps for removal of tooth fragment from their socket.
- **Rongeur forceps** = for removing the bone.
- **Blumenthal rongeur** = side cutting/end cutting forceps–can be inserted into the sockets for remaining inter-radicular bone also.
- **Chisel and mallet** = for bone removal.

- **Monobevel chisel** = used for bone removal.
- **Bibevel chisel** = used for tooth splitting.
- **Difference b/w chisel and osteotome** = chisel is monobevel instrument and osteotome is bibeveled.
- **Bone files** = for final smoothening of bone before suturing; used with PULL motion only.
- **Needle holder** = its beak is shorter and stronger than that of hemostat; face of the beak is cross-hatched for a positive grasp of needle and suture.
- **Needle** = is held approx at 2/3rd of the distance between the tip and end of needle.
- **Suture** = size most commonly used to suture oral mucose is 3–0, black silk, poly-filament (which is easy to tie).
- Most commonly used suture scissor is the **DEAN scissors**.
- **Austin retractors** = are cheek and soft tissue retractors; has a right angle.
- **Minnesota retractor** = is an offset broad retraction.
- **Rubber bite blocks** = to help hold the mouth open, e.g. in Rx of ankylosis, hypomobility, etc.
- **Molt mouth prop** or side action mouth prop for opening the mouth wider.
- **CO_2 laser** = latest method of cutting; efficient cutting; good hemostasis; better healing.

Dental elevators = its 3 parts are handle + Shank + Blade

3 types of elevators
- Straight/gouge type = Most common used.
- Triangle/penant shape type = CRYER.
- Pick type = CRANE pick; apex elevator.

Principle of elevators

Lever principle = mechanical mdvantage is 3.

- **Most commonly used principle.**
- Here the elevator is a lever of first class.
- Effort arm is longer than resistance arm.

- Mechanical advantage = output force/input force = 3 for each pound of pressure.

Wedge principle = Mech. Adv. is 2.5 for each pound of pressure.

- e.g. apexo-elevators.
- Is like a movable inclined plane.
- Used to remove the apices of roots from the sockets.

Wheel and Axle principle = Mech. Adv. is 4.6 for each pound of pressure.

- Should be used carefully as it applies maximum pressure.
- May cause fracture of bone if used improperly.

EXODONTIA

Definition: The ideal tooth extraction is the painless removal of whole tooth or root with minimal trauma to the investing tissues, so that the wound heals uneventfully and no post-operative prosthetic problems are created.

METHODS: There are 2 methods of extraction:

1. Forceps extraction = also known as intra-alveolar extraction.
2. Surgical method = also known as trans-alveolar extraction or open method.

MECHANICAL PRINCIPLES OF EXTRACTIONS

1. Expansion of bony socket.
2. Use of a lever and fulcrum to remove a tooth.
3. Insertion of wedge or wedges–to help the tooth/root to rise in the socket.

Analgesia = loss of pain sensation; without loss of other forms of sensations (e.g. pressure; temperature, etc.).

Anaesthesia = loss of all forms of consciousness and also a loss of motor functions.

EXTRACTIONS

- ♦ For md teeth = chair should be as low as possible.

- For Mx teeth = upper jaw of patient should be at the height of operator's shoulder.
- Patient should be in SEMI-RECUMBENT POSITION.
- Autoclaving = best way for sterilization.
- Molt's curet is used to check the anaesthesia for severing the soft tissues.
- Palatal/lingual beak of the forceps is placed first on the tooth.
- Long axis of forceps should be parallel to the long axis of tooth.
- First pressure is placed towards the apex of the tooth to set the forceps at CEJ.
- No more than 4 ml of LA solution with 1:1 lac conc. of adrenaline for a total dose of 0.04 mg in any 30 min. interval should be injected in a patient having angina.

Contra indications of extractions

- Irradiated jaws may develop an acute radio-osteomyelitis after extraction due to lack of BLOOD SUPPLY.
- Uncontrolled D.M. = wound infection and healing problems.
- Cardiac problems = a post-infection patient is not subjected to surgery within 6 MONTHS of his infarction.
- Hemophilia, leukemia.
- ADDISION'S DIS (i.e. STEROID deficiency) is an absolute C.I. They can't withstand the STRESS of an extraction without taking any steroids. (Read Pts. on STEROID TREATMENT).
- PUO (pyrexia of unknown origin), SABE.
- **Pregnancy** = 2nd trimester is SAFEST.
- Senility is a relative C/I = patient may have a negative N_2 balance.

Relative contra-indications to extractions

1. Uncontrolled diabetes.
2. Acute blood dyscrasias.
3. Untreated coagulopathies.
4. Adrenal insufficiency.

5. Teeth should be removed only 6 mos after myocardial infarction.
6. In previously irradiated jaws, at least 1 year is allowed for maximum recovery of circulation. It helps in proper healing.
7. Acute infections in the floor of mouth is a C/I to any form of anesthesia (GA/LA) in an outdoor patient.
8. Mimp C/I to LA is the po acute infection at the site of operation. It may lead to spread of infections and LA is not effective due to acidic nature of pus.
9. PO of hemangioma is C/I for LA.
10. Disease which impairs patency of airway or respiratory efficiency is C/I for GA.
11. Adr/N Adr should not be injected in patients taking tricyclic anti-depressant drugs; as then hypertension or cardiac arrythmia may occur. The effects of Adr and N Adr get potentiated with them.
12. In such patients, prilocaine with felypressin, i.e. a no-amine vasoconstrictor should be used.
13. Patients with H/O hypersensitivity to sulphonamides should not receive LA with PABA rings.

ABSOLUTE C/I of EXODONTICS

1. Arterio-venous or sinusoidal aneurysms.
2. Central hemangiomas.

DEFINITIONS

- **ODONTOTOMY** = i.e. cutting of the tooth apart.
- **Odontectomy** = removal for partly erupted/unerupted tooth by surgical excision.
- **Replantation** = replacing the tooth after extraction and RCT; it is know as elective/intentional replantation.
- **Ankylosis** = i.e. bone fuses directly to the root surface.
- **Replacement resorption** = i.e. after replantation, ankylosis occurs and progressive replacement of root occurs by bone.
- **Auto-transplantation** = also known as **tooth autograft**. It is the transplantation from one position to another position within the same mouth.

- **Allogenic tooth transplant** = also known as **tooth allograft**; is a tooth transplanted from one patient to another.
- **Curettage** = is the removal of pathologic tissues from around the root.
- **Hemi-section/odontosection** = is the cutting of the tooth in half and removal of root with overlying crown part.
- **Amputation/radisectomy** = is the root removal with the coronal tooth structure remaining intact.
- **Gingival curettage** = is the scrapping of soft tissues walls of the pocket.
- **Gingivectomy** = is the removal of soft tissue wall of the pocket to the point at which the tissue is attached.
- **Gingivoplasty** = is the contouring of gingival tissues.
- **Osteoplasty** = is the reshaping of alveolar process, without removal of the supporting bone.
- **Ostectomy** = is the removal of supporting bone.
- **Apicoectomy** = is the removal of a part of the root end.

Principles of apicoectomy (Refer to the section on endodontics Vol. I.)

- While cutting the apical part of the root, the cut should be placed in an oblique direction to maintain the length of the root, rather than in the horizontal direction, which then reduces the length of the root.
- Retrograde filling material should be bio-compatible.
- A hermetic seal is a must with obturation.

Important points

- PA granulation tissue should be removed with a small curet. But it is not done in MAXILLARY INCISOR AREA, because the veins here have no valves and so the infected material and thrombi may ascend into the cranial cavity to form CAVERNOUS SINUS THROMBOSIS.
- Socket must be compressed after extraction
    - To re-establish the normal width of the alveolar ridge.

- Brings gingival margins near to each other.
- Helps maintain the clot in position.

♦ In un-complicated cases, the remaining posterior teeth in maxilla and mandible on ONE side can be removed in one visit.

♦ If maxillary tuberosity fractures during extractions; every effort should be made to retain it, as it is important for denture retention.

♦ **Mechanism of action of cold** at surgical site = cold acts by producing vasoconstriction and so decreases the exudation of fluid and blood into tissue spaces.

♦ **Mechanism of heat** = leads to vaso-dilation and increases circulation, more rapid removal of tissue breakdown products and greater influx of defensive cells and anti-bodies.

♦ **Mechanism of action of saline rinses** = since the saline water is hypertonic, and the exudate is having less conc. of salts but more water, there exists an osmotic gradient to expel out the excess fluids from the inflammed tissues under the influence of hypertonic saline rinses.

♦ **Prophylactic odontectomy of 3rd molars** = best time is when the R/G shows the roots of 3rd molars to be half to 2/3rd formed. It is generally at 16–17 yrs of age.

♦ Mesio-angular impaction is easiest and disto-angular impaction is most difficult to remove.

Other points

♦ While removing the apical 3rd of root/tip, the tip of apexo-elevator is placed between the socket well and the highest side of the fragment (which is closest to the rim of alveolar socket).

♦ Long **Winter's elevators** are used for removing mand. molar roots and are never used elsewhere.

♦ A **root apex** = is defined as a root fragment < 5 mm in its greatest dimension.

♦ If 2, 3, 4 no. of teeth are to be removed at one visit, the chances of fracture of labial plate are reduced if canine is removed first.

♦ Root displaced in max antrum is mainly of max premolars and molars and most often the palatal root.

- **Tannic acid** powder placed on a pack adj to the bleeding socket helps to arrest the bleeding.

Position of the operator

- For extraction of right mand 3 –8 teeth, the operator should stand behind the patient.
- For rest of the teeth, he stands on right side of the patient.
- For removal of maxillary teeth, the chair is adjusted s.t the site of operation is **8 cm, i.e. 3 inches below the shoulder** level of the operator.
- For mand teeth, the chair is adjusted s.t the tooth to be removed is **16 cm/6 inches below** the level of operator's **elbow**.
- **Hearing** is the **last sense lost** under GA and first to be regained as the consciousness returns.
- When average extractions are being done, limit the extractions to the **equivalent of 12 roots** on one occasion.
- If patient is allergic to procaine, then lidocaine may be given
- Vasoconstrictor action of LA with adrenaline is useful to control bleeding.
- In GA–more bleeding occurs, as it has no vasoconstriction property.
- Extraction of teeth should be done from posterior to anterior, if multiple extractions are to be done.

Forceps principles

1. Beaks should be placed as far apically as possible.
2. Beaks should be placed as parallel as possible to the long axis of the tooth.
3. Applications of excessive forces should be avoided.
4. First direction of placement of forceps is in apical direction.

Order of extraction

Teeth should be removed in a systematic fashion, i.e.

1. Very loose and painful teeth are extracted first.
2. Roots are extracted before whole tooth.

3. Lower teeth are removed before the upper teeth.
4. Posterior teeth are removed before the anterior teeth, so that the vision is not obstructed by bleeding.
5. All extractions of one side should be completed before starting on other side.
   - Since anesthesia becomes effective in maxilla first, so the maxillary teeth are extracted first.
   - Most posterior teeth are removed first for better vision.
   - First molars and canine are removed after their adjacent teeth are removed, so that better purchase can be obtained and also advantage of earlier alveolar plate expansion is gained.
   - **8 7 5 6 4 2 3** is the order of removal.
   - More difficult and more posterior teeth should be removed first during multiple extractions b'coz Hemorrhage from earlier extraction will not hamper the vision and field of work of these teeth.

Types of extraction

1. Trans-alveolar (open, surgical) extraction.
2. Intra-alveolar (closed) extraction.

Alveoloplasty—or alveolectomy is the surgical removal of a part of the alveolar process.

- ♦ Most of the initial resorption will be completed in 3 weeks after extractions.

Types

1. **Simple alveoloplasty.**
2. **Radical alveoloplasty** = e.g. in cases of extreme overjet, labial plates are removed for satisfactory prostheses replacements.
3. **Inter-radicular alveoloplasty** = no flap/periosteum is raised and so less resorption/post-operative pain occurs.

Complications of exodontics

- ♦ **Post-operative hemorrhage** is the **most common** complication of exodontia.

- **Oro-antral fistula;** mostly in case of palatal root.
- Buccal roots of M and PM are pushed laterally through the wall of maxilla and lie **above the attachment of the BUCCINATOR** ms.
- **Infratemporal space** lies directly posterior and superior to the tuberosity of maxilla, where lie the neurovascular structures. Avoid any dislodgement of tooth, root, etc. in this area.
- If hemorrhage is coming from a bone bleeder, the dull side curet is used to **burnish** the bone in the area of hemorrhage or socket may be packed with **"Gelfoam soaked in Thrombin".**

Dry socket/localized osteitis

- Also known as alveolar osteitis; localised osteitis.
- It is due to loss of blood clot form the sockets.
- Develops on 3–5th post-operative day and has severe, continuous pain and necrotic odor.
- Develops in mandible more frequently than maxilla. It is mainly due to less blood supply in mandible.
- Vasoconstrictor in LA may be a cause as they interfere with blood supply to the bone.
- No pus but foul odor and severe radiating pain is there.
- A septic alveolus is a denuded bone surface.
- Dry socket repair usually takes 2–3 weeks.
- Dry socket aka ALVEOLITIS SICCA DOLOROSA, i.e. (Inflammation of alveolus/Dryness/Pain).
- CURETTAGE is C/I in dry socket, as it leads to spread of infection.
- Treatment of dry socket is PALLIATIVE, i.e. packing with THYMOL IODINE POWDER and BENZOCAINE CRYSTALS dissolved in EUGENOL.
- **Trypsin** also applied = to stop bacterial growth.

Exodontia in children

- Bones are softer in children and more pliable.
- Maxillary sinus is small or absent.

- Mand canal is lower i.r.t. the teeth.
- Healing is more rapid; greater remodelling capacity.
- Greater porosity of bone in child, there is better penetration of LA and so infiltration anaesthesia can be used in molar region of mandible and in other parts of maxilla and mandible.
- Position of inferior alveolar foramen i.r.t. to the OP varies in children, so the block should be given accordingly.
- **Inferior alveolar nerve block level** varies in children with age in very young patients, as related to the level of OP; the injection is to be given at or above the level of OP in young children; as cp to adults; in which it is given below the OP.
- With nerve block, patient should be instructed/cautioned against/ about biting the numb lip/buccal mucosa/tongue, which is the **most common injury** to the child after LA.
- Bilateral inferior alveolar block is not C/I, but tongue may fall back posteriorly in the larynx and may cause problem in breathing.
- **Cowhorn forceps** should never be used to remove deciduous teeth as it may lead to avulsion of premolars.
- **Cryers elevators** should never be used in children to remove deciduous roots as it may lead to the damage to tooth buds.

Surgical Flaps (Refer to section of perio also).

Principles of flap designing

- **Base of flap should be broader** than the free end, to maintain the BLOOD SUPPLY.
- Should be sufficiently large for **adequate vision** and area of operation.
- Incision should be made over the bone not to be removed, i.e. flap should be well supported by bone on repositioning. Flap margins should **rest on the sound bone**.
- Incision should not be started at the tip of interdental papilla but at the proximal line angle of the tooth. Integrity of I/D papilla should be maintained.

- Avoid tearing of periosteum.
- Should be no sharp angles in the flap.
- Vertical/oblique incisions should not be placed over a root eminence.

Types of incisions

Types of flaps: e.g. envelop flap; 2 sided triangular flap; 3 sided rhomboid flap; semilunar flap; pedicle flap.

- **horizontal**
- **semilunar/elliptical/curved** = helps to maintain the attached gingival.
- **vertical** = most desirable to be used; it may be single, i.e. triangular flap or double, i.e. trapezoidal flap has vertical incision extending from the mucobuccal fold to horizontal gingival incision–around the neck of the teeth, incision should be directed away at 45 degrees from the tooth to be removed.
- **Ochsenbein–Luebke flap** = is a combination of semilunar and vertical incisions.
- **Envelop flap** = has no vertical releasing incision; used for posterior mandibular and palatal surgery; also known as **Bayonet shaped flap**.

Pre-medication/relaxation of patient pre-surgically.

- 0.1 gm of pento barbital sodium oral.
- 2 ml of pento barbital sodium oral.
- 20 mg of diazepam I/V to achieve Verrill's sign, which may be supplemented with meperidine (Demorol) or $N_2O–O_2$.

IMPACTED TEETH

- **Impacted tooth** = A tooth which is completely or partially unerupted and is inhibited by bone/tooth/soft tissue s.t. its further eruption is unlikely.
- **Malposed tooth** = A tooth, erupted or unerupted, which is in an abnormal position.

- **Unerupted tooth** = A tooth which has not perforated the oral mucosa.
- **Oxycephaly** = known as steeple head; top of head is pointed.
- **Chair position** = low enough so that the operator's right elbow is opposite the pt's (R) shoulder.
- An impacted tooth is more easily removed, if it is displaced to a buccal position (as cp to lingual) and if it is at a higher occlusal level.
- Disto-angular impaction is more difficult to remove.
- **Cow-horn forceps** (No. 16) is **not used for extraction of lower deci**. molars b'coz sharp beaks of this forceps can cause damage to the unerupted premolars.
- During extraction of Max. primary. Anterior teeth = No/little pressure should be placed lingually, because permanent teeth lie lingual to them.
- A very young patient is BEST managed under GA, usually of INHALATIONAL TYPE.
- In p.o. infection, LA is not always profound and is less effective.
- Nerve block is most effective and allows injection in a non-infected area. As it is given at a distant site other than the localised infection, it can be used to remove the tooth in p.o. of infection without the fear of spread of infection by injection. However, antibiotic coverage is necessary in such cases to avoid bacteremia/ septicemia.
- Injection in an infected area may cause SPREAD OF INFECTION. So GA may be used in p.o. ACUTE INFECTION.
- **TRISMUS** = i.e. inability of patient to open his mouth. ETHYL CHLORIDE spray on the ms in spasm can help open the mouth.
- Oral procedures taking > 30 min. should be done under "LA with pre-medication". Pre-medication help in removing the anxiety and fear of the patient.

IOPA–**WAR lines/Winter's lines**: For mandibular 3rd molar impactions.

Line	Details
White line	• Joins the buccal cusps of erupted molars and extended posteriorly. • Indicates the **relative depth** of 3rd molars.
Amber line	• Runs at the level of the crest of inter-dental septum b/w the molars. • Represents the **bone level covering** the impacted tooth.
Red line	• Is a **perpendicular** drawn on the amber line from an imaginary point, where the elevator will be applied. • Indicates the **amount of resistance** and difficulty encountered during extraction.

Difficulty index for removal of impacted mandibular third molars:

Classification spatial relationship	**Value**
Mesioangular	1
Horizontal/transverse	2
Vertical	3
Distoangular	4
Depth	
Level A	1
Level B	2
Level C	3

Ramus relationship/space available	
Class I	1
Class II	2
Class III	3

Difficulty index

- Very difficult 7–10
- Moderately difficult 5–7
- Minimally difficult 3–4

CLASSIFICATION OF IMPACTED Mandibular third Molars: By Pell and Gregory.

(A) According to the relation of tooth to ramus of mandibular and 2nd molars

Class I	There is sufficient amount of space between ramus and distal of M_2 for accommodation of MD crown diameter of M_3.
Class II	Space between ramus and M_2 is less than MD diameter of M_3.
Class III	All or most of the M_3 is located within the ramus.

(B) Relative depth of M_3 in bone

Position A	Highest position of tooth is on a level with or above the O.P.
Position B	Highest position of tooth is below OP, but above the cervical line of M_2.
Position C	Highest position of tooth is below the cervical line of M_2.

(C) Position of long axis of impacted M_3 i.r.t. the long axis of M_2 (Winter's classification)

- Vertical; Horizontal; Inverted;
- Mesio angular
- Disto angular
- Bucco angular
- Linguo angular
- Buccal version
- Lingual version
- Torso version

Relationship of impacted maxillary M_3 to the maxillary sinus

1. Sinus approximation (SA)—no bone or a thin portion of bone between the impacted maxillary 3rd molar and maxillary sinus.
2. No sinus approximation (NSA)—2 mm or more of bone between M_3 and maxillary sinus.

Classification of impacted maxillary canines

Class I	Impacted canines located in palate (1) Horizontal (2) Vertical (3) Semivertical
Class II	Canines located on labial /buccal surface of maxillary (1) Horizontal (2) Vertical (3) Semivertical
Class III	Impacted canines located in both the palatal process and labial or buccal maxillary bone.
Class IV	Canines located in alveolar process, usually vertically between incisor and first PM.
Class V	Canine located in an edentulous maxillary.

Haemorrhage

- Definition = it is an acute loss of circulating blood.
- Total blood is = 7% of the body wt.
- Most effective method of control haemorrhage for almost all intra-oral wounds = PRESSURE.

Hypotensive anaesthesia—i.e. during GA, the patient's BP is decreased with hypotensive agents to decrease the bleeding.

- Adr. (in LA, etc.) can produce cardiac-arrhythmias if used with Halogenated GA and may also cause post-operative reactive hyperemia.
- But felypressin (0.03 IU/ml) with Prilocaine 3% used during HALOTHANE GA does not cause reactive hyperemia.

Classification

1. **Primary** = occurs as a normal part of surgery.
2. **Reactionary** = i.e. after few hours post-operatively.
3. **Secondary** = i.e. after 7–10 days of extraction.

Types of haemorrhage

1. **Arterial Hg** = pulsating nature; vigorous flow of blood; bright red colour of blood.
2. **Venous Hg** = no pulsating nature; flow is slow; dark red colour.
3. **Capillary Hg** = oozing, non-pulsating; intermediate, red in colour.

- **Intravascular Hg** = i.e. due to deficiency of clotting factors.
- **Extravascular Hg** = i.e. there is a normal clotting system.
- **Stick ties** = it is the suture placed in the soft tissues lateral to the free end of vessels, which has been clamped, to prevent the Hg. The knot is tightend to occlude the vessels by compression of the adj. tissues, after removal of hemostat.

Methods to control extravascular Hg

- Pressure.
- Direct occlusion with hemostats.
- Coagulation by precipitation of proteins.
- Production of artificial clots.

Class I haemorrhage	Loss of upto 15% blood
Class II haemorrhage	Loss of upto 16–30% blood
Class III haemorrhage	Loss of upto 30–40% blood
Class IV haemorrhage	Loss of > 40% blood

Feature	Class I	Class II	Class III	Class IV
Blood loss	< 750 ml	750–1500	1500–2000	> 2000 ml
Blood loss	< 15 %	15–30 %	30–40	> 40 %
Pulse rate	< 100	> 100	> 120	> 140
B.P.	Normal	Normal	Decrease	Decrease
Pulse pressure	Normal/ increased	Decreased	Decreased	Decreased
Respiratory rate	14–20	20–30	30–40	> 35
Urine output	> 30 ml/hr	20–30	5–15	Negligible

- Provision of an artificial fibrin network.
- Hastening coagulation to produce vasoconstriction.
- Production of an adherent.
- Administration of systemic agents.

Coagulation of proteins can be done by:

- Electro-coagulation.
- Cryotherapy
- Styptic and astringents = e.g. ferric subsulfate; Monsel's solution; tannic acid; tea-bags.
- Thrombin and absorbable gelatin sponge.

Hemostatic agents—e.g.

- Gelfoam.
- Topical thrombin.
- Oxidized cellulose.
- Avitene.
- Local pressure.
- Adrenaline pack.
- Turpentine or tannic acid; but cause skin burns.
- Thrombin; it is expensive.
- Russel-viper venom; it is very expensive.
- Oxidized regenerated cellulose (**Surgicel**) = is absorbable; **acts as a fibrin trap**.
- Horsley's bone wax (Bees wax + olive oil + phenol in the ratio of 7:2:1).

    - **Bone wax** (Bees wax + salicylic acid).
    - Artificial clot may be produced by OXIDIZED = cellulose and regenerated **oxidized cellulose (surgicel).** It attracts RBCs and produces artificial clot.
    - **Absorbable gelatin sponge** (gelfoam) = forms artificial fibrin network by disrupting platelets.

- **Thrombin** = topical use, clots fibrinogen to produce rapid hemostasis.
- **Epinephrin** = causes vasoconstriction; topical solution is 1:1000; or Inj. 1.8 ml of 1:100,000 Adr can also control primary Hg.
- **Cyano-acrylate** Adhesive Monomers = it bonds to oral tissues and coagulum, and so produces a protective dressing on the surgical site.

Hemophilia (Also refer to the oral patho/pedodontics section.)

- Due to deficiency of factor VIII (AHG) in plasma.
- Defective gene is on X-chromosome; it is sex-linked inheritance.
- At levels of 25–50% of AHG in blood = no trouble to patient unless major trauma occurs.
- At 10–25% = bleeding even on minor cuts.
- At < 10% = **bleeding occurs in joints** and Ms esp. **knee joint.**
- Blood CT is normal with factor 8 levels above 1–2 %.
- CT is not prolonged until the level of AHG falls below 1%.

Hemophilia

1. Most common bleeding problem in hemophilics = spontaneous bleeding in the joints.
2. Most frequently affected joint = elbow/knee.
3. In cases of haemarthrosis, the factor VIII levels should be raised upto = 30–50%
4. In cases of haematoma, the factor VIII levels should be raised upto = 50%.
5. In cases of GI bleeding, the factor VIII levels should be raised upto = > 50%.
6. In cases of lacerations, the factor VIII levels should be raised upto = 30–50 % and supplemented by eACA or transemic acid.
7. In cases of head injury, the factor VIII levels should be raised upto = 100 %.

8. In cases of infilteration anaesthesia in the maxillary jaw, the factor VIII levels should be raised upto = 30 %.
9. In cases of extraction, deep scaling, IAN block, the factor VIII levels should be raised upto = 50%.
10. In cases of surgical extractions, the factor VIII levels should be raised upto = 100 %.
11. For major elective surgeries = 50–70 % level for 2 days.
12. For normal hemostasis = 70–100 % level + EACA or Tranexamic acid should be given.
13. Prophylactic Rx is = gene therapy.
14. 4 things can be given to such patients = FFP (fresh frozen plasma), cryoprecipitates, DDAVP, and factor 8 concentrates. The Rx can be started with FFP.
15. Relative specific activity of factor 8 as compared to other plasma proteins is = 1 in FFP; 30 in cryoprecipitates; 3 lac in highly purified factor 8 preparations.
16. BEST is = purified factor 8 concentrate as it does not cause LOADING.
17. Development of recombinant factor 8 represents one of the milestones in biotechnology.
18. DDAVP = has vasopressin like action; should not be given to < 1 yr old child; not useful in head trauma and intra cranial bleeding; helps release of VWF (von willebrand factor), which is a carrier of factor 8. It can be given if factor 8 levels in blood is > 10%.

Preparations which contains factor 8 are:

1. Fresh whole blood = 5–7% level.
2. Fresh/frozen plasma = 15–20% level.
3. Cryoprecipitates prepared from frozen plasma.
4. Freeze-dried animal AHG = 60–100% level.
5. Freeze-dried human AHG = 50–60% level.
   - Cryoprecipitates and fresh frozen plasma are mainly used during exodontia.
   - Cryoprecipitates is 5–15 times more concentrated.

- For minor injuries and single tooth extractions 5–20 % of AHG levels required.
- For multiple extractions = 10–40% levels AHG required.
- For major trauma or surgery = 100% AHG is required.
- **Endo-tracheal intubation should not be done**, as it may lead to bleeding in the region of glottis.
- **Mandibular block injections (of LA) are absolutely C/I**– because it may cause persistent Haemorrhage into the parapharyngeal tissues.
- **Only absolute safe site for injection is PDL**. (Not even infiltration).
- **Socket should not be sutured** after extraction b'coz otherwise blood collected in the socket may seep down the fascial planes of the neck.
- **Aspirin is absolutely C/I**, as it impairs platelet functions. Paracetamol/dihydrocodeine may be given.
- **EACA**—is anti-fibrinolytic substance; used for treatment during hemophilia.
- **Tranexamic acid** = decreased plasminogen activity by **competitive inhibition** and also decrease activity of plasmin; safer than EACA.

Christmas disease: deficiency of factor IX.

Cryoprecipitates does not contain factor IX and so is not used for Rx of Christmas disease.

- Vitamin K is required for production of 2, 7, 9, 10–factors in LIVER.
- **Von-Willebrand's dis** = also known as pseudo-hemophilia; increased BT

Ehlers Danlos syndrome

1. Fragile skin = hyper–elastic; **difficult to suture;** gaping wounds.
2. Scarring = scar instead of contracting, **tend to spread.**
3. Hyper-mobile joints = also in Marfan's syndrome.
4. Excessive bruising.

Hereditary Haermorrhagic Telangiectasia

Also known as **Osler-Weber-Rendu** disease.

- Triad of Telangiectatic lesions
- Hereditary
- Haemorrhagic diathesis
  - Is due to **purely mechanical defect** in vessels.
  - **Fragile vessels** are liable to RUPTURE.

Haemorrhagic lesions

- Astero-venous (AV) or sinusoidal aneurysms and central hemangiomas are absolute C/I for exodontics/surgical procedures.
- Aspirate any radiolucent lesion before surgery.
- If undiagnosed central venous lesion is exposed by extraction immediately REPLACE the tooth to act as stopper.
- Management of central aneurysm and hemangiomas includes surgical excision, irradiation, curettage and embolization.
- Haemorrhages from soft tissue lesions, e.g. ranula and mucocele can also occurs.
- Treatment of soft tissue hemangiomas and aneurysms is CRYOTHERAPY; **Fibrosing solutions** like sodium morrhuate; resection, etc.
- LYMPHANGIOMAS usually **do not cause a haemorrhagic threat**. It may be treated by surgical excision or by cryotherapy.
- **Bone bleeding** = controlled by Burnishing the bleeding bone; crushing the areas with hemostat; using bone wax; gelatin sponge pack with thrombin.

SHOCK

Definition = it is an abnormality of circulatory system, which results in inadequate organ perfusion, e.g. skin, kidneys, CNS.

Compensatory mechanisms may prevent a measurable fall in systolic pressure until 30% of blood volume is lost.

Types

- Hypovolemic
- Cardiogenic
- Septic
- Neurogenic
- Vasovagal
    - Septic and neurogenic shocks are due to peripheral pooling and decreased venous return and decreased cellular uptake.
    - Shock is mainly due to either **poor oxygen delivery** or poor oxygen use at cellular level. So due to anaerobic metabolism, **lactic acid is produced** leading to increased serum lactate level. So **primary metabolic acidosis** and compensatory **respiratory alkalosis**.
    - There occurs passing of Na and H_2O into the cells and K^+ into the serum.
    - Fluid from extra-cellular compartment shifts to the vascular compartment.
    - So use **CRYSTALOID SOLUTIONS as primary treatment** of shock to restore homeostasis.
    - Vascular space = 5% of total body weight.
    - Extracellular space = 20% of total body weight = (5% intravascular/plasma + 15 % of extravascular/interstitial).

S/S of hypovolemic shock

1. **Decreased cardiac output** = is due to decreased various returns in hypovolemic shock.
2. **Cool, clammy extremities** = due to vasoconstriction.
3. **Tachycardia and Tachypnoea** = both are EARLY symptoms of shock, and represent a compensatory increase in O_2 delivery.
4. **Arterial BP** = **postural hypotension** is the most sensitive sign of early hypovolemic shock.
5. **Central venous pressure decreased** due to poor venous return.
6. **Arterial blood gases.**

- PO_2 should not be allowed to drop below 60.
- Fair reserves exist with PO_2 = 60–90.

7. **Renal function:** normal GFR = 125 ml/min.
   - Renal blood flow decreases with fall in GFR and urine output.
8. **Hematocrit** = to monitor continuous blood loss and progress of shock.

Treatment

- O_2
- Replenish vascular volume, e.g. Ringer's lactate.
  - No place for glucose, so water and artificial plasma expanders, eg dextran.
  - **Position of the patient** – Body supine
    – Legs elevated
    – Head down
  - Monitoring.

  1. BP; HR, Resp. rate, temperature.
  2. Renal flow should be more than 20 ml/hr.
  3. Arterial blood gases-PO_2 > 60.
  4. CVP.
  5. Hematocrit.

8 measurements for the follow up of shock

1. Arterial BP = (120/80 mm Hg)
2. Pulse rate = (80/min)
3. CVP = (5 cm H_2O)
4. Urine flow = (50 ml/hr).
5. Cardiac index = (3.2 liters/min/m^2).
6. Arterial blood - PO_2 = 100 mg Hg
   PCO_2 = 40 mg Hg
   PH = 7.4
7. Arterial blood lactate = 12 mg/100 ml.
8. Hematocrit = 35–45%.

TISSUE TRANSPLANTATION

Autogenous grafts = tissue taken from same individual.

Allogeneic graft/allograft: tissue taken from an individual of same species, who is not genetically related to the recepient.

Isograft/syngenesio plastic graft = taken from an individual of same species genetically related to recepient.

Xerograft = tissue taken from donor of other species, e.g. animal.

Graft = is the true transplantation of living tissue.

Implant = transplantation of non-viable tissue, e.g. freeze–dried allogenic bone; xenogenic implants of animal bone.

Alloplasts = are synthetic materials of non-animal origin, e.g. Hydroxyapatite, POP; etc.

Antigen = invading agent causing initiation of immune response.

Antibody = specific protein developed in the body in response to the Ag.

Humoral immunity = plasma cells, large lymphocytes and reticulum cells produce Abs and release them in circulatory body fluids. It lasts for as long as the specific Ab persists in body fluids.

Cells mediated immunity/tissue immunity = certain cells do not release Abs, but react with foreign materials. It may last indefinitely.

Allograft response = is rejection of tissue graft between unrelated members of same species. It occurs due to cellular reaction of host to the graft.

White grafts = high resistance gets developed in a donor after rejection of first allograft. Now if a 2nd allograft is placed from same donor, it gets destroyed even more RAPIDLY. These 2nd grafts are know as White grafts.

Autogenous grafts = also known as autografts; self-grafts.

- Obtained from the same individual.
- Only type of graft which provides living and immuno-competent cells.
- **Block grafts** = are solid pieces of both cortical and cancellous bone, e.g. iliac crest; and ribs.

- **Particulate marrow-cancellous bone**/PMCB grafts = are obtained by harvesting the medullary bone and associated endosteum and hematopoietic marrow. It provides greatest concentration of osteogenic cells; obtained mostly from ilium.
- **Composite grafts** = they contain both soft tissues and osseous elements, e.g. pedicle grafts, i.e. some blood supply to graft is maintained with the original site.
- **Free graft** = graft is totally removed from its site and immediately replaced. The blood supply is restored by reconnection of blood vessels.

Allogenic grafts

- Aka allografts/homografts.
- Are taken from another individual of same species.
- e.g. freeze dried.
- Cannot participate in phase I of osteogenesis, b'coz osteogenic cells get destroyed by freeze drying, etc.
- Offers a hard tissue matrix for phase II induction of osteogenesis.

Xenogenic graft

- Aka heterograft/xenograft.
- Taken from a different species.
- Antigenic dissimilarity of these grafts are greater than allogenic grafts.
- It is rarely used.
- Does not provide viable cells for osteogenesis.

3 methods to attenuate immune response

1. Modify host's immune mechanism
   - Thymectomy
   - Irradiation
   - Immuno sppressive drugs = it is generally used in major organ transplant.

2. Alter the inherent graft ANTIGENIC properties
   - Irradiation
   - Freezing
   - Freeze drying

   It is mostly used is ORAL SURGERY.
3. By storing transplant organ in INTERMEDIARY HOST

Storage of allergenic bone for transplantation

- Best = Cryobiological, i.e. by cooling, freezing or freeze–drying.
- Grafts are more completely REVASCULARIZED and remodeled.

Bone and cartilage have less cellular content, but a LARGE amounts of calcified/uncalcified matrix which is NON-VIABLE.

- During cryogeny–**only cellular death occurs**, without altering the remaining osseous structure of graft, which is the essential part for the development of an effective graft substance.
- **Osteo-genic process** is purely PASSIVE.
- Extracellular matrix of the graft acts as a system of ABSORBABLE surface on which new bone can grow.
- **Sterilization** can be done by ETHYLENE OXIDE and Beta propiolactone.
- **Autogenous bone graft** is MATERIAL of choice in most orthognathic surgical sites.
- Autogenous **iliac crest bone** is recommended for rebuilding the HEIGHT of deficient alveolar ridge.

Purpose of decalcification of allogenic bone is to release more BONE–MORPHOGENETIC–Proteins (BMP) as a stimulator of osteo-induction in appropriate progenitor cell substrates.

Other graft materials are

- Partially decalcified allogenic bone.
- Completely decalcified allogenic bone.
- Allogenic banked cartilage.
- Xenogenic bone graft = it

- Stimulates an immune response.
- Major antigenic component of animal bone is contained within the organic fraction of the tissues; e.g. calf bone.

Autogenous grafts

- Usually used to restore large areas of lost mandibular bone.
- Costo-chondral RIB graft is employed to reconstruct the disarticulated mandible, as the cartilage part stimulates the TMJ and condyle.
- RIB graft.
- Iliac graft.

Autogenous particulate marrow cancellous bone graft (PMCB)

- Autogenous hematopoietic marrow and cancellous bone containing marrow are the only type of bone graft materials capable of ACTIVELY inducting osteogenesis.
- Particulate marrow graft are better than the solid grafts in RAPID regeneration of large defects. It is easy to obtain through a small opening.

In Cleft Lip and Palate

- Autogenous cancellous bone grafts are most effective.
- Grafting is done between 5–12 yrs age.
- Canine is moved in occlusion between 8–12 wks after grafting (at 9–11 yrs age).

COMPOSITE GRAFTS

- They contain both hard tissue and soft tissue.
- Obtained from chest wall or iliac crest (with superior iliac circumflex A attached).

WOUNDS AND INJURIES

Soft tissues injuries: e.g. abrasion; contusion; laceration.

Contusion

- Is also known as bruise.
- Produced by an impact **from blunt object.**
- Without breaking the skin or mucous membrane.
- Submucosal or s/c haemorrhage occurs.
- Ecchymosis is seen after 48 hrs.
- Skin continuity is usually not broken.

Abrasion

- Painful due to involvement of nerve terminals.
- Is produced by rubbing or **scraping off** of the covering surface; exposes NERVE endings.
- It results **from friction**.
- Wound is superficial and produces RAW BLEEDING surface.
- Bleeding is capillary in nature.

Laceration

- It is a tear in the epithelial and sub-epithelial tissues.
- It is most frequent type of injury.
- Wound **resulting from tear**, with sharp margin.
- Produced **by SHARP object.**

BURNS–"RULE of 9"

- **First degree** = which produces **erythema** of skin.
- **Second degree** = which produces **vesicle formation.**
- **Third degree** = which causes **complete destruction** of epidermis and dermis, extending into or beyond the S/C tissue.
- Major **systemic problem** with burns = shock esp OLIGEMIC/ HYPOVOLEMIC shock, due to fluid/colloid loss.

Estimated **need for replacement** in first 24 hrs is

1. Colloid = % of body burned × Body weight × 0.25.
2. Electrolyte = % of body burned × body weight × 0.50.

3. Glucose in water = 2000 ml.
   - Requirements for second 24 hrs. = half the amount required for first 24 hrs. + 2000 ml. of glucose in water.

Closure of wound

1. **Objective = accurate co-adaptation/**approximation of layers of tissues with elimination of all dead spaces.
2. Handle the tissue **Gently**.
3. Suture to form water–tight seal.
4. Deeper ms and S/C tissue should be **closed by inverted buried interrupted sutures** with absorbable (plain gut/PGA) sutures.
5. Under tension should not be placed.
6. Sutures should be **placed at equal distance** and **equal depth** on either side of the wound.
7. Slight **eversion of skin margins** should be produced to avoid contracture scars.

Prophylaxis against Tetanus

- ♦ Caused by clostridium tetani
- ♦ Active immunization is long tasting
- ♦ Given as 0.5 ml in 3 doses.
  - First dose = zero day
  - Second dose = 6 wks.
  - Third dose = 6–12 mos.
  - Booster dose = every year.

Passive Immunity—By I/M inj. 250 units of Human Anti-tetanus globulin (ATG).

Traumatic injuries to teeth and associated structures: Please refer to the section on pedodontics for details.

Repair of displaced tooth

1. **Hematoma phase** = upto 24–72 hrs.
   - Blood clot formed.
   - Early organization.

2. Fibrous repair phase

- 3rd day–3 weeks.
- Prevent additional injury to blood clot.

3. Final bone forming phase

- For 4–6 weeks.
- Bone formation completed.
- Undesirable movement/traumatic stress leads to surgical failure. So avoid it.
- Most traumatic wounds of oral cavity are OPEN and all such injuries should be treated as infected wounds.

FRACTURE OF JAWS

Classifications and definitions

Pathological fracture = bone gets weakened by some underlying pathology and get fractured under very less stresses than it can bear normally.

Simple fracture = is in which the overlying integument is intact; bone is broken completely but not exposed to air.

Green-stick fracture

- One side of bone/cortical plate is broken and other is bent.
- Seen often in children as their bones are soft.
- Time required for healing is minimal.

Compound fracture

- Here an external wound is associated with break in the bone.
- Fracture is open to out-side air.
- Almost all jaw fractures in the teeth region are compounded through PDL.

Comminuted fracture = is one in which the bone is splintered or crushed.

Displaced/undisplaced fracture

Favorable/unfavorable fracture

FACTORS

Bones get easily fractured due to weakening under certain systemic conditions

1. Endocrine disorders
   - Hyper parathyroidism
   - Post menopausal osteoporosis.
2. Developmental disorders
   - Osteopetrosis
3. Systemic disorders
   - Reticulo-endothelial diseases
   - Paget's disease
   - Osteomalacia
   - Mediterranean anemia
4. Local disorders
   - Fibrous dysplasia
   - Tumors and cysts

Healing of BONE

3 phases

1. Haemorrhage = clot organization and proliferation of blood vessels; lasts upto 10 days.
2. Callus formation
   - Woven bone/**primary callus** formed.
   - Lasts from 10–20 days.
   - **Secondary callus** = haversian systems formed.
   - From 20–60 days.
3. FUNCTIONAL/Reconstruction phase
   - Mechanical forces are required.
   - Haversian systems line up according to STRESS–LINES, as according to **Wolff's law of trabeculation.**
   - Bony shape molded with functional use.
   - Runs for 2–3 yrs.

Healing of fracture-studied by Weinmann and Sicher, occurs in 6 phases

1. Clotting of blood of hematoma = 6–8 hrs.
2. Organisation of blood of hematoma
   - Capillaries invade = 24–48 hrs.
   - Fibroblasts invade = 24–48 hrs.
   - Proliferation of blood vessels.
3. Formation of fibrous callus–10 days
   - Fibroblasts are most important cells.
   - Decreased number of white cells.
   - Partial obliteration of capillaries.
   - End of hyperemic phase.
4. Formation of primary bony callus
   - 10–30 days.
   - Very low calcium content.
   - Woven bone is formed.
   - Can't be seen on R/G.

PRIMARY CALLUS– 4 types

(a) Anchoring callus

- Develops on outer surface of bone near periosteum.
- Spongy bone, produced by OSTEOBLASTS.
- Extends some distance away from fracture.

(b) Sealing callus

- Develops on INSIDE surface across the fractured ends.
- Fills the marrow spaces.
- Forms from ENDOSTEAL PROLIFERATION.

(c) Bridging callus

- Develops on outer surface between the anchoring callus on the 2 #ed ends.
- It is the ONLY one, which is **primarily CARTILAGINOUS.**

(d) Uniting callus

- Between the ends of bones and between the areas of other primary calluses.
- It forms only after the development of other calluses.

5. **Secondary Callus** = is the MATURE bone, which replaces the immature bone of primary callus.
   - More **heavily calcified.**
   - **Can be seen on R/G.**
   - Haversian system not formed UNIFORMLY.
   - HAS LAMINATED bone, which can withstand the active force.
   - 20–60 days.
6. **FUNCTIONAL reconstruction of fractured bone**
   - Bone subjected to functional stresses.
   - Haversian systems get uniformly oriented.

MAXILLARY FRACTURES

Le Fort's Classification

Le Fort I – Horizontal fracture/Floating Jaw/Low level fracture/Guerin fracture.

Le Fort II – Pyramidal fracture/Sub-zygomatic fracture.

Le Fort III – Transverse fracture/Cranio-facial dysjunction/High level fracture/Supra-zygomatic fracture.

Modified Le Fort classification

Le Fort I	Low Mx fracture
Ia	Low Mx II/multiple segment
Le Fort II	Pyramidal fracture
IIa	Pyramidal and nasal fracture
IIb	Pyramidal and Naso-orbito-ethmoidal (NOE) fracture

Le Fort III		Cranio-facial dysjunction
	IIIa	Cranio-facial + nasal fracture
	IIIb	Cranio-facial + NOE
Le Fort IV		Le Fort II or III fracture and cranial base fracture
	IVa	Supra orbital rim fracture
	IVb	Ant. Cranial fossa + SOR fracture
	IVc	Ant. Cranial fossa + orbital wall fracture

Orbital blow-out fracture

- When an object of slightly greater diameter than the orbital rim strikes protruding eyeball,
- The rapid rise in the intra-orbital pressure fractures the orbital floor.
- The contents get displaced in the antral cavity like a trap-door.
- It is seen as **hanging-drop sign** in the Water's view R/G.
- It interferes with the IO/IR ms and so diplopia occurs in the vertical/upward gaze.
- It causes enophthalmos.

Blow-in fracture

- i.e. an inward buckling of the orbital floor and so decrease in volume of orbit occurs.

CSF Rhinorrhoea

- It occurs with the fracture of cribriform plate of ethmoid bone.
- Mucus associated with cold will dry with the starching of the handkerchief.
- But **CSF dries without starching.**
- CSF produces **TRAM LINE pattern** on face and **a halo–effect** on the sheet and pillow.
- CSF has **much higher glucose content.**

- Associated with Le Fort II, and III; ethmoid bone fracture; cribriform plate and severe nasal fractures.
- Patient with head injury **should not be given MORPHINE,** as it may depress the respiratory centre.

Various s/s associated with fractures

CSF rhinorrhoea	Le Fort II, and III; ethmoid bone fracture; cribriform plate and severe nasal fractures.
Damage to infra-orbital and zygomatic nerves	Le Fort II and zygomatic fractures.
Cranial N damage in orbit	In Le Fort II and III; zygomatic fracture.
Hooding of eye	In zygomatic fracture; in Le Fort III fracture. Level of globe drops and upper eyelid comes down. Occurs when fracture **passes above** the Whitnall's tubercle.
Diplopia	Mainly due to interference in the activity of ocular ms especially IO/IR/LR; it should be recorded in all the nine gauges.
Epiphora	Increased lacrimation; occurs in Le Fort II and III fractures.
Telecanthus	Increased distance b/w canthi of eyes; due to severe naso-ethmoidal fractures.
Circum-orbital ecchymosis	Seen in zygomatic fractures; Le Fort II and III fracture
Sub-conjunctival hacmorrhage	
Black cyc	

Neurological evaluation after trauma

Battle's sign	Area of ecchymosis behind the ear in mastoid area, e.g. in basilar skull fracture esp. middle cranial fossa.
Raccoon eye	Area of ecchymosis around the eye, e.g. in anterior cranial fossa fracture.
Marcus–Gunn pupil	It is an afferent pupillary defect due to optic N damage; the involved eye constricts to the light in the opposite eye and dilates as the light is brought into the involved eye.
3rd nerve palsy	Unilaterally dilated pupil, which does not react to the light and appears displaced laterally due to paresis of Medial Rectus ms.
Epidural hematoma	Haemorrhage b/w dura and inner table of skull; caused by tear of middle meningeal A by fracture in the temporal area, pressure on 3rd n and so dilated pupils Lucid interval is present.

Difference between epidural and subdural hematoma

- Lucid interval
- **Subdural hematoma** = occurs when veins bridging the cortex to the venous sinuses are torn.
- **Concussion** = is the temporary loss of consciousness with no permanent organic brain damage.
- **Contusion** = is a bruising of the brain.
- **Jafferson fracture** = is a comminuted fracture of the ring of vertebra C–1.
- **Hangman's fracture** = is a fracture through the pedicles and laminae of C–2.
- **Most frequently damaged**/injured cranial n in fractures = 6th N.

- **Optic N** is protected by a ring of compact bone. The fracture line involving orbit goes around that foramen rather than thro it.
- **Crow's foot** skin creases are present on the outer corner of the eyes; the incision should be given in these creases to avoid significant scar formation.
- If the fractured zygomatic arch impinges on coronoid process of mandible, then it interferes with normal range of excursion of mandible.
- Do not use morphine in patients of fracture and head injury as it:
  - Depresses the cough reflex.
  - Causes pupil constriction.
  - Depresses level of consciousness.
  - Depresses respiration.
  - Drug of choice here is diazepam (sedative) and pentazocine (analgesic).
- Haemorrhage anterior to orbital septum causes lid–ecchymosis.
- Haemorrhage posterior to orbital septum includes sub-conjuctival haemorrhage; it is sharply limited by septum and tarsal plate.
- **Retro-bulbar haemorrhage** = if decompression is not done, it may lead to blindness by ischemia of optic N due to occlusion of **short posterior ciliary As**.

Suspensory ligament of lockwood

- Maintains the level of eye globe.
- Passes from medial attachment of lacrimal bone to Whitnall's tubercle, which is present on inner aspect of zygomatic bone just below fronto-zygomatic suture.
- If fracture occurs below Whitnall's tubercle, there is no alteration in the level of eye globe.

Signs and symptoms of Le Fort I fractures

- **Ecchymosis** in the buccal sulcus below zygomatic arch.
- Disturbed occlusion.

- Mobility of teeth bearing segment is ascertained by = grasping the teeth and applying slight and firm movement.
- **Cracked–pot sound** = occurs on percussion of upper teeth.

Signs and symptoms of Le Fort II and III fractures

- Massive oedema of face is a characteristic feature = **moon–face appearance.**
- Bilateral circum-orbital ecchymosis.
- Subconjunctival ecchymosis.
- Maxilla is displaced down and backward = **dish-face deformity.**
- Gagging of occlusion and anterior open bite.
- Floating maxilla.
- Cracked pot sound on teeth percussion.

Signs and symptoms peculiar of Le Fort II fractures

- Step deformity and mobility at infra-orbital margin.
- No change in the pupil level because line of fracture passes below the lateral attachment of suspensory ligament.
- Hematoma in upper buccal sulcus in first and second molar region = as the fracture line passes across the zygomatic buttress.
- CSF rhinorrhoea is not a constant finding.
- **Sub-conjunctival Haemorrhage.**
- **Black eyes.**
- CSF rhinorrhoe if cirbriform plate of ethmoid bone gets fractureed.
- H/O unconsciousness
- Lesions of cranial Ns **(esp 6, 7th).**
- **Battle's sign** (ecchymosis in line of the posterior auricular A in MASTOID area) after 24 hrs of fracture.

Signs and symptoms peculiar of Le Fort III fractures

- **Aka High level fracture.**
- Tenderness and separation at fronto-zygomatic suture.

- Fracture line passes above the Whitnall's tubercle and so ocular level is lowered and **hooding of eye** occurs.
- Profuse CSF rhinorrhoea.
- Results in depressed posterior end due to pterygoid ms attachment and so Ant open bite.
- Dish face/transverse fracture.
- Orbit separated at zygomatico–frontal suture.
- Bleeding from ear (shows middle cranial fossa fracture).

Diplopia: i.e. double vision

- due to injury to **inferior oblique ms** or due to depressed orbital fracture.
- In NOE fracture.
- In zygomatic complex fracture.
- In orbital blow-out fracture.

Zygomatic arch fracture

- Seen best by **JUG HANDLE/Water's view.**
- Treatment by **Gillies approach.**

Ophthalmoplegia and ptosis = due to involvement of **3, 4,** 6th **Ns.**

Fixed and dilated pupils = due to **disturbances in p-sympathetic Ns**.

Proptosis = by paresis of **extra-occular ms**, which normally exert a retracting influence on the globe.

Sensory disturbance = due to **ophthalmic div of 5th N.**

McGregor and Campbell's lines: Seen in OMV/ PNS view.

- **First line** = path from zygomatico-frontal suture to superior orbital margin across the glabella region to superior orbital margin and zygomatico-frontal suture of the other side.
- **Second line** = from zygomatic tubercle to continuous line of zygomatic arch till it blends into zygomatic bone and the line continues along inferior orbital margin, across the frontal process

of maxilla and lateral wall of nose through septum and then same course on the opposite side.

- **Third line** = from condyle across the mandibular notch, coronoid process of the mandible to lateral wall of antrum and continuous through the medial wall of antrum or lateral wall of nose at the nasal floor level and the same course on the opposite side.
- **Fourth line** = occlusal curve of the U/L arches.
- **Fifth line** = lower border of mandible from one angle to other side angle.

TREATMENT

- If maxillary tuberosity is attached to the periosteum = it can be left alone with or without splinting.
- Rx of zygomatic arch and/or complex fracture = by **Gillies temporal approach; Bristow's elevator** is use.
- Fixation of zygomatic arch fracture is not required because temporalis fascia attached along the superior aspect of the arch effectively immobilizes the segments.
- For reducing nasal complex fracture—**Walsham's and Asch's forceps** are used.
- Delayed Rx of zygomatic complex fracture may lead to interference of mandibular movements. So coronoidectomy should be done.
- Delayed Rx of nasal complex fracture and dish face deformity may require osteotomy and alloplastic implants.
- Damage to naso-lacrimal duct may occur in Le Fort II and nasal complex fracture. So epiphora may develop.
- Improperly reduced Le Fort 1, 2, 3, fractures may cause posterior gagging of occlusion and anterior open bite.

Steps of treatment of a fracture

1. Reduction
2. Fixation and immobilization

Immobilization

Internal fixation	External fixation
	By
• direct osteosynthesis	• craniomandibular
• suspension	• craniomaxillary
• support	• suspension from cranial vault
Direct osteo-synthesis:	Suspension from cranial vault
• trans-osseous wiring	• circumzygomatic
• bone plate and screws	• zygomatico-mandibular
• kirschner wire	• inferior orbital border–mandibular
• steinmann pins	• fronto-mandibular
	• pyriform fossa-mandibular

WHAT ARE THE ABC'S OF PATIENT MANAGEMENT?

A	Airway maintenance with cervical spine control
B	Breathing and ventillation
C	Circulation and control of haemorrhage
D	Disability and neurological status
E	Exposure

AVPU method of patient's level of consciousness

A	Alert
V	Responds to verbal stimuli
P	Responds to pain
U	Unresponsive

Glasgow coma scale

- Evaluated for a patient of head injury.
- It has 3 areas of assessment, i.e. eye response, verbal response and motor response (EVM).
- Maximum GCS index = 15.
- Minimum GCS index = 3.

Grade response	Motor response	Verbal response	Eye
6	Obeys command	–	–
5	Localizes pain	Oriented	–
4	Withdraws from pain	Confused conversation	Spontaneous opening
3	Abnormal flexion	Inappropriate words	Opens to speech
2	Extensor response	Incomprehensible words	Opens to pain
1	No response	None	None
Mnemonic	OLWFEN	OCIIN	SSPN

MANDIBULAR FRACTURES

- Mandible is the strongest and most rigid component of the facial skeleton.
- Are the most common fractures of the facial skeleton, followed by maxilla, zygoma and nasal bones.
- Fracture of mandible requires high forces (425 lbs); while fracture of maxilla requires low forces (140 lbs).
- Fracture of neck of condyle acts as a safety mechanism and prevents the middle cranial fossa fracture.
- Relative lines of weakness in mandible are = 3rd molar region and canine regions due to its long root.

- **Civilian type fracture** = mandibular fracture with no gross comminution of bone.
- **Gun shot type fracture** = mandibular fracture with gross comminution of bone and with extensive loss of hard and soft tissues.

Types of fracture

- **Simple** = not associated with outside atmosphere but in oral cavity, the fracture is associated through PDL to outer environment and so becomes compound.
- **Green-stick type** = mostly found in children; bones are very slender and elastic; one cortex is bent and other is intact.
- **Compound** = fracture associated with outer atmosphere through PDL in tooth bearing segment.
- **Comminuted** = multiple fragments of bone at the same fracture site.
- Displaced and undisplaced fracture.
- Favorable and unfavorable fractures.
- Horizontal and vertical fractures.
- **Pathological** = bone weakened by pathological conditions, e.g. neoplasm, osteomyelitis.
- **Complicated** = severe fracture involving vessels, nerves, etc.
- **Impacted** = 2 segments of fractures are inter-digitated and cannot be dislodged.
- **Atrophic** = thickness or size of bone gets decreased very much.
- **Multiple fracture** = involving more than one bone or at multiple sites of the same bone.
- Most common fracture of mandible = **angle.**

Guardsman fracture

- Is a multiple fracture.
- Is due to fall on the midpoint of chin with fracture of both condyles and the symphysis, e.g. in epileptics, soldiers, elderly patients.

Displaced fracture = Due to **muscular sling of the mandible,** i.e. masseter and medial pterygoid ms. It displaces posterior fragment of jaw UPWARD, aided by TEMPORALIS.

- Anterior segment is displaced DOWNWARD by suprahyoid ms.
- Posterior segment also displaced MEDIALLY, by especially medial pterygoid m. and aided of SUPERIOR constrictor m.

Symphysis fracture = displaced by the bilateral POSTERIOR and SLIGHT LATERAL pull of SUPRAHYOID and DG ms.

Condyle fracture = displaced by the pull of lateral pterygoid m in an upward, anterior and medial direction.

Direction of fracture line

- **Horizontal favorable** = line of fracture **extends in a distal direction** towards the alveolar ridge while the fracture at inferior border is located ANTERIORLY.
- **Horizontal unfavorable** = fracture extends **forward towards the alveolar ridge** from a posterior point on the inferior border.
- **Vertical unfavorable** = line extends **from a postero-lateral point to an antero-medial** point.
- **Vertical favorable** = fracture line extends **from an antero-lateral to the postero-medial** point.

Condyle fracture: Shift of midline occurs towards the fractured side.

- Premature posterior occlusion (open-bite).
- Condyle dislocated forward/medially due to LATERAL PTERYGOID Ms.

M/m of condylar fracture SHOULD BE CONSERVATIVE, i.e. closed treatment especially in unilateral case.

- Main growth centre of mandible is located in the CONDYLAR region.
- Main mandibular growth occurs between 1–5 years of age in human; followed by a period of quiescence at 5–10 years age and then active mandibular growth from 10–15 years age.

- Growth during 10–15 years age is mainly due to muscular functions more than the growth centre. (functional matrix theory of growth by MOSS).
- So the most **critical period** for condylar fracture is 1–5 years.
- So the most **critical situation** is a fracture dislocation in a child of 2 ½ years old or less.
- **Wolff's law** = i.e. the shape of the bone conforms to the stresses placed on it during function.
- In children
  1. Condylar fractures are Rxed CONSERVATIVELY mostly.
  2. IMF is placed for 2 weeks.

Time for repair

- Most md. fractures heal well enough to allow removal of fixation in 6 weeks.
- Young adults = 4–4½ weeks.
- Children = 3–4 weeks.

Classification of the fractures based on the presence of dentition by Kazanjian and Converse

Class	Teeth present/absent
I	If teeth are present on both sides of the fracture line.
II	If one tooth is missing on one side of the fracture line.
III	If no tooth is present on either side of the fracture line, e.g. edentulous mandible.

Fracture at the angle

- Influenced by the medial pterygoid-masseter sling.
- Can be vertically and horizontally–favorable or unfavorable.
- Medial pterygoid is stronger m than the masseter.

- Pull of masseter is in upward and forward direction.
- Pull of MT is in U, F, medial/lingual direction.
- In vertically unfavorable fracture—the fracture line runs in U and F directions, i.e. site of fracture line at lower border is distal and on alveolar border it is mesial. The posterior fragment is pulled U, F and lingually.
- If fracture line runs U and B towards the alveolar border—it is vertically favorable fracture.
- In horizontally unfavorable fracture = the fracture line runs in bucco-lingual direction, parallel to the pull of ms. The line starts distally on buccal surface and comes mesially on the lingual surface.
- In horizontal favorable fracture—the line starts mesially on buccal surface and comes distally on the lingual surface.

Fracture at symphysis and parasymphysis

- Mylohyoid and geniohyoid ms form a diaphragm at the floor of mouth.
- Transverse midline fracture of symphysis are not displaced.
- Oblique fracture tends to overlap. The fracture part with genial tubercle is displaced lingually by ms pull.
- Bilateral parasymphyseal fracture gets displaced posteriorly under the influence of genioglossus mainly.
- Tongue falls in oro-pharynx only if patient's level of consciousness is depressed in bilateral parasymphysis, e.g. in head inury.
- In severe cases, detachment of genio-glossus m. may lead to loss of tongue control and airway obstruction.
- Displacement of condyle occurs mainly in the antero-medial direction, i.e. upward; forward and medially, under the influence of lateral pterygoid m.
- Fracture of coronoid process occurs by reflex contraction of temporalis m; displacement occurs upwards; a rare fracture; limited mandibular movements especially on protrusion occurs.

Fracture of edentulous mandible

- Bilateral fracture occurs mostly near the posterior attachment of mylohyoid m.
- Anterior fragment gets extreme displacement (because there is no dental interference/inter-locking) in D and B direction; which is due to digastric and myloyoid ms. It is known as **bucket-handle displacement**. It may cause respiratory distress.
- Mandible is weak due to bony resorption.
- With ageing—the periosteal blood supply becomes increasingly important. So the periosteum should be preserved as much as possible as it helps in healing. Healing problems occur due to decreased blood supply.
- No precise reduction of fracture is required.
- Modified Gunning splint is used mainly.
- Primary bone graft, e.g. ribs, iliac crest, etc. used in ultra-thin mandible. 5 cm long rib graft is sufficient.
- Open reduction of fracture in aged patients may lead to loss of periosteum.
- Clinical examination = ecchymosis/hematoma in lingual sulcus is pathognomonic. It is because on the lingual side, the mucosa of the floor of mouth overlies the periosteum of mandible.

CONDYLAR FRACTURES

1. Intracapsular and extra capsular.
2. Unilateral and bilateral.
3. Displaced and undisplaced.
4. Intracapsular are rare; extracapsular are most common.
5. Displacement is due to pull of lateral pterygoid m, which is attached at antero-medial aspect of condyle.
6. Bleeding from the middle ear may due to the fracture of petrous temporal bone and with CSF otorrhoea. It is a significant finding and should be immediately dealt with.
7. **Battle's sign** = ecchymosis of skin just below the mastoid process; especially seen with fracture of base of the skull.

8. Gagging of molars on the same side of fracture.
9. Mandibular deviation on opening towards the side of the fracture.
10. If bilateral displaced fracture is there, then anterior open bite develops.

Treatment

- Immobilization is must for adequate healing.
- Mal-union is more common than non-union.
- Minimum period = for 3 weeks, i.e.

If in a **young adult** with fracture of **angle of mandible** taking **early** treatment, in which the **tooth is removed** from the fracture line.

- It requires **3 weeks** for treatment.
- If tooth is retained in the fracture line = add 1 week.
- If fracture is at symphysis = add 1 week.
- If age is > 40 yrs = add 1–2 weeks.
- If child/adolescent = subtract 1 week.
- Active movements are must for intracapsular fracture in children; immobilization is contra-indicated, to avoid analysis.

SUMMARY	Intracapsular		Extracapsular	
	Unilateral	Bilateral	Unilateral	Bilateral
Children	Zero	Zero	7–10 days	7–10 days
Adults	2 weeks	2–3 weeks; elastics for 4 weeks	4 weeks	4–6 weeks

Intracapsular fracture in children

1. Disturbance of growth occurs because condylar cartilage which is growth site in mandible gets involved.
2. Fibrous/bony ankylosis may occur.
3. It should be Rxed by active movements only to avoid the ankylosis, no immobilization is recommended.

Extracapsular fracture in children

1. Should be Rxed conservatively.
2. Risk of ankylosis is less.
3. Early movement is done.
4. But if painful, then 7–10 days of immobilization can be done.

Unilateral intracapsular fracture in adults

1. Occlusion is undisturbed.
2. No immobilization of mandible done.
3. If painful, then IMF done for upto 2 wks only.

Unilateral extracapsular fracture in adults

1. IMF is done for 4 wks if occlusion is disturbed due to fracture-dislocation.
2. If not displaced, then no active Rx required.

Bilateral intracapsular fracture in adults

1. IMF should not be done for more than 2 weeks/2–3 weeks, otherwise ankylosis or stiffness may occur.
2. Intermaxillary elastic forces used at night for 6 weeks after removing IMF.

Bilateral extracapsular fracture in adults

1. Dislocation is anteromedially by lateral pterygoid ms.
2. Occlusal gagging and anterior open bite.
3. IMF done for 4–6 weeks.
4. Open reduction may be required.

Fracture of mandible in children

- May interfere with growth.
- Difficulty in IMF because of loose deciduous teeth and young permanent teeth.
- Morphology of deciduous molars is also troublesome during IMF.
- Gunning splint may be required.

- Unerupted teeth may get damaged if trans-osseous wires, bone plates and pins are used. So these are contra-indicated in children.
- Healing is very rapid.
- Slight imperfections in reduction get compensated by growth and remodelling.
- Prolonged follow up is required.

TREATMENT OF MANDIBULAR FRACTURES

- Different methods of immobilization can be used depending on demand.
- Fractures must always be tested clinically before releasing the IMF.

Methods	**Details**
Dental wiring	Direct wiring done by Gilmer; 0.45 mm/ 26 gauge soft s.s wire is used; wire should be stretched by 10% before use.
Eye lets	Ivy Hearley 5 eyelets used in each arch.
Arch bars	e.g. a Winter's; Jelenko; Erich bars best if the patient has insufficient no. of teeth for effective inter-dental eyelets. Mostly, Erich arch bar is used. Upper and lower bars are fixed and then tied with wires to close the mouth in occlusion. It is know as inter-maxillary fixation (IMF).
Cap splints	Especially used when there are multiple loose/damaged teeth, which have to be retained, e.g. Gunning splint for edentulous mandible.
Trans-osseous wiring	
Circumferential wiring	
Fig-of-8 wiring	

(*Contd.*)

Methods	Details
Bone plating	Simple bone plates, compression bone plates/EDCP/2-hole/4-hole plates, etc. • The screws should engage the inner cortical plate of mandible. • The holes in compression plates are such that their widest diameter lies nearest the fracture line.
External pin fixation	• Pins of s.s. or Ti are used. • Are approx 3 mm or 1/8 inches in diameter. • Are not parallel to each other but diverge. • Are attached by cross bars.
Bone clamps	• e.g. Brenthrust splints.
Kirschner wires	• For transfixation; are of 2 mm diameter.

ACUTE INFECTIONS OF ORAL CAVITY

Pus producing bacteria = **Staphylococcus**

Deep cervical fascia has 4 part

- Investing layer/superficial layer
- Carotid sheath
- Pre-tracheal layer
- Pre-vertebral layer

1. Superficial/**investing layer** splits and encloses
   - 2 ms = SCM m and trapezius
   - 2 glands = Parotid and submandibular
   - Forms suprasternal space.

   Associated with 3 fascial compartments, i.e. submandibular, submental and parotid.

2. **Carotid sheath** = contains CCA/ICA/IJV/Vagus N.

3. **Pre-tracheal layer** forms investment for THYROID GLAND.
4. **Visceral space** = lies between pre-tracheal and pre-vertebral layers; is continuous with mediastinum of thorax.

Masticator Space

- Formed by splitting of investing layer of deep cervical fascia at lower border of mandible, which runs both medially and laterally to ramus enclosing masseter, temporalis, ramus, medial and lateral pterygoid ms.
- Continuous with space of body of mandible subperiosteally.
- Involved after dental extractions especially of **third Molars.**
- **Subperiosteal abscess** occurs, so incision should be given till bone.
- **Trismus** = due to masseter-medial pterygoid sling irritation.

Temporal pouches

- 2 = superficial and deep.
- Superficial pouch lies between temporal fascia and temporalis m.
- Deep pouch lies deep to temporalis m between the muscle and skull.
- Communicate with infra-temporal and pterygo-palatine fossae.

Submental space = contains **Submental lymph nodes,** which drain median part of lower lip, tip to tongue and floor of mouth.

- Floor formed by **mylohyoid m.**

Submandibular/Digastric space

- Floor formed by **MH and hyoglossus M.**
- Contains **superficial part of submandibular gland.**
- **Deep part of SMG** continues posterior to mylohyoid m. **into sublingual space.**

Sublingual space = lies **above the mylohyoid** and laterally bound by inner surface of body of mandible **above the MH line.**

- Floor is formed **by MH m.**
- Contains **sublingual gland**, SM duct, **deep part of SMG**, lingual N, 12th N. and terminal branch of lingual A.

Lateral pharyngeal space–aka parapharyngeal space

- Extends from BASE of skull to level of HYOID bone.
- Subdivided into **2 parts by STYLOID process**—Anterior and Posterior.
- Carotid sheath is in **posterior compartment** (containing ICA/IJV/9, 10, 11, 12 Ns and cervical sympathetic TRUNK).
- Posterior compartment has NO LYMPH NODES.
- Most often involved by spread of infection from masticator space; palatine tonsil, parotid gland; etc.
- Especially by infection of **max. 3rd molar.**

PAROTID SPACE

- Formed by splitting of investing layer of deep fascia.
- **Stylomandibular ligament** separates parotid from the submandibular space.
- Stylomandibular ligament is formed by Investing Fascia.
- Br. of 7th N lies **deep to the superficial part** of parotid gland.
- Not involved directly by dental infections.

Pterygo-palatine/and Infra-temporal Fossae

- Involved by **infections of upper molars especially M_3.**
- PPF fossa communicates with **infra-temporal Fossa** through pterygo-maxillary fissure (PMF).
- PMF is continuous with inferior orbital fissure (IOF).
- IOF has infra orbital N (which is a continuation of Mx N).
- ION gives br. = Ant. and middle superior Alveolar N, which supply Mx 1–5 and upper gums).
- PPF also communicates with pterygoid canal.

- Pterygoid canal has VIDIAN N. (made of gr. Petrosal br. of 7th N). + Deep petrosal N.
- Gr. Petrosal N = gives preganglionic para-sympathetic fibers to pterygopalatine ganglion.
- Deep petrosal n = has posterior ganglionic sympathetic fibers from superior cervical sympathetic ganglion.
- Foramen ovale and F. Spinosum are in Greater Wing of sphenoid bone.

Ludwig's Angina

- From mandibular Molars infection.
- **Roots of mand. Molars lie BELOW the attachment of MYLOHYOID** m.
    - 3 fascial spaces are involved bilaterally = submand + sublingual + :ubmental.
    - Eilateral involvement.
    - **Open-mouth appearance** of patient—due to elevated floor of mouth and tongue is protruded and elevated.
    - Cause = **Hemolytic streptococci.**

Cavernous sinus thrombosis

- **STAPHYLOCOCAL** infection.
- Due to extraction of **acute infected maxillary anteriors** and curettage of the sockets.
- Infected thrombus ascends in the veins **due to absence of valves in angular/facial and ophthalmic vs.**
- Paresis of **3, 4, 6th Ns.**
- Venous obstruction in retina; conjunctiva or eyelid occurs.
- Meningeal irritation occurs.

Miscellaneous points

- Osteolytic lesions in cancellous bone can't be detected on R/G. It is only seen if a part of cortical bone is destroyed.

- Attachment of buccinator and mylohyoid ms determine the path of pus eruption, i.e. intra-oral or through the skin.
- To search for broken needle in the tissues, it should be searched in a direction perpendicular to the direction of insertion.

CYSTS (Also refer to the sections of oral pathology Vol. 1.)

Congenital cysts	**Others**	**Developmental cysts (Inclusion type)**		**Odontogenic cysts**
		Retention	**Fissural**	
Thyroglossal duct cyst	Haemorrhagic	Mucocele	Nasoalveolar cyst	Dentigerous
Branchiogenic cyst	Traumatic	Ranula	Median cyst	Periodontal
Dermoid cyst			Incisive canal/ nasopalatine cyst Globulo-maxillary cyst	Primordial/ fissural Keratocyst; OKC

Important points

- If protein level in aspirated fluid of cyst is less than 4 mg %, its is OKC.

Aspiration of fluid and its inference

Light straw coloured fluid with cholesterol crystals	Cyst
Creamy white fluid with keratin suspensions	OKC
Brick red fluid No fluid	Hemorrhagic cyst Solid growth

Congenital cysts: or branchial cleft type.

1. **Thyroglossal duct cysts**
    - Are in MIDLINE.
    - Lie between thyroid gland and foramen cecum.
    - Move upward with swallowing.
2. **Branchiogenic cyst**
    - Arise from persistancies of 2nd branchial cleft.
    - Present along the **anterior border of SCM m.**
3. **Dermoid cyst**
    - Occurs along the **natural lines of union.**
    - Causes **Bony Erosion** beneath them.
    - Contains hair, sebaceous glands, sweat glands and tooth structure.
    - In floor of mouth–cause swelling in the same location as RANULA but it has a **yellow** colour.
    - More superficial to branchiogenic cleft cysts and not attached to lateral pharyngeal wall.

Developmental cysts–(Inclusion cysts)

(a) Fissural type

1. **Nasoalveolar**
    - At the junction of globular, lateral nasal and maxillary processes.
    - Swelling at the attachment of ALA of nose.
    - They are not central bony lesions.
    - R/G = negative findings.
2. **Median cysts**
    - Forms in median fissure of palate from embryonic remnants.
    - Occurs more posteriorly in the palate as cp. To INCISIVE CANAL CYST.
3. **Incisive canal/Nasopalatine cysts**
    - Located **in the centre** of the bone.

4. **Globulomaxillary cyst**
   - At the junction of globular and maxillary process.
   - Between L.I. and canine teeth.
   - Cause divergence of roots of these teeth.
   - **Pear - shaped radiolucency in R/G**.
   - Teeth are VITAL.

(b) Retention cysts

Mucocele

- Due to obstruction of ducts of minor salivary glands.
- Lie just **below the oral mucosa**.
- Present especially on lips/buccal mucosa, etc.
- Treatment = **complete excision with involved gland** and duct.

Ranula

- Arise from sublingual gland.
- Bluish colour due to thinning of mucosa. Seen as the belly of the frog, and hence is the name.
- Larger size than mucocele.
- Tongue may be raised.
- Does not pit on pressure.
- Contain stringy–mucoid material.
- Best treatment is MARSUPIALIZATION.
- **Partsch operation** is also known as MARSUPIALIZATION.
- **Waldron's operation** = is a 2-stage operation, which consists of marsupialization first and then the ENUCLEATION of cyst membrane at a later stage.

CRYOSURGERY

It involves the application of cold solutions to tissue to freeze and destroy it. *ROBERT BOYLE* observed that the freezing of tissues produced necrosis.

EFFECTS OF FREEZING

- The events that are involved in cellular necrosis during freezing are as follows.
- Formation of extracellular ice.
- Concentration of extracellular solutes.
- Decrease in intracellular water.
- Cell shrinkage.
- Concentration of intracellular solutes.
- Cell membrane damage.
- Formation of intracellular, ice.
- The most expensive type utilizes **liquid nitrogen** to freeze the surgical site through an insulated probe. Liquid nitrogen can be used to achieve temperatures of **–196°C.**
- Other refrigerant media are **carbon dioxide, nitrous oxide** and **freon.** This may reach temperatures of **–20°C to –89°C.**
- Generally **4-5 minutes** of freezing at –80°C will result in sufficient tissue necrosis to eradicate most intraoral mucosal lesions.

MAXILLARY SINUS

- aka **Antrum of Highmore.**
- It is the first paranasal sinus to develop; it grows laterally from middle meatus of nasal cavity at approx 17th day IU; start developing at 3 mo IU.
- Expands by pneumatization into developing alveolar process.
- It Vol. is 10–15 ml is the capacity of adult sinus; size is 34 × 33 × 23 mm (L , H, W).
- It is largest of all the 4 PNS.
- **Pyramidal** in shape = **apex in root of the zygoma/zygomatic process of maxilla.**
- Grows during 7–15 years age.
- It is lined by respiratory epithelium, i.e. pseudostratified ciliated columnar epithelium and periosteum.

- It opens at OSTIUM MAXILLAE in the **middle meatus of nasal** wall.
- Opening/ostium lies 2/3rd of the distance up from the inferior part of the medial wall and drains into nasal cavity; is at a higher level than the floor and so there is drainage problem.
- It opens in the posterior end of hiatus semilunaris in middle meatus of nasal cavity b/w middle and inferior nasal conchae.
- Covered inside by **ciliated** epithelium know as **Schnedrian membrane.**
- In infants and children = floor of sinus is always higher than the floor of nose and so better drainage due to gravity is possible from window operation.
- In adults = the floor of sinus is lower than nasal floor.
- **Nasal antrostomy** = opening is made in the **inferior meatus**, where bone is very thin.
- Postero-superior alveolar br of Mx nerve (br of **5th N)** supply the lining of membrane.
- **Blood supply** = from infra orbital A (br of Mx A).
- Lymph drainage = submandibular LN.
- Best r/g view for diagnosis = water's view; OPG.
- If acute sinusitis = r/g shows air filled levels.
- In chronic sinusitis = r/g shows opacifications, polyps and mucosal thickenings.
- Normal flora of sinus = aerobic streptococci; anearobic G (ve) rods, e.g. bacteroides and fusobacterium.
- Sinusitis of non-odontogenic origin = mainly aerobes especially *Strept pneumonial*, *H. influenzae* and *Staph. aureus*. The anerobes are bacteroides, peptococcus, fusobacterium.
- Sinusitis of odontogenic origin = main anaerobes, e.g. peptococcus; peptostrept; bacteroides and eubacterium and aerobic strept.
- Penicillin, erythromycin and clindamycin are effective vs odontogenic sinusitis.

Functions

- Gives resonance of the voice.
- Warms the air.
- Lightens the skull
  - **Water's view** (PNS view) of R/G shows all sinuses.
  - During acute sinusitis, teeth may be painful, as their roots approximate the lining of sinus.
  - Lining becomes thick due to cellular proliferation in chronic Mx sinusitis.
  - Fractured root of molars may enter the sinus.
  - Mx 3rd molar may slip in INFRATEMPORAL FOSSA during extraction.

Caldwell–Luc operation

- Cuspid–2nd molar area is exposed.
- **Opening** is made in the facial wall of antrum ABOVE THE BICUSPID ROOTS.

ORO-ANTRAL FISTULA = an opening communicating between the sinus and the oral cavity. It may get formed by entry of roots of the maxillary molars due to improper extractions.

DANKER'S OPERATION = i.e. joining the antero-lateral nasal opening with canine fossa opening (piriform aperture).

Salivary glands (Also refer to the section on anatomy; oral pathology.)

- Minor salivary glands are mucus type.
- Parotid = largest; serous.
- 7th n lies deep to parotid's superficial lobe and passes between the lobes rather than within the parotid substance.
- Parotid duct passes anteriorly and medially; open at the level of mx 2nd molar in buccal vestibule.
- Submandibular gland is muco-serous/mixed.
- At the post border of mylohyoid m–SMG enters the sublingual space and gives off its excretory duct, i.e. Wharton's duct. The

duct opens at the caruncle lateral to lingual frenum. It crosses beneath the lingual N at the level of 3rd molar and above the lingual N at the level of 2nd molar.

- Sublingual gland = is mucus; lies above the mylohyoid m; its landmark is plica sublingualis; has got multiple ducts; it has **simple ductal system.**
- Minor glands = are mucous in nature; has got **simple ductal system.**
- Ductal pattern of SMG and parotid glands resembles the **leafless tree.**

Anatomical weaknesses

- SMG lies in dependant position; may cause retrograde infections.
- Lumen of the duct of SMG and parotid glands are broader than their opening and may get blocked by the obstructions formed by the setting of epithelial cells and salivary fluid contents.
- Duct of SMG and parotid glands take a radical turn along their course, which acts as favorite point for lodgement of obstructions.
- Retention cysts develop due to rupture of a duct into the gland parenchyma and then filling with salivary secretions. It does not fill with radiopaque solutions in sialography.
- **Branchial cleft cyst** = It arises from the epithelium between the branchial arches, occurs as the swelling on the lateral aspect of the neck or in the floor of the mouth.
- **Mixed tumor** = Also known as **pleomorphic adenoma**; most commonly occurs in parotid and minor glands, ball-in-hand appearance in sialogram, does not respond to radiations; so surgical excision with the normal part of gland supporting it has to be done, recurrence is possible.
- **Muco-epidermoid tumors** = Are malignant, occur most frequently in parotid gland; involve ductal and acinar structures of the gland.
- **Stones/sialolithiasis** = **Most common in submandibular** glands and ducts (83%), parotid (10%), sublingual (7%), best Rx for stone is **trans-oral sialo-lithotomy** for SMG, save lingual N.

- Secretions of SMG contains more calcium.
- Relation of 7th ns and it s branches with parotid gland.

Consistency

Abscess	Fluctuant
Dermoid cyst	Doughy
Stones	Dense/stellate
Infected/obstructed gland	Firm/tense
Tumor	Fixed/painless

Definitions

- **Sialodochitis** = i.e. inflammation of salivary duct; it is the dilation of salivary duct secondary to epithelial atrophy with irregular narrowing caused by reparative fibrosis.
- **Sialadenitis** = inflammation of salivary gland.
- **Sialolithiasis** = stone in salivary gland.
- **Sialo-angiectasis** = gland and duct system is vastly dilated by stasis of the salivary secretions.
- **Sialogogues** = agents which increase the salivary flow.

SIALOGRAMS

- **Sialography** = radiographic study after injecting radiopaque oil in the ductal system. The r/g obtained is know as **sialogram**.
- **Lipiodol** as the radiopaque solution is used. Iodised oil has antiseptic action also.
- **Water-based** contrast medium is better than the oil based media; why, because oil irritates the soft tissues; and its clearance is slow as compared to water based medium.
- Sialadenitis = **leafy-tree appearance.**
- Sialolith = **link sausage appearance.**
- Mixed tumor of parotid = **ball-in-hand** deformity in many cases.
- Sjogren's syndrome = **branchless-fruit- laden tree/cherry–blossom** appearance.

Leafless tree	Normal acinar structure of parotid
Leafy tree	Sialadenitis; terminal acini of parotid gland are dilated
Link-sausage dilation	Sialolith; blocking collecting ducts; sialodochitis
Ball in hand deformity	Mixed tumor of parotid

Summary

Parotid	Serous	Stenson's duct; opens near max 2nd molar	Lies superficial to masseter ms
Subman-dibular	Mixed	Wharton's duct; opens in floor of mouth	Posterior border of mylohyoid m
Sublingual	Mucus	Bartholin's duct; has 8–20 small ducts of Rivinus	Lies on superior surface of mylohyoid ms

TEMPORO-MANDIBULAR JOINT (Also refer to the sections of anatomy; orthodontics, oral pathology.)

It is a type of Ginglymo-arthroidal joint.

- Condylar type of synovial joint (complex).
- Articulating surfaces covered with AVASCULAR fibrous tissues rather than HYALINE cartilage.
- Articular surface of condyle faces U and F. Neck of condyle appears to be bent anteriorly.
- Articular disc has comcavo–convex upper surface and concave lower surface. It divides TMJ in superior and inferior compartments.
- Disc is very thin and **avascular in centre**, so healing is a problem in disc.
- Lateral pterygoid M attached to disc and pterygoid fovea at the anterior of the condyle of mandible.

Capsule

- Superior portion of capsule is loose and permits anterior gliding movement.
- Inferior portion is TIGHTER and allows HINGE movement.

Temporo-mandibular ligament = runs D and B from zygomatic arch to condylar neck.

- It gives DIRECT SUPPORT TO THE CAPSULE. It is the main ligament of the joint.
- Nerve supply: Auriculo-temporal and masseteric br. of 5th N; prioprioceptive.
- Blood supply: superficial temporal br of ECA.
- Movement in upper compartment = GLIDING.
- Movement in lower compartment = Rotation + Gliding.

TMJ pain = Jaw deviates to the affected side during normal opening motion.

- **Injection therapy** of TMJ pain by **Hydrocortisone** helps in reducing the inflammation. Drug is deposited **in superior compartment**.

Sclerosing solutions

- For treatment of hypermobility/subluxation/luxation.
- Injection is given **in capsule** overlying the upper condylar neck only to aid in fibrosis and tightening of that structure.
- Solutions should not be injected into JOINT.

- High condylectomy/**condylar shaving** is done in cases of extensive proliferative changes or erosion of condylar head.
- **Costo chondral graft** are useful in children with agenesis of condyle, as they can help during growth spurt for growth of mandible.
- Treatment of luxated condyle-downward and backward pressure on the mandibular posterior teeth and the mandible is then moved in a downward/backward and upward direction to place it in condylar fossa.

- **Ankylosis** = most common cause is trauma; it may lead to micrognathia/**bird-facies** due to lack of condylar growth in children.
- Ankylosis can be bony/fibrous; unilateral/bilateral; intra-articular/extra-articular; complete/partial.

Movement	Muscles
Depression	Lateral pterygoid.
Elevation	Masseter medial pterygoid temporalis.
Protrusion	Lateral and medial pterygoid ms.
Retrusion	Posterior fibers of temporalis.
Lateral	Medial and lateral pterygoids of each side acting alternately.

Arthrosis

- Initial stage of arthritis.
- No R/g findings seen.

NEUROLOGICAL DISORDERS

Definitions

Paralysis	• Loss of or impairment of motor function in a body part.
Paresis	• Is incomplete paralysis.
Anesthesia	• Is the loss of any and all sensations.
Ageusia	• Loss of specific sensations of taste.
Analgesia	• Loss of sensitivity to painful stimuli.
Hyperesthesia	• Excessive sensitivity.
Hypoesthesia	• Decreased sensitivity especially to touch.

Definitions (*Contd.*)

Hyperalgesia	• An increased sensitivity to pain.
Hypoalgesia	• Decreased sensitivity to pain.
Pain detection threshold	• Is the lowest level, at which a given stimulus is considered painful.
Pain tolerance threshold	• Is the level of maximally tolerated stimulus and is highly variable; it is altered by pharmacological and hypnotic techniques.
Sensory dissociation	• Loss of certain senses with simultaneous maintenance of other senses.
Paresthesia	• Any altered sensation.
Dysesthesia	• Is a painful paresthesia, e.g. burning, boring, stabbing or phantom pain.
Referred pain	• In which symptoms are felt in distant tissues and are unrelated to the true pathological site.
Phantom pain	• Is the awareness of a previously extracted tooth or a burning tongue after glossectomy, why?

- **Phantom bite syndrome** = it is the situation where a patient cannot find a position of comfort despite having worn dentures for many years.
- **Components of pain** = 3, perception; affect/emotion; and reaction.
- **Nociceptors** = 1–5 micron nerve fibers; are unmyelinated/thinly myelinated; are A–delta and C–type fibers; activated by serotonin, prostaglandins AG.
- **Gate-control theory** = given by **Melzack and Wall;** the gate is located in the **caudal portion of the brain stem trigeminal**

synaptic regions especially in subnucleus caudalis of the descending trigeminal tract.

- **Somatic sensations** = trigeminal nerve; max and mand divisions; 5th n. contains the largest proportion of myelinated axons and smallest proportions of unmyelinated axons on the entire somatic sensory system.
- **Multiple sclerosis** = is a demyelinating disease (Also refer to section on oral pathology).
- In *D mellitus*, polynephropathy of 5th nerve may occur, which is symptomatic degeneration of many nerves.
- Sympathetic nerve supply to maxillofacial region arises in cervical spinal cord and after synapse in the superior cervical chain ganglion, it is distributed along the arteries to glands and smooth ms.
- Para-sympathetic neurons arise in brain stem cells columns of 3, 7, 9th cranial ns , which then synapse in ciliary, sphenopalatine otic and submandibular ganglia and is distributed to smooth ms, salivary glands and lacrimal glands.
- **Gustatory sweating/auriculo-temporal nerve syndrome** = is due to severence of auriculotemporal n and its associated autonomic fibers; and then the inappropriate regrowth of 9th n para-sympathetic fibers along the vacant sympathetic paths, which then terminate in sweat glands rather than salivary acini.
- **Motor supply** = originate in upper motor neurons; comes to lower motor neurons; from LMN the peripheral extracranial processes go to skeletal ms and form the cranial nerves.
- All the lower motor cranial ns except 4th nerve are completely UNCROSSED in their courses to skeletal ms, so any lesion of LMN produces a deficit in all the ms supplied by that nerve.
- Lesions of UMN of 7th n cause a deficit in lower facial ms only; it is due to some crossing of UMNs, which cause double innervation to some parts of facial motor nucleus.
- Lesions of LMNs of 7th n produce a deficit in all the ms supplied by this nerve, i.e. upper and lower facial ms.
- **Diagnostic nerve blocks** = it is a simple and most revealing technique for locating and characterizing neurological lesions.

Tests of cranial N functions

3, 4, 6 ns 5 7 9, 10 11 12	Extraocular ms functions Masticaroty ms functions Facial ms functions Palatal; pharyngeal; laryngeal functions Sternomastoid; trapezius ms Tongue functions
Somatosensory functions	5, 7, 9 ns
Special functions	
1 2 7, 9 8	Smell Vision Taste Hearing
Autonomic functions	
Sympathetic	Pupillary dilation, eye lid tone; sweating; vaso-constriction; salivation
Para-sympathetic	Pupillary constriction; serous salivation

Idiopathic trigeminal neuralgia

- Aka tic douloureus, because of ms spasm.
- Unilateral; does not cross the midline.
- Commonest mainly on RHS; in females; in 6th decade age.
- There are trigger zones.
- Fibres of 5th n does not cross the midline of face; so it is unilateral.
- Expression less face known as starey face.
- Segmental demyelination of the sensory root of 5th nerve, may occur due to the anomaly of superior cerebellar A may be the cause.

- Rx = carbamazepine; phenytoin; decompression and complete resection of ganglionic posterior root fibers; peripheral neurectomy, etc.

Different neurological diseases

Vago-glossopharyngeal neuralgia	9, 10th nerves; sensory, autonomic and motor fibers involved more on LHS pain in the base of tongue, tonsillar pillars, soft palate and external auditory canal syncope, hypotension; bradycardia = are due to effect on N of HERING, which is responsible for initiating carotid sinus reflex activity.
Eagle's syndrome	Due to elongated, ossified stylohyoid ligament, which causes pressure on the nerves in the area of F spinosum Rx = intracranial rhizotomy of posterior roots of 9th and 10th nerves; no use of peripheral neurectomy.
Geniculated neuralgia; nerve; aka intermedius neuralgia	Due to sensory/intermedius part of 7th N. Unilateral entity is known as Ramsey-Hunt syndrome. Pain in deep external auditory meatus; auricle and soft palate.
Migraine	Unilateral pain in temporal area, appears before 16 yrs of age, is due to excess vasodilation of extracranial vessels, e.g. maxillary A and dural part of (MMA), middle meningeal A. Rapid pain relief by digital pressure of CCA/ ECARx = ergotamine tartarate (a vasoconstrictor agent)
Cluster headache	Also known as periodic migrainous, neuralgia, histamine, cephalgia.

Different neurological diseases (*Contd.*)

	Invloves ciliary neuralgia, vidian neuralgia and sphenopalatine (sluder's neuralgia). No trigger points; problem is along the course of greater superficial petrosal n. Rx = ergotamine tartarate, methysergide (serotonin antagonist).
Atypical facial neuralgia	Pain does not follow the distribution of somatic sensory trigeminal nerves. Palpable tenderness at the carotid bifurcation and along the ECA branches. 5, 7, 9, 10 and cervical afferent fibers are involved distribution of pain is along the maxillary A and its terminal branches, i.e. middle meningeal; deep temporal; and sphenopalatine division.
Bell's palsy	Due to neuritis of 7th nerve within the facial canal. If chorda tympani n is involved, then impaired taste sensation over anterior 2/3rd tongue occurs. If nerve to stapedius ms involved = then loud noise intensification occurs. If upper motor neuron lesions = the upper facial ms are spared lower facial ms are involved. In lower motor neuron lesions = whole face is involved.
Orbital edema	3rd, 4th and 6th nerves get involved, 1. 3rd n neuritis = Horner's syndrome, i.e. ptosis, anhidrosis and pupillary constriction; deficient upward gaze.

Different neurological diseases (*Contd.*)

	2. 4th n neuritis = inability to rotate the eye ball down and out ward. 3. 6th n paralysis = impaired lateral gaze.
Causalgia	Is due to injury to mixed peripheral nerves; is a deep burning pain of post-traumatic nature. It is caused by the excitation of demyelinated sensory nerve segments by adjacent unmyelinated sympathetic fibers, i.e. artificial synapsing of efferent sympathetic fibers with somatic sensory fibers. In regenerated fibers—the distance b/w nodes of Ranvier is shorter and conduction velocity is decreased; they are poorly myelinated.
Phantom pain	Patient who have got amputation of a body part often experience a sense of awareness of the missing part known as phantom phenomenon; complain of phantom teeth is a usual phenomenon.

- **Pulpal ns** are poorly myelinated.
- **Leprosy** is thc only known direct infection of peripheral fibers.
- H. zoster is the only definite viral infection of peripheral nervous system. It occurs in sensory N distribution of 5, 7, 9, 10 nerves; mostly involves ophthalmic div of 5th n; it occurs due to VZ virus latent in the larger neuron cell bodies of sensory ganglia.
- **Raynaud's phenomenon** = fingers and toes respond to cold and emotional stress with pallor, cyanosis, and trophic skin changes due to vasospasm.
- Most common disease associated with connective tissue disease neuropathies = diabetes mellitus.

- **Nutritional neuropathy** = mainly occurs in branches of nerves most acutely affecting vibratory and position senses.
- **Wernicke's encephalopathy** = occurs by thiamin deficiency in chronic alcoholism.
- **TENS** = i.e. transcutaneious electronic nerve stimulation = it is based on the gate control theory, where stimulation of large cutaneous fibers thro transcutaneous electronic stimulation may be responsible for over-riding the pain input from structures, e.g. TMJ and ms.
- **Syringobulbia** = degenerative disease of medulla oblongata; there is dissociated sensroy loss of pain and temperature but not of touch; occurs due to cavitation and gliosis.

Traumatic nerve injuries

Inferior alveolar N	With fracture of mandibular body; ostectomy, etc.
Infraorbital N	Zygomatico-maxillary complex fracture.
Lingual N	Mandibular 3rd molar surgery.
Long buccal N	By raising the buccal flap for 3rd molar surgery, mandibular osteotomy, etc.
Nasopalatine N	Impacted maxillary canine surgery.
Mental N	Skin graft, vestibuloplasty of mandible, periapical surgery of mandibular premolar region.

Degeneration

1. **Segmental demyelination** = is selective dissolution of the myelin sheath segments; slowing of conduction velocity occurs.
2. **Wallerian degeneration** = it is the disintegration of peripheral nerve fibers and myelin sheaths, which spreads distally from the point of injury.
3. **Dying back neuropathy** = degeneration begins in the most peripheral nerve tissues and progresses centrally from that point.

It occurs due to metabolic intoxications; anesthesia and paresthesia appear peripherally and progresses centrally.

CLEFT LIP AND PALATE (Also refer to orthodontics and pedodontics.)

Classifications and causes: hereditary/congenital.

- **Cleft lip CL.**
- **Cleft lip and alveolus CLA.**
- **Cleft lip and palate CLP = unilateral/bilateral; partial/ complete.**
- **Midline CL** are rare.
- **Soft palate cleft.**
- **Incomplete cleft palate** = i.e. only secondary plate is involved.
- **Complete cleft** = involves alveolar ridge and hard and soft palates.
- **Occult cleft palate** = are submucosal clefts, i.e. muscle slings of soft palate are not united. No cleft is seen intraorally.
  - Cleft lip is know as **cheiloschisis.**
  - Cleft plate is know as **palatoschisis.**
  - CLP are congenital.
  - Incidence = 1:800 live births.
  - CL are more frequent in males.
  - Isolated CP more frequent in females.
  - Cleft develops b/w 6–10th weeks of IUL.
  - CL are more common on LHS than RHS.
  - Lip forms by fusion of fronto-nasal and lateral maxillary processes.
  - Palatine shelves contact at the MIDLINE and fuse from anterior to posterior forming the palate.
  - Point of fusion of future hard palate with septum is the site of ossification of future VOMER.
  - Cleft occurs due to lack of mesodermal proliferation along the lines of fusion of embryonic processes.
  - With increased maternal age–there are increased chances of cleft.

- **Cheilorrhaphy** = cleft lip repair; done at 3 weeks to 3 months age.
  - Lip is corrected as early as is medically possible.
  - **Millard's rule of ten** = **wt** = 10 lbs; **age** 10 wks; **Hb** 10 gm%; **WBCs** 10,000.
- **Staphylorrhaphy** = aka soft palate closure. Soft palate cleft is closed b/w 18–24 mos, leaving the hard palate open.
- **Palatorrhaphy** = i.e. palate repair.
  - For normal speech and swallowing.
  - Bony union of hard palate area is not achieved and the hard palate defect is covered with obturator till 5–6 yrs age **for proper maxillary growth to occur.**
  - At 2 yrs age = soft palate is repaired for proper velo-pharyngeal function.
- **Uranorrhaphy** = is the hard palate closure.
- **Alveolar bone grafting**
  - Provides support for the teeth.
  - Helps to improve arch contour.
  - Stabilises mobile premaxilla in bilateral clefts.

Early alveolar grafting has adverse influences on maxillary growth and development.

In bilateral clefts = the premaxilla is excessively thrust forward due to septal-premaxillary ligament, which influences the amount of anterior and upward rotation and due to the influences of septum and vomer.

In bilateral complete clefts = the blood supply to pre-maxilla is from the vomer and septal midline source only. So there are no collateral anastomosis and there may be interference in blood supply and growth after surgical setback.

- 70% of adult premaxilla is the alveolar bone, so if teeth are lost, there is alveolar atrophy and lip support is lost. So save the teeth.
- 9–12 yrs of age is the BEST time for the graft, when the canines root is 1/4th to 1/2 formed.

- Bone graft used is of **cancellous particulate** type and helps to form a bridge, which will unite maxilla.
- Grafting is done after orthodontic expansion of maxillary arch, coordinating with the mandibular arch.
- For Rx of malposed premaxilla–the surgical correction to normal position and bone grafts are best done between 8–14 yrs age.

Speech AID appliances, e.g. obturator.

- ♦ To cover the velopharyngeal insufficiency.
- ♦ Help in developing the muscle action.

Speech difficulties in CLP cases

- ♦ Retardation of consonant sounds = B, D, K, P, T, G.
- ♦ Hypernasality.
- ♦ Articulation problems.
- ♦ Hearing problems.
- ♦ Velopharyngeal mechanism is disturbed due to discontinuity of ms from one side to the other side, i.e. velopharyngeal insufficiency.
- ♦ Compensatory mechanism occurs by development of Passavant's ridge.

ACQUIRED DEFECTS

Grafts

Graft = a tissue which is transplanted and expected to become a part of the host to which it is transplanted.

Type of response the immune system of the body mounts against the foreign grafts is primarily a **cell mediated response by T– lymphocytes.**

Free/pedicled.

Spilt thickness/full thickness.

Spilt thickness graft

- ♦ Good assurances of a "take".
- ♦ But have marked tendency to contract.

- Also known as **Thiersch's graft.**

  Best for the defects oral/nasal cavity and orbits.

Full thickness graft

- Also known as **Wolfe's Graft.**
- Less tendency to contract.
- Superior to spilt thickness graft as far as matching the face colour is concerned.
- Decreased chances of graft survival as cp to split thickness graft.

Local flaps

- Use the contiguous tissues and include advancement, rotation and transposition.
- Aka **French flap.**

Rotation flap

Transposition flap = is one that is rotated at an angle, jumping an area of normal tissue to reach the defect.

Inturned flap = here, the margins of a dcfcct are inside, undermined, and turned in to form the back side of the defect if a double lining is required.

Pedicle flaps: Has s/c tissue and skin both.

- **Z-plasty** is a double rotation flap; most effective method for releasing tension on a tissue contrature.

  Rotation of flap allows the direction of tension to be changed.
- **V-Y flap**
  - Is a type of advancement flap.
  - Acts as a lengthening procedure.
- **Y-V Flap** = acts as a shortening procedure.
- **Abbe or Estlander flap** = is used for repairs of full thickness losses of lip; achieved by rotation of flap from one lip to the other.
- **Musculo-cutaneous flap** = for extensive defects of head and neck.

- **Distant or pedicle flaps** = are those carried over an area of normal skin on a pedicle, which later sectioned and returned to the donor site.
- **Bone grafts.**
  - Fresh autogenous bone, e.g. iliac bone.
  - Large spaces within the substances of cancellous iliac bone allow rapid revascularization with survival of many of the graft cells.
  - Dense bone has low osteogenic power, because of the increased need for its resorption and replacement, e.g. tibia; rib.
  - Spilt rib graft are better as they have open specs present for revascularization.
  - Iliac bone is much more resistant in PO infection.
  - Greater the area of graft-recipient bone contact, the more certain and more rapid regeneration.

ARTIFICIAL IMPLANTS

1. **Alloplasts** are inert foreign body implants.

METALS

1. Vitalum = Co + Cr + Mo
2. Tantalum
3. 18–8—SMO steel = 18 Cr + 8 Ni + 4 Mo.

Titanium

- Is RADIOLUCENT.
- Extreme light.
- High degree of strength.
- Resistant to corrosion.
- Tantalum and vitallium—both are RADIOPAQUE.

Synthetic resins = e.g.

- Methyl methacrylate MMA.
- Polyethylene.

- Polyvinyl alcohol.
- Telon/PTFE = most chemically-inert and least irritating to tissue autoclavable.

Rubber silicones/silastics

- Autoclavable.
- Contourable.
- Non-irritating to the tissues.

Proplast = is a composite of PTFE and carbon fibers.

- **Microprosity** = pore vol. 70–90 vol%, pore size 80–400 nm; helps in tissue-ingrowth.
- Used for contour correction.
- Autoclavable.

PROPLAST-II

- Composite of PTFE and **aluminum oxide**; white colour.
- Used below thin skin, e.g. nasal bridge.

Reconstruction of mandible

- Plates for correction of continuity defect for adequate functions and esthetics.
- Also maintain the position of bone fragments till grafting is done.
- Autogenous bone graft is the material of choice (osteo-genic effect).
- Grafts may be in the form of Block/chips/osteo-periosteal/pedicle.
- Osteo-periosteal graft contains all the elements required for osteogesis of bone.
- Sliding bone graft for Rx of defects is also a method.

Advantage of Iliac bone GRAFTS

- Cancellous.
- Allows rapid transmission of tissue fluids and nutritive elements.
- Provide pathway for the ingrowth of cells.

- Readily contoured to desired shape.
- Resistant to infection.
- Rapid vascularization and consolidation.
- **Composite graft** of autogones iliac cancellous bone marrow and frozen lyophilized cortical allogenic bank bone can be used for larger bone defects.
- **Costochondral graft is best** for the reposition of mandibular joint in both the growth period and later in life.

TUMORS (Refer to the section of oral pathology for details.)

- **Block resection** = of the involved bone should extend into and include 10 mm of the normal peripheral bone surroundings the tumor mass.
- **Enostoses** = i.e. osteomas arising from the INNER surface of bone cortex also known as **central osteomas**.
- **Exostoses** = i.e. locally circumscribed bony growths developing outside the cortical plates. Also known as **peripheral osteomas**.
- **Myxoma** = honey-camb appearance in R/G.
- **Osteogenic sarcoma** arise from bone forming cells, generally occur in children **during periods of active growth.**
- **Sun-ray appearance** of osteoblastic sarcoma is due to the radiating spicules of bone extending outward from the cortex.
- All types of **sarcomas metastasize to LUNGS** through the bloodstream.

Fibro osteoma

- Occurs mainly in females and in maxilla.
- Tumor may obliterate the maxillary sinus.
- Does not invade nasal structures.
- In hyper ostosis and Paget's disease, the nasal meati are obliterated.

Ewing's tumor

- Arises from endothelial lining of the blood or lymph vessels.
- Growth is radio–sensitive, so treated by x-rays.
- s/s = elevation of body temperature pain; swelling.

Multiple myeloma

- Arise from bone marrow cells.
- **"Pain of wandering type"** is an outstanding symptom.
- **Bence-Jones proteinuria.**
- Alk Pase level is normal.
- R/G = **multiple punched out round lesions** in multiple bones, which are the sites of bone marrow.

Central giant cell tumor

- Arise in bone of cartilaginous origin.
- e.g. symphysis, angle of mandible, canine fossa of maxilla.
- Root resorption of teeth.
- Perforation of cortices.
- Highly vascular and haemorrhagic.

Peripheral giant cell tumor

- Also known as giant cell epulid.
- Arise from connective tissue of dental periodontium.

Biopsy

- It is the removal of tissues form a living individual for diagnosis by microscopic and histopathologic examination.
- It has got the **most diagnostic value.**
- It is of following **types** = excisional; incisional; aspiration; punch; exfoliative cytology; fine needle aspiration cytology.
- Specimen should be immediately placed in **10% formalin** or 4% formaldehyde solution, which is **20 times the volume of the surgical specimen.**
- **Oral cytology** = used for monitoring of dysplastic changes in mucosa; unreliable method; lesion is scraped and placed in fixing solution.
- **Aspiration biopsy** = i.e. to aspirate fluid/air from the lesion for examination; e.g. straw coloured fluid (cyst); pus (inflammatory/

infectious lesion); air (traumatic bone cavity); blood (hemangioma, aneurysmal bone cyst, central giant cell granuloma).

- **Incisional biopsy** = is done if lesion is of bigger size, e.g. larger than 1 cm; a part of normal tissue is also included in the sample for comparison purpose; a deep/narrow biopsy should be taken.
- **Excisional biopsy** = removal of entire lesion is done; normal tissue is also involved for comparison and to ensure total removal; done for smaller lesions < 1 cm diameter.

Procedure for removal of jaw tumors

- **Enucleation/curettage** = local removal of tumor by instrumentation in direct contact with lesion. It is used for very benign lesions.
- **Resection** = also known as **en-bloc resection**; it is the removal of a tumor by incising through uninvolved tissue around the tumor, thus removing the tumor without direct contact during instrumentation.
- **Marginal/segmental resection** = resection of a tumor without disruption of the continuity of bone.
- **Partial resection** = resection of tumor by removing a full–thickness part of the jaw; here jaw continuity is disrupted.
- **Total resection** = resection of a tumor by removal of the involved bone, e.g. maxillectomy; manidbulectomy.
- **Composite resection** = resection of a tumor with bone, adjacent soft tissues and contiguous lymph node channels.

ODONTOGENIC INFECTIONS

- Normal flora of oral cavity are = aerobic G (+) cocci; anaerobic G (+) cocci; anaerobic G (–) rods.
- Most common aerobic bacteria are G (+) strept and staph.
- Anaerobic G (+) cocci are strept; peptostrept; and peptococci.
- G (+) rods are eubacterium and lactobacilli.
- G (–) anaerobic rods are bacteroides and fusobacterium.
- Most of infections are mixed, i.e. aerobic–anearobic 60%.

- Most common odontogenic infections is a vestibular abscess.
- Infections spreads along the line of least resistance in the bone.

Maxillary spaces	Mandibular spaces
Canine spaces	Submental space
Buccal spaces	Sublingual and submandibular space
Infratemporal spaces	Masseteric Temporal Pterygo-mandibular

SITE OF LOCALIZATION OF ACUTE DENTAL INFECTIONS

Tooth	Usual exit from bone	Relation of exit to ms attachment	Which m/ms involved	Site of localisation
Max CI	Labial	Below	**Orbicularis oris**	Oral vestibule
Max LI	Labial Palatal	Below –	**Orbicularis oris** –	Oral vestibule Palate
Max 3	Labial	Below **Above**	**Levator anguli oris** –do–	Oral vestibule **Canine space**
Max 4, 5	Buccal Palatal	Below –	**Buccinator/ Zygomaticus major/minor ms; levator labii superioris** –	Oral vestibule Palate
Max 6–8	Buccal Buccal Palatal	Below **Above** –	**Buccinator** **Buccinator** –	Oral vestibule **Buccal space** Palate

EXTENSION OF LOCALIZED MAXILLARY ABSCESSES

1. Mx 1, 2 = Labial cortical plate; upper lip swells.
2. Mx 3, 4, 5, 6, 7 = Swelling of cheek upto eye. Infection can spread to pterygoid plexus, cavenous sinus or IJV.
3. Md 1, 2, 3 = **Apices lie above the origin of inferior incisive and mental ms.**
   - If it spreads on lingual side = it involves **SUBLINGUAL space ABOVE the mylohyoid ms**, which has its origin close to lower border of mandible.
4. Md 4, 5 = depressor anguli oris, the triangularis and quadrate m, arise near the lower border of mandible, BELOW the apices of PM. PA abscess localizes frist into the VESTIBULE, on labial side.
   - Lingual perforation will infect **SUBLINGUAL SPACE above mylohyoid m.**
5. Md 6, 7.

If buccal perforation

- Swelling in SULCUS if roots are short.
- If roots are LONG = below the buccinator m insertion and so S/C tissue is involved.

If lingual/perforation

- If below the mylohyoid m = abscess of sub-mandibular space.
- If **above the mylohyoid m = abscess of sublingual space.**

6. Md 8.
   - Mostly perforates the LINGUAL Plate and so SUBMANDIBULAR space involved.
   - Origin of buccinator m at oblique line directs the spreading abscess D and F of M3 in the buccal vestibule.
   - Mand 1–5 teeth usually erode through labial–buccal plate and above the attached ms.

Tooth	Usual exit from bone	Relation of exit to ms	Which m./ms involved attachment	Site of localisation
Mand CI,	Labial	Below	**Mentalis**	**Submental space**
LI	Labial	Above	**Mentalis**	Oral vestibule
Mand 3	Labial	Above	**Depressor labii inferioris; depressor anguli oris; platysma**	Oral vestibule
Mand 4, 5	Buccal Above	Below **Buccinator**	**Depressor labii inferioris; depressor anguli oris; platysma** Buccal vestibule	Oral vestibule
Mand 6	Buccal Buccal Lingual	Above Below Above	**Buccinator** **Buccinator** **Mylohyoid**	Oral vestibule **Buccal space** **Sublingual space**
Mand 7	Buccal Buccal Lingual Lingual	Above Below Above Below	**Buccinator** **Buccinator** **Mylohyoid** **Mylohyoid**	Oral vestibule **Buccal space** **Sublingual space** **Submandibular space**
Mand 8	Lingual	Below	**Mylohyoid**	**Submandibular/ pterygopalatine spaces**

- Molar infections erode through lingual plate more frequently than the anterior teeth.
- 3rd molars infections almost always erode lingually.
- If the root apices of mand first molar are above the origin of buccinator, then infections is in oral vestibule.
- If apices are below the buccinator, then buccal space abscess occurs.
- Apices of 4, 5, 6 are almost always above the attachment of mylohyoid and so result in sublingual space abscess.
- Mand 7, 8 infections give rise to submandibular space infections as it perforates below mylohyoid ms.

Differences b/w cellulitis and abscess

Characteristic	**Cellulitis**	**Abscess**
Duration	Acute	Chronic
Pain	Severe and generalized	Localised
Size	Large	Small
Localisation	Diffuse borders	Well circumscribed
Palpation	Doughy to induration; board like	Fluctuant
po pus	No	Yes
Bacteria	Aerobic	Anaerobic

CANINE SPACE

- Lies **between levator anguli oris and levator labii superioris** ms.
- Involved due to **maxillary canine infections.**
- Canine is the only tooth with long root to allow bony **erosion superior to ms** of facial expression.
- Infection erodes superior to origin of levator anguli oris and below levator labii superioris ms.

- Swelling obliterates naso-labial folds.
- Spontanecus drainage occurs just inferior to medial canthus of eye.

Buccal space

- Involved when infection **erodes superior to buccinator m.**
- Due to infections of maxillary molars and premolars and mandibular molars.
- Swelling below zygomatic arch and above the inferior border of mandible.

Infratemporal space

- Involved by infections of **maxillary 3rd molars.**

Cavernous sinus thrombosis

- Infections spreads through pterygoid plexus and emissary vs or via angular veins and inferior or superior ophthalmic vs to cavernous sinus.
- These vains **do not have valves.**

Submental space

- Infected by the **infections of mandibular incisors.**
- Infection erodes **apical to mentalis m** and spreads under the inferior border of mandible.

Sublingual and submandibular spaces

- Involved by **lingual perforation** of infection of molars and premolars.
- Location of infected space is **determined by mylohyoid m attachment.**
- If **infections is above MH m, then sublingual space** is involved and occurs with premolars and first molars; intraoral swelling and raised tongue.
- If infection is **below MH m, then submandibular space** is involved; mainly involved by infections of 3rd molars.

- Mand 2nd molar may involve either of the space depending on its root length.
- **Sublingual space lies above MH m and submandibular space lies below MHm.**

Ludwig's angina

- **Bilateral** involvement of **submental; sublingual and submandibular** spaces.
- Due to streptococcal odontogenic infections.
- Breathing problems, trismus, elevated tongue, difficulty in swallowing.

Masseteric space

- Involved by the spread of **infections from buccal space.**
- Mand 3rd molar infections may spread.
- Severe trismus.
- Swelling over the angle and ramus of jaw.

Pterygomandibular space

- Lies **lateral to medial pterygoid** ms.
- **LA solution is injected** in this space during inferior alveolar block.
- **Little or *no facial swelling* seen, but significant trismus.**
- Significant diagnostic feature = *trismus without swelling.*

Temporal space

- Divided in 2 parts by temporalis m.
- Swelling occurs in temporal area **superior to zygomatic arch** and posterior to the lateral orbital rim.

Masticator space: Has 3 spaces, i.e. **masseteric, pterygomandibular and temporal** spaces; bounded by the ms of mastications.

Lateral pharyngeal space

- Involved **by infections of pterygomandibular space.**
- Medial to medial pterygoid ms and lateral to superior pharyngeal constrictor ms.
- Severe trismus; difficulty in swallowing.
- Swelling of lateral neck especially inferior to the angle of mandible.
- May lead to **thrombosis of IJV; erosion of carotid A;** interference with the functions of 9–12th Ns.

Retro-pharyngeal space

- Extends from the base of skull to C7 or T1 vertebra.
- Infections can spread to mediastinum.

Pre-vertebral space

- Extends from pharyngeal tubercle on the base of skull to the diaphragm.
- Involved by retro-pharyngeal space infections.

FASCIAL SPACES

Masticatory spaces: 3 SPACES.

1. **Buccal space:** Is between buccinator and masseter m. Connected posteriorly to PTERYGOMANDIBULAR Space and connected superiorly to zygomatico-temporal space.

2. **Pterygomandibular space**
   - Lateral boundary = medial surface of mandibular Ramus.
   - Medial boundary = medial pterygoid m.
   - Above = lateral pterygoid m.

- Its infection occurs most commonly ***by extraction of lower molars.***
- Abscess in this space points at the anterior aspect of masseter.

3. **Zygomatico temporal/Retrozygomatic/Infratemporal space**

- ♦ Space lies directly behind maxilla and zygomatic bones.
- ♦ Medial to insertion of temporal m.
- ♦ ***Infection of mx. Teeth*** drains through the cortical bone above the BUCCINATOR m. may spread to this space.

Parapharyngeal space (also known as lateral pharyngeal space) is continuous with RETRO-PHARYNGEAL space.

Pterygomandibular space communicates with the parapharyngeal space around the anterior and posterior borders of medial pterygoid m.

Sub-mandibular space = is **divided by mylohyoid** m in sublingual (above the MH m) and submental (below the m.)

Submental space = lies between mylohyoid and platysma ms. It contains Ant. Belly of DG m; **PA infection of md. 1, 2, 3, 4, 5, perforate lingually below t**he origin of mylohyoid m.

Sublingual space

- Lies below the mucosa (i.e. roof).
- Floor is mylohyoid m.
- Medially by = GH and genioglossus m.

♦ Sublingual cellulitis can spread across the midline.

Cavernous sinus thrombophlebitis: Infection can spread via 2 paths:

1. From anterior facial V to sup. ophthalmic V
2. From posterior facial V to pterygoid venous plexus.

- In first type–orbit is involved, danger signals are seen.
- In 2nd type–intra-cranial/meningeal symptoms appear; no warning s/s seen. More dangerous.
- Antibiotics may increase the chances of failure of birth control pills to prevent pregnancy.
- Bactericidal antibiotics should be used than the bacteriostatic antibiotics.

Antibiotics for the odontogenic infections

Penicillin	Drug of choice; has a narrow spectrum and is bactericidal; only given "After Sensitivity Test" AST.
Erythromycin Clindamycin	If patient is allergic to penicillins.
Cephalexin Cefaclor	For broad spectrum.
Metronidazole; ornidazole, etc.	Only for anaerobes.
Tetracycline especially doxycycline	For gingival infections.
Clindamycin	May cause pseudomembranous colitis by Clostridium difficile.
Tetracycline	May cause photosensitivity and tooth discoloration.
Metronidazole	May cause disulfiram effect with alcohol.
Aminoglycoside	Kidney damage and 8th nerve damage antibiotics.
Chloramphenicol	Aplastic anemia.

- Bactericidal antibiotics interfere with cell wall formation of new bacteria, while bacteriostatic interfere with bacterial reproduction and growth.
- Usual recommended duration of antibiotics therapy is 2–3 days after the infection has resolved.

METASTATIC INFECTIONS

- Is the infection which occurs at a location physically separate from the portal of entry of bacteria, e.g. bacterial endocarditis.
- BE is mainly due to **alpha-hemolytic streptococci viridans.**

- Antibiotic prophylaxis should be given as = 3 gms of amoxicillin 1 hr before the procedure and 1.5 gm 6 hrs after the initial dose.
- Amoxicillin is the drug of choice than penicillin–V, because it is better absorbed from GIT; provides more sustained and higher plasma levels; and is effective killer of alpha–hemolytic viridans streptococci.
- Erythromycin and clindamycin are alternatives for patients allergic to penicillin.
- Erythromycin = 1 gms 2 hrs before and 500 mg 6 hrs after the surgery.
- Clindamycin = 300 mg 1 hrs before and 150 mg 6 hrs after the surgery.
- Clindamycin = is the alternative if patient cannot tolerate erythromycin.

OSTEOMYELITIS (Also refer to oral pathology.)

- Inflammation of bone marrow. It is the **infection of cancellous/ medullary part** of the bone.
- **Starts in medullary cavity**, involves cancellous bone, spreads to cortical bone and periosteum.
- It is due to compromise of blood supply and ischemia.
- **Mandible is more commonly involved** than maxilla, because blood supply of maxilla is much richer than mandible.
- Acute osteomyelitis occurs **most frequently in mandible** than in maxilla.
- **Bacteria** = streptococci; anaerobiccocci, e.g. peptostreptococci; G (–) rods fusobacterium and bacteroides.
- R/G = 10–12 days are required to be seen on it.
- Chronic osteomyelitis is seen as radiolucent **moth eaten appearance** on R/G.
- **Devitalised part of the bone is called as SEQUESTRUM.**
- Radiopaque areas are also seen in radiolucent areas know as **sequestra.**
- **Sequestra** are seen radiopaque due to osteitis–type reaction, in which bone production increases due to inflammatory reactions.

- Sequestrum becomes a site for **precipitation of ionized calcium,** which has been mobilized by the secondary osteolytic process and so it **appears more RADIOPAQUE** than the normal bone.
- **Involucrum** = is **radiolucent**, new bone.
- **Drug of choice** = penicillin; as it is effective veins strept and anaerobes.
- Drug of 2nd choice = clindamycin, if penicillin allergy is there.
- Surgical m/m = all tissue with compromised vascularity must be removed, i.e. sequestrectomy; decortication and saucerization.
- Mostly due to **M_3 infections.**
- R/G = early destruction of bone is not evident, until cortical bone is involved.
- Seen as **wormy appearance** on R/G.
- Curettage should not be done.
- **Saucerization** = after removal of sequestrum, the overhanging margins of bone are rongeured back to the cortical bone, which then rest on the intact medullary bone.
- Antibiotics should be given for 4–6 weeks.

Actinomycosis

- Is a bacterial infection; caused by *Actinomyces israelii; A. naeslundii; A viscosus;* G (+) branching rods; **anaerobic.**
- It does **not follow usual anatomic planes** as other infections, but burrows through them and becomes a lobular **pseudotumor.**
- **Multiple sinuses** on skin for drainage.
- **Sulfur granules** in exudate, which are **colonies of bacteria;** 1–2 mm in size.
- Multiple episodes of recurrent infections.
- Surgery = incision and drainage; excision of all sinuses.
- **Antibiotic** of choice = penicillin; 10 million units/day for 3–14 days I/V.
- And then long term **maintenance dose** = 500 mg qid for 3 mos.
- Drug of 2nd choice = tetracycline or doxycycline or minocycline as these can be given once/day.

HOST DEFENCE MECHANISMS OF THE BODY

Local defense	Humoral	Cellular defense
Anatomical barriers	Is a non-cellular type, e.g. by	It is cellular type, e.g.
• Skin	• Immunoglobulins	• Phagocytes; granulo – and monocytes
• Mucosa indigenous bacteria	• Complements	• Lymphocytes

Immunoglobulins (Also refer to the section of microbiology.)

- Are antibodies; help in phagocytosis of bacteria by leucocytes; produced by plasma cells/B-lymphocytes; are of 5 types:

IgG	75 %; defensive veins G + bacteria.
IgA	12 %; secretory Ig; prevents adhesion of bacteria to surface mucosa.
IgM	7 %; defends veins G (–) bacteria.
IgE	For delayed hypersensitivity reactions.
IgD	

- Primary phagocytes in early phase of infections are PMN leucocytes cells.
- Monocytes are seen in later stages and chronic infections
- T-lymphocytes play role in graft rejection and tumor surveillance.
- B-lymphocytes produce plasma cells and so the Ig antibodies.

RADIOTHERAPY (Also refer to the sections of oral pathology and radiology.)

- Used for the Rx of malignancies.
- Short wavelength x-rays or gamma rays of radium are used. Radioactive–Co is used to irradiate the tumor site. X-rays are used to sterilize the tumor from a distance.

- Rays destroy the neoplastic cells by interfering with the nuclear material required for reproduction, cell maintenance or both.
- Faster the cellular turnover, the more the susceptible is the tissue to the rays. (Which stage of mitosis is most vulnerable?)
- Tumor cells in stages of active growth are more susceptible.
- The more undifferentiated these cells appear, the more radiosensitive the tumor is.
- Normal cells, e.g. hematopoietic cells, epithelial cells and endothelial cells are also very susceptible.
- Salivary glands as such are radio-resistant, but their **finer vasculature gets destroyed** by rays. It causes atrophy, fibrosis and degenration and **xerostomia**.
- **Xerostomia** leads to rampant **' RADIATION CARIES'** of teeth; caries is seen around the entire circumference of the cervical part of tooth.
- OSTEO-RADIO-NECROSIS; ORN = is the devitalization of bone by radiations. It occurs **due to endarteritis; fibrosis of the blood vessels** and loss of fine vasculature. Turnover and repair rates of bone are slow. **Mandible is more affected than maxilla** due to higher density and poor blood supply.
- Irrigation with **dil hypochlorite solutions** help to oxygenate the areas of devital bone in Rx of ORN.
- **Hyperbaric O_2** gas increases the osteogenesis by **increasing the capillary proliferation** and leucocyte activity in irradiated bone. **150–750 mm Hg of O_2 is used for 2 hrs daily for 6–14 days**.
- Oral flora get altered; anaerobes and candida overgrow; 0.1% of Chlorhexidine and Nystatine are advised for Rx.
- All teeth with poor prognosis should be extracted before radiotherapy.
- Extractions should be done with removal of good portion of alveolar bone and atraumatic handling of flaps for better healing.
- Healing capacity greatly reduces with radiotherapy.
- Radiation dose = larger doses lead to more damage of normal tissues. If total dose is less than 5000 rads, the long term side effects are less.

- For squamous cell carcinoma, the most common tumor of oral cavity = > 6000 rads dose is required.
- Radiotherapy should be started 3 weeks after the extractions to give time for proper healing.
- RCT is difficult due to progressive sclerosis of pulp chambers in irradiated teeth.
- Hyperbaric $O_2 = O_2$ is given in the area before and after extractions under pressure. It increases local tissues oxygenation and vascular ingrowth in the hypoxic tissues and thus decreases the chances of ORN.
- Denture fabrication should be deferred for at least 6 months after the radiotherapy for those patients who were previously edentulous.

CHEMOTHERAPY

- Destroy or retards the division of rapidly growing/proliferating cells.
- Normal cells with high mitotic index are also affected, e.g. bone marrow, epithelium of GIT and oral cavity.
- Hematopoietic system—myelosuppression occurs, i.e. leukopenia; neutropenic anemia; infections occur in oral cavity; spontaneous bleeding; gets corrected after 3 weeks of cessation of chemotherapy.
- Overgrowth of candida and G (–) bacilli occurs in oral cavity. It is Rxed with nystatine and chlorohexidine.
- 3 stages of chemotherapy.

IMPLANTS (Also refer to the section on prostho.)

Bone implant interface:

- Fibro-osseous integration = i.e. collagen fibers in between the interface.
- Osseo-integration = i.e. direct contact with bone occurs; bone ingrows through thc implants.

Important points

- Bone temperature should be kept below 56°C during drilling to avoid bone damage.
- A low speed (1500–2000 rpm) should be used to drill the bone for implant placement.
- Areas of jaws with high % age of cortical bone, e.g. anterior mandible anchor the implant successfully.
- Areas of jaws with high % age of cancellous bone makes initial stability of implant more difficult.
- Minimum vertical dimension of bone for endosteal implant placement is 8 mm.
- Leave at least 2 mm bone between apical end of implant and inferior alveolar canal.
- Implant should have at least 1 mm of bone on buccal and lingual aspects.
- Maxilla has more cancellous bone, so a longer healing period is required.
- Peri-implant soft tissues environment and biomechanical overload of implant are the **2 most common factors** associated with breakdown of osseo-integrations.
- Uncontaminated surface oxide layer of implant is necessary to obtain osseo-integrations of implant in the bone.
- Immediate placement of implant can be done after extraction if site is not infected. Implant is placed at least 4 mm apical to the apex of the tooth. It should be placed 2 mm below the alveolar crest to allow bone resorption after extractions.
- How to sterilize an implant, if it falls on floor from its container by infra-red radiations?

Sub-periosteal implants

- Fits on the top of supporting areas in maxilla and mandible under mucoperiosteum for support.
- Maxillary subperiosteal implants have **lower success rate** than mandible.

Transosteal implants

- Projections penetrate the mandible from its inferior border and rests on the inferior border.
- Can only be **used in anterior mandible.**
- Used in very atrophic mandible.

Endosteal implants

- Placed in alveolar and basal bone.
- Root form and blade form type of implants.
- **Root form implants** = cylindrical shape; 3–5 mm in diameter; and 7–20 mm long.
- **Blade implants** = wedge shape/rectangular; 2.5 mm wide; 8–15 mm depth; 15–30 mm length.
- **One stage implants** = placed in bone and projected immediately through oral mucosa.
- **2–stage implants** = first placed in bone to the level of cortical plate; healing period of 3–6–9 mos. for osseo-integration; then a second surgery is done to fit abutment, which projects in the oral cavity.
- **Threaded and non-threaded** implants.
- Implants are made of biocompatible materials, e.g. titanium; Ti-Al-V; with/without hydroxy-apatite coating.
- **Self–tapping implants** = used in maxilla where bone is soft.

COMPONENTS OF IMPLANTS

1. Implant
2. Sealing screw
3. Healing cap
4. Abutment
5. Impression post
6. Laboratory analogue
7. Waxing sleeve
8. Prosthesis retaining screw.

Implant	is placed in bone during first stage surgery.
Sealing screw	Placed in implant during healing phase after stage–one surgery. It is removed at stage–two surgery.
Healing cap	It is placed after stage–two surgery and before prosthesis placement to allow soft tissue healing.
Abutment	It screws directly into the implant. It supports the prosthesis.
Impression post	It helps the transfer of intra–oral location of fixture or abutment in the cast.
Laboratory analogue	It exactly represents implant or abutment in the lab cast. It is screwed into the impression post to be placed into impression before pouring.
Waxing sleeve	It is attached to abutment by prosthesis retaining screws on the cast and it becomes part of prosthesis upon the casting.
Prosthesis retaining screw	It penetrate the fixed restoration and secures it to the abutment.

Minimum distance b/w implant and anatomic structures

Buccal plate	0.5 mm
Lingual plate	1.0 mm
Max sinus floor	1.0 mm
Nasal cavity	1.0 mm
Incisive canal	Avoid midline; place away from the midline.

Minimum distance b/w implant and anatomic structures (*Contd.*)

Mental N	5.0 mm anterior to the mental foramen to avoid injury to the nerve.
Inferior alveolar canal	2.0 mm above the canal.
Adj. natural tooth	0.5 mm
Inter-implant distance	3.0 mm
Inferior border	1.0 mm

Minimum integration time

Anterior mandible	3 mos.
Posterior mandible	4 mos.
Anterior maxilla	6 mos; due to more cancellous bone.
Posterior maxilla	6 mos; due to more cancellous bone.
Into bone graft	6–9 mos.

Rehabilitation options

(A) For completely edentulous cases

1. ***Implant and tissue–supported overdenture***
   - Esp for mand denture.
   - **2 implants** are placed in mandibular symphysis area between mental foramina.
2. ***All–implant supported overdenture***
   - a minimum of **4 implants in lower jaw** and ***6 in upper jaw*** should be placed.
3. ***Fixed–detachable restoration***
   - **5 implants in mandible** and ***6 in maxilla*** are required.
   - Best for recently extracted cases with minimum bone loss.
   - Gives best psychological advantage to the patients.

(B) For partially edentulous patients: 2 main indications are:

- Free end–distal extension bases.
- Long edentulous span.

BIOMEDICAL WASTE/BMW MANAGEMENT

Categories of BMWs

Category	Type	Rx and disposal
1.	Human anatomical wastes	Incineration/deep burial
2.	Animal wastes	–do–
3.	Microbiology and biotechnology wastes	Local autoclave/ incineration.
4.	Waste sharps	Disinfection/autoclave, etc.
5.	Discarded medicines and cytotoxic drugs.	Incineration/destruction
6.	Soiled wastes	Incineration/autoclave.
7.	Solid wastes	Chemical disinfection, etc.
8.	Liquid wastes	Chemical disinfection/ discharge in drains, etc.
9.	Incineration ash	Dispose in municipal landfill
10.	Chemical wastes	Chemical Rx and discharge in drains.

Colour coding and type of container

Colour	Nature of waste	Category
Separately to be packed in **yellow** bags	Anatomical wastes like placenta, biopsies and all other human tissues including amputation material, surgical resection, etc.	1, 2, 3, 6
Yellow bags	Infectious wastes like waste from OT, emergency room, labor rooms, dressing of wounds, swabs, etc.	6

Colour coding and type of container (*Contd.*)

Colour	Nature of waste	Category
Red bags	Used syringes, I/V tubing, gloves, urine bags, catheters, etc. and all plastic materials.	3, 6, 7
Red bags separately.	All glass bottles.	7
Blue/white translucent puncture proof containers	All needles, sharps, scalpels, broken ampoules, etc.	4, 7
Black bags	All non-infectious BMW.	5, 9, 10

Note

1. **Plastic wastes** are not to be placed in yellow bags. They are to go **into red bags only**.
2. All bags shall be labeled as per **schedule IV (rule 6) of BMW (management and handling) rules 1998**.
3. General municipal wastes should not be packed in any of the yellow or red bags.

SCHEDULES OF DRUGS

Schedules	Properties
I.	• These drugs are not available for clinical use in US. • e.g. heroin, marijuana.
II.	• These drugs have high abuse liability. • Require written prescription and DEA no. • Prescription cannot be refilled without a new prescription. • e.g. morphine, meperidine, plain codeine, pentobarbital, oxycodone compounds.
III.	• These have lower abuse potential.

SCHEDULES OF DRUGS (*Contd.*)

Schedules	Properties
	• Prescription can be phoned in the pharmacy but require DEA no. • Prescription can be refilled upto 5 times in 6 months. • e.g. codeine and hydrocodone compounds; dihydrocodeine compounds; pentazocine.
IV.	Non-narcotic drugs with lower abuse potential DEA no. is required, e.g. chloral hydrate, diasepam etc.
V.	These are in low–dose preparation for OTC sales. primarily for cough syrup and anti-diarrheal purposes. NSAIDs are not scheduled drugs.

Stabilisation periods for dento-alveolar injuries

Injury	Duration
Mobile tooth	3–4 wks
Tooth displacement	3–4 wks
Root fracture	2–4 mos
Replanted tooth mature	7–10 days
Replanted tooth immature	3–4 wks

Physical types of lesions

Bulla	Loculated fluid in or under epithelium of skin/mucosa; a large blister.
Crusts	Dried/clotted serum proteins on the surface of skin/mucosa.
Erosions	Superficial ulcer/excoriations.
Macule	Circumscribed area of colour change without elevation.
Nodule	Large palpable mass, elevated above the epithelium surface.

Physical types of lesions (*Contd.*)

Papule	Small palpable mass, elevated above the epithelium surface.
Plaque	Flat, elevated lesion; the confluence of papules.
Pustule	Cloudy/white vesicle, the colour of which results from the p.o. PMN cells/pus.
Scale	Macroscopic accumulation of keratin.
Ulcer	Loss of epithelium.
Vesicle	Small loculation of fluid in or under the epithelium; a small blister.

Characteristics of lesions that raise the suspicion of malignancy

Erythroplasia	Lesion is totally red or has a speckled red and white appearance.
Ulceration	Lesion is ulcerated or present as an ulcer.
Duration	Lesion has persisted for more than 2 wks.
Growth rate	Lesion exhibits rapid growth.
Bleeding	Lesion bleeds on gentle manipulation.
Induration	Lesion and adjacent tissues are firm to the touch.
Fixation	Lesion feels attached to adjacent structures.

COMPOSITIONS AND INDICATIONS OF FLUIDS

Isotonic saline, NS	NaCl = 0.9 gms, water for injection	Hyponatremia, hypochlorine, metabolic alkalosis, post-op maintenance
1/5 isotonic saline + 5 % dextrose	• Dextrose anhydrous = 5 gms • Dibasic K-phosphate = 0.13 g	Same as above

COMPOSITIONS AND INDICATIONS OF FLUIDS (*Contd.*)

	• Sodium chloride = 0.091 g • Na acetate = 0.28 g • Na metabisulphite = 0.021 g • K chloride = 0.15 g	
Dextrose 5%	Anhydrous dextrose = 5 g Water for injection	Early post-op period women Na excretion is less
DNS	Anhydrous dextrose = 5 g, Nacl = 0.9 g Water for injection	Intraoperative period; late post-op period
Darrow's solution	Anhydrous dextrose = 5 g KCl = 0.12 g Dibasic K phosphate = 0.12 g	Hypokalemia; started from 3rd post-op day toeplenish K loss Sod. Acetate = 0.026 g Sod metabisulphite = 0.021 g
Haemaccel	Polymer from degraded gelatin = 3.5 g Electrolytes and sterile distilled water to 100 ml Polypeptides are added for isotonicity.	Burns; extensive trauma.
Ringer's lactate/ hartmann's solution	Sod hydroxide; sod lactate; sod chloride; pot chloride; calcium chloride	GI losses, ECF volume deficit-hypovolumic shock; good results in intraoperative use.

R/G VIEWS (v) BEST FOR

Subcondylar fracture; condylar neck	Towne's view
Medially displaced condylar neck fracture	PA view

R/G VIEWS (v) BEST FOR (*Contd.*)

Ramus/body of mandible	LO at 15 degrees
Horizontal favorable/ unfavorable mand fracture	LO at 30 degrees
Frac. body mand, base of skull, zygomatic arch	SMV view
Max sinus	Water's/PNS view
Rim/floor of orbit	30 degree OMV
Coronoid	PA skull
Base of skull	Towne's and SMV
Zygoma; fracture of max-zygomatic complex	OMV
Sialolith of submand gland	Cross-sectional occlusal view
Impacted mand 3rd molar	Occlusal and IOPA
Zygomatic arch; base of skull	SMV/jug-handle view
Herniation and perforation of TMJ disk	Arthrography
Stenson's and wharton's duct sialoliths	OPG
Condyle neck fracture in TMJ view	Infracranial/ transpharyngeal view
Internal derangement of TMJ	MRI
Difference b/w CSF and blood	CT scan
Middle face fracture	Water's view
Fracture of mand condylar neck	Fronto-occipital; OPG
Medial wall, orbital roof	OM; lateral skull
Coronoid process	OM, PA view

R/G VIEWS BEST FOR (*Contd.*)

Palate	Oblique upper occlusal
Frontal sinus	Caldwell's view
Middle face fracture; BEST view	Water's view
TMJ space	Reverse towne's view; fronto-occipital

FRACTURES

- Le Fort I = guerin fracture/horizontal/floating palate/low-level fracture.
- Le Fort II = pyramidal/floating maxilla.
- Le Fort III = transverse; crániofacial dysjunction; high level fracture.
- **Panda facies** = in Le Fort fractures = it is bilateral black eyes due to circumorbital ecchymosis and facial edema.
- **Blow–out fracture** = hinged/trap door effect in R/G.
- Most common fracture of mid face = nasal bone.
- 2nd most common fracture of mid face = zygomatic bone.
- Most common fracture of face = nasal bone.
- 2nd most common fracture of face = mandible.
- Least common fracture of mandible = coronoid process; 1%.

SYNONYMS

1. JUG HANDLE V = oblique axial v/SMV = for zygoma.
2. Key-hole v = transpharyngeal/infracranial/Parma/McQueen projection v = TMJ.
3. Water's v = occipitomental view; OMV = PNS.
4. Caldwell luc v = PA v = frontal sinus.
5. Rheese v = oblique/optic foramen view.
6. Towne's v = occipitofrontal v = TMJ space.
7. Reverse Towne's = fronto-occipital view.

8. Transcranial v = posterior auricular approach of Lindblom = TMJ.
9. Transorbital v = zimmer projection = TMJ.
10. PA at–10 degrees = caldwell view.

McGregor and Campbell's lines: Seen in OMV/ PNS view.

- **First line** = path from zygomatico-frontal suture to superior orbital margin across the glabella region to superior orbital margin and zygomatico-frontal suture of the other side.
- **Second line** = from zygomatic tubercle to continuous line of zygomatic arch till it blends into zygomatic bone and the line continues along inferior orbital margin, across the frontal process of maxilla and lateral wall of nose through septum and then same course on the opposite side.
- **Third line** = from condyle across the mandibular notch, coronoid process of the mandible to lateral wall of antrum and continuous through the medial wall of antrum or lateral wall of nose at the nasal floor level and the same course on the opposite side.
- **Fourth line** = occlusal curve of the U/L arches.
- **Fifth line** = lower border of mandible from one angle to other side angle.

R/G lines on IOPA for impacted teeth: know as Winter's lines/ WAR lines

- **White line** = line joining the buccal cusps of erupted molars and going posterior over the third molar region. A perpendicular line drawn to the occlusal plane of second molar represents the long axis of this tooth. It shows axial inclination of impacted molar i.r.t. the second molar. The relation to white line shows the relative depth of the third molar.
- **Amber line** = runs at the level of the crest of interdental septum between the molars and represents the bone level covering the impacted tooth.
- **Red line** = a line perpendicular from the amber line to an imaginary point where the elevator will be applied. It indicates the amount of the resistance and difficulty encountered during removal of third molars.

SIALOGRAMS

Sialodochitis = inflammation of salivary duct.

- Sialadenitis = leafy-tree appearance.
- Sialolith = link sausage appearance.
- Mixed tumor of parotid = ball-in-hand deformity in many cases.
- Sjogren's syndrome = branchless-fruit-laden tree/cherry-blossom appearance.

GRAFTS: Transplantation of LIVING tissues.

Autografts	From same patient.
Allografts/ homologus	Same species, i.e. from alleles.
Isografts	Same species, but genetically related to patient, e.g. monozygotic twin.
Xenografts	Another species, e.g. animals.
Alloplast	Synthetic material, non-animal origin, e.g. POP, hydroxyapatite.
Implant	Transplantation of NON-LIVING tissues, e.g. POP, HA.
Partial thickness	Aka Thiersch graft.
Full thickness	Aka Wolfe's graft.
Graft rejection	Occurs due to CMI; it leaves the reciepient in a condition of increased resistance. So when a second graft known as white graft is placed it is rejected much more rapidly than the first one.

DEFINE FOLLOWING

- Displaced fractures.
- Degloving injuries.
- Bucket handle displacement.
- Blow out and blow in fractures.
- Suspensory ligament of lockwood attachments.

Absolute C/I for using steroids

- Active/healed/incompletely healed TB.
- Ocular herpes simplex.
- Primary glaucoma.
- Acute psychosis.
- Allergy.

Relative C/I to steroids use

- Peptic ulcers.
- Cushing's syndrome.
- HT, DM.
- Osteoporosis.
- First trimester.
- Acute/chronic infections.
- Thromboembolic tendencies.

Only **3 emergency situations,** in which drug is administered before the oxygen are:

1. Acute allergy/anaphylaxis.
2. Insulin shock/hypoglycemia.
3. Narcotic overdose.

Others require prior oxygen therapy, i.e. ABCs and CPR.

Proper measure taken by the dentist if anaphylaxis reaction occurs = CPR immediately, Oxygen and Adrenaline.

Shock of adrenaline insufficiency is a problem= because it is not reversed by vasoconstrictors, e.g. adrenaline, etc.

Appropriate therapy for bronchospasm = I/V succinylcholine and oxygen by face mask.

Mechanical advantages

- Lever principle = 3.0.
- Wedge principle = 2.5.
- Wheel and axle principle = 4.6.

Stages of GA = details

- Stage I = stage of analgesia, concious sedation.
- Stage II = stage of delirium.
- Stage III = stage of anaesthesia; surgical.
- Plane 1
- Plane 2
- Plane 3
- Plane 4
- Stage IV = stage of medullary depression; dangerous; death.

NERVE INJURIES

1. Neuritis = acute, reversible irritation of nerves.
2. **Neuropraxia/type I/first degree injury** = least severe injury; axonal conduction is interrupted; the nerve is intact; anatomic continuity of connective tissues sheaths and nerve axons is maintained; occurs due to blunt trauma, nerve manipulation/compression. Recovery is rapid, i.e. repaired within 4–8 weeks; no Wallerian degeneration occurs.
3. **Axonotmesis/type II/second degree injury** = occurs by tensile/crushing force; loss of axonal blood supply with potential demyelination; Wallerian degeneration occurs; necrosis and loss of nerve axons distal to the point of injury occurs; all layers of nerve are intact; gets repaired in 12–18 months.
4. **Neurotmesis/3rd, 4th, 5th degree injury** = loss of CT continuity to varying degrees; caused by blunt mechanical, e.g. strech, contusion. The Wallerian degeneration occurs distal to the nerve trunk.
5. **Compression** is the most common mechanism of peripheral nerve injuries.
6. **Anesthetic injury** = associated with sever stretch or disruptive injuries; prognosis is unfavourable; prognosis of extraosseous nerve repair is worse than intraosseous nerve injury.

7. **Paresthesia** = nerve is intact clinically; best prognosis for spontaneous recovery.
8. **Dysesthesias** = seen later in post–injury/post–surgical phases; may be seen with both divisions and incontinuity nerve injury; C/O pain in anatomic distribution of divided nerve and anaesthesia in that dermatome clinically (ka anaesthesia dolorosa). The pain should be controlled to prevent wide-range neuron sensitization on priority basis.

Pattern of spread of odontogenic abscesses

Maxillary tooth	**Potential spread sites**
Molars/PMs	Swelling or sinus in buccal sulcus may spread to buccal space, i.e. lateral to buccinator.
Canine	Canine fossa-facial nasolabial fold area.
LI	May track to palate due to distal inclination of root, but usually labial.
CI	Labially, can give a swollen lip.

Mandibular tooth

3rd molars; (pericoronitis may track buccally along the inner aspect of buccinator to present in 5, 6 region), and 2nd molars.	Both have a potential to spread in many directions; submandibular space via lingual plate. Pterygomandibular space, lateral pharyngeal space and on down the neck. Spreading laterally, infection from the 3rd molar may give severe trismus with an extension in submasseteric space.

Mandibular tooth (*Contd.*)

First molar	Buccally, if lingual may be submental or submandibular depending on level of drainage and mylohyoid attachment.
PMs and Canines	Buccally.
Incisors	Labially.

Glasgow coma scale

Scale	Best motor response	Best verbal response	Eyes open
6	Obeys commands	—	—
5	Localises pain	Oriented	—
4	Normal flexion to pain	Confused conversation	Spontaneously
3	Abnormal flexion to pain	Inappropriate words	To speech
2	Extension to pain	Incomprehensible	To pain
1	None	None	Do not open

Score	CODE
15–15	5
11–13	4
8–10	3
5–7	2
5–5	1

Immunological features of vesiculo-bullous disorders

Disease	**Direct immunofluorescence**	**Indirect immunofluorescence**
Pemphigus	Intercellular IgG and C3	Titre correlates with disease severity
Mucous membrane pemphigoid	Linear IgG and C3 at basement membrane zone	Negative
Bullous pemphigoid	Linear IgG and C3 at basement membrane	Positive in 75% cases zone
Linear IgA disease	Linear IgA and C3 at basement membrane zone	Negative
Dermatitis herpetiformis	Granular deposits of IgA and C3 at the tips of dermal papillae	Negative

Classification of white patches

Genetic	• White sponge nevus • Darier's disease • Dyskeratosis congenita • Pachyonychia congenita • Hereditary intraepithelial dyskeratosis
Traumatic	• Chemical burns • Mechanical • Thermal burns = smoker's keratosis; nicotinic stomatitis
Infection	• Caniddosis/pseudomembranous and hyperplastic types; • Hairy leukoplakia • Syphilitic leukoplakia
Idiopathic	• Leukoplakia

Classification of white patches (*Contd.*)

Dermatological	• Lichen planusLupus erythematosus
Metabolic	• Associated with renal failure
Neoplastic	• Squamous cell carcinoma

Different types of nerve fibers

Fibre type	Diameter, microns	Velocity; m/sec.
A–alpha	13–22; **thickest**	70–120; **fastest**
A–beta	8–13	40–70
A–gamma	4–8	15–40
A–delta	1–4	5–15
B	1–3	3–14
C	0.51; **thinnest**	0.5–2; **slowest**

Nociceptors are unmyelinated or thinly myelinated fibers of slow conduction A–delta and C–type fibers.

Cranial nerve testings

Nerve	Abnormal tests results
1.	Unable to identify odours.
2.	Failure of pupil to constrict or presence of non-consensual gaze.
3.	Failure of pupil to constrict or presence of ptosis.
4.	Inability of eye to look to ipsilateral shoulder.
5.	Inability to feel light touch, i.e. sensory part; weakness of masseter ms, i.e. motor part.
6.	Inability of eye to look to ipsilateral side.
7.	Inability to raise eyebrows, hold eyelid closed; symmetrically smile; pucker.
8.	Poor hearing or symptoms of vertigo.

Cranial nerve testings (*Contd.*)

Nerve	Abnormal tests results
9.	Failure of uvula to elevate on the stroked side.
10.	Weakness in turning head against resistance.
11.	Deviation of tongue to one side on that side factors of extrinsic pathways = 1, 2, 5, 7, 10 = tested by PT.

- Factors of intrinsic pathways = tested by PTT.
- Vitamin K dependent factors = 2, 7, 9, 10 = tested by PT/PTT.
- Platelet inadequacy = tested by BT/platelet count.

SIGNS NOTED IN TRAUMA

Guerian's sign	Seen in Le Fort 1 fractures, near the greater palatine foramen.
Battle's sign	Seen in fracture of middle cranial fossa, near the mastoid area. (post-auricular region).
Sublingual hematoma	Seen in mandibular symphysial and parasymphysial fracture.
Subconjunctival haemorrage	Is red in colour due to the free oxygen influx and eflux (has no posterior limit).
Black eye	As compared to SUBCONJUNCTIVAL HAEMORRAGE has a posterior limit.
Periorbita breach	Leads to subconjunctival haemorrage.
Verill's sign	Partial ptosis, partial hooding of the eyes.
Mongoloid slant	Seen in naso-ethmoid fractures.
Anti-mongoloid slant	Seen in zygomatic complex fractures.
Tinnel's sign	Seen in nerve injuries.
Vertigo	Dizziness.
Nystagmus	Uncoordinated movement of the eyeball.

DIPLOPIA

LEFT SIDE PARALYSED RIGHT SIDE PARALYSED

LATERAL RECTUS

Diplopia on looking towards the paralysed side

MEDIAL RECTUS

Diplopia on looking towards the sound side

SUPERIOR RECTUS

Diplopia on looking up

INFERIOR RECTUS

Diplopia on looking down

SUPERIOR OBLIQUE

Diplopia on looking down

INFERIOR OBLIQUE

Diplopia on looking up

SUMMARY OF ANTIBACTERIAL PROPHYLAXIS

Prevention of endocarditis in patients with heart valve lesions, septal defects, patent ductus or prosthetic valve.

(A) Dental procedures under local or no anaesthesia

- Patients who have not received more than a single dose of a penicillin in the previous month, including those with a prosthetic valve (but not those who have had endocarditis).
  - **Oral Amoxicillin** 3 g 1 hr before procedure.
  - CHILD UNDER 5 YEAR—QUARTER ADULT DOSE.
  - 5–10 YEARS—HALF ADULT DOSE.
- Patients who are **penicillin-allergic** or have received more than a single dose of a penicillin in the previous month.
  - **Oral clindamycin** 600 mg 1 hr before procedure.
  - CHILD UNDER 5 YEARS—QUARTER ADULT DOSE.
  - 5–10 YEARS—HALF ADULT DOSE.
- Patients who have had endocarditis.
  - **Amoxicillin + Gentamycin**, as under general anaesthesia.

(B) Dental procedures under local general anaesthesia

No special risk (including patients who have not received more than a single dose of a penicillin in the previous month).

- Either i/v **Amoxicillin** 1 g at induction, and then oral amoxicillin 500 mg 6 hours later.
- CHILD UNDER 5 YEARS—QUARTER ADULT DOSE.
- 5–10 YEARS—HALF ADULT DOSE.

OR

1. **Oral Amoxicillin** 3 g 4 hours before induction and then **oral amoxicillin** 3 g as soon as possible after procedure.
2. CHILD UNDER 5 YEARS—QUARTER ADULT DOSE.
3. 5–10 YEARS—HALF ADULT DOSE.
4. or **oral amoxicillin** 3 g + **oral probenecid** 1 g 4 hours before procedure.

♦ **Special risk** (patients with a prosthetic valve or who have had endocarditis).

1. **i/v Amoxicillin** 1 g + **i/v gentamycin** 120 mg at induction, then **oral amoxicillin** 500 mg 6 hours later.
2. CHILD UNDER 5 YEARS—AMOXICILLIN QUARTER ADULT DOSE, GENTAMYCIN 2 mg/kg.
3. 10 YEARS—AMOXICILLIN HALF ADULT DOSE, GENTAMYCIN 2 mg/kg .

♦ **Patients who are penicillin allergic** or who have received more than a single dose of a penicillin in the previous month.

Either **i/v vancomycin** 1 g over at least 100 minutes then **i/v gentamycin** 120 mg at induction or 15 minutes before procedure.

CHILD under 10 year—**vancomycin** 20 mg /kg,
—**gentamycin** 2 mg /kg,
or **i/v teicoplanin** 400 mg + **gentamycin** 120 mg at induction or 15 minutes before procedure.

CHILD under 14 years—**teicoplanin** 6 mg/kg,
gentamycin 2 mg/kg

Or **i/v clindamycin** 300 mg over at least 10 minutes at induction or 15 minutes before procedure then oral or i/v clindamycin 150 mg 6 hours later.

CHILD under 5 years—QUARTER ADULT DOSE.

5–10 years—HALF ADULT DOSE.

VACCINATIONS

BIRTH	BCG OPV (1) HBV (1)
6 weeks	DPT–1 OPV–2 HBV–2
10 weeks	DPT–2 OPV–3
14 weeks	DPT–3 OPV–4
6–9 mths	OPV–5 HBV–3
9 mths	MEASLES
15–18 mths	MMR DPT 1st booster OPV–6
5 years	DPP 2nd booster OPV–7
10 years	TT–3rd booster HBV–booster
15 –16 years	TT–4th booster
OPTIONAL	typhoid fever Hemoph influenza type–B Hepatitis A Varicella vaccine

TNM STAGING OF HEAD AND NECK CANCER

PRIMARY TUMOUR

Tx primary tumour cannot be assessed.

To no evidence of primary tumour.

Tis carcinoma in situ.

T1 tumour 2 cm or less in greatest dimension.

T2 tumour > 2 cm but < 4 cm in greatest dimension.

T3 tumour > 4 cm in greatest dimension.

T4 tumour invades adjacent structures (e.g. through cortical bone, skin, etc.).

LYMPH NODE

Nx regional lymph nodes cannot be assessed.

No no regional lymph node metastasis.

N1 metastasis in a single ipsilateral lymph node 3 cm or less in greatest dimension.

N2a metastasis in a single ipsilateral lymph node more than 3 cm but not more than 6 cm in greatest dimension.

N2b metastasis in multiple ipsilateral lymph nodes none more than 6 cm in greatest dimension.

N2c metastasis in bilateral or contralateral lymph nodes none more than 6 cm in greatest dimension.

N3 metastasis more than 6 cm in greatest dimension.

DISTANT METASTASIS

Mx presence of distant metastasis cannot be assessed.

Mo no distant metastasis.

M1 distant metastasis.

STAGE GROUPING

STAGE				
STAGE	O	T is	No	Mo
	1	T1	No	Mo
	11	T2	No	Mo
	111	T3	No	Mo
		T1	N1	Mo
		T2	N1	Mo
		T3	NI	Mo
	IV	T4	No	Mo
		T4	N1	Mo
		ANY T	ANY N	M1

EMERGENCIES IN THE DENTAL OFFICE

1. **Syncope/fainting is the most common** emergency. It is due to cerebral hypoxia. Dilation of the SPLANCHNIC VESSELS causes a fall in BP with a decrease in cerebral blood flow.

   Treatment is = placing the patient SUPINE.

   - Head lower than rest of the body.
   - Spirit of ammonia as RESPIRATORY STIMULANT.
   - O_2 administration.
   - Airway maintenance.
   - **Trendelenburg's position.**

2. **Toxic reactions of.LA** = initial excitation followed by marked depression.

   - Patient is talkative and anxious.
   - If given I/V–may lead to convulsions. It can be Rxed by I/V Diazepam; give adequate O_2 and **aspirate** before injecting.
   - If **Anaphylaxis** occurs due to LA—give **Adr,** which is vaso-pressor/bronchodilator and anti histaminic, it is the **drug of choice.** Dose in adults is 0.3–1.0 mg S/c or I/m. O_2, antihistaminics and corticosteroids are also given.
   - If BP is low–give vasopressor, e.g. phenyl-ephrine 1–5 mg I/m.

- If tooth goes inside the larynx/tracheo-bronchial tree = the ABDOMINAL THRUST PROCEDURE/HEIMLEICH'S procedure to dislodge large objects from tracheo-bronchial tree is recommended.
- If tooth is not dislodged from the larynx—then CRICOTHYROIDOTOMY is done.

Tracheostomy/Cricothyroidotomy

Tracheostomy = is the surgical creation of an opening into trachea through neck, for insertion of a tube to facilitate respiration.

Tracheotomy = is the incision of trachea through skin and muscles of neck, for exploration, removal of foreign body or obtaining biopsy sample.

Emergency cricothyrotomy = is surgical creation of an opening into the larynx between the anterior inferior border of thyroid cartilage and anterior superior border of cricoid cartiloge (in cricothyroid space). It is most accessible point inferior to the glott's.

Important points

- Molt's curet no. 5/Moon's probe is used to ascertain the depth of anesthesia.
- Parade ground fracture.
- Knock out fracture.

S/s of Hypothyroidism

- Fatigue
- Constipation
- Dry brittle skin/hair/nails
- **Wt gain**
- Edema

DISTRACTION OSTEOGENESIS (DO)

♦ It is a slow application of force to a bone cut thereby widening the gap and resulting in production of new bone as well as soft tissues.

- Used for Rx of growth deficiencies.
- Based on the principle of "LAW OF TENSION-STRESS".
- It is also called CALLOTASIS.
- Tensile forces are used for stimulation of callus and generation of new bone.
- There is simulteneous expansion of functional soft tissue matrix. It is called as distraction histogenesis.
- First decreased by codivilla and then propagated by Ilizarov.
- Synder et. al. (1972) used an mandible using extra-oral device.
- Michielli and Miotti (1977) used intra-oral device.

Advantages–are long term stability; simple; physiologic bone generation; 3D destruction; no grafts required; early result, etc.

6 types of DO

1. Unifocal distraction Re—to lengthen the mandible.
2. Monobloc advancement—to advance the midface.
3. Bifocal distraction—bone segment-transplantation.
4. Trifocal destraction—e.g. to reconstruct mandibular symphyseal defects.
5. Alveolar augmentation.
6. Distraction implantology.

Biological priciples of DO

1. Atraumatre corticotomy/osteotomy.
2. Healing period or latency period or delay—is the time internal when corticotomy is done; untill the time the DO is started. It is 4–7 days.
3. **Rate of DO**—i.e. the no. of mm/day at which bone surfaces are stretened @ 1 mm/day is normal.
4. **Rhythm**—no. of distractions/day divided in equal increments, e.g. 0.35 mm four times a day.
5. Healing index/consolidation period = 6–10 weeks.

Stages of bone formation in DO gap

1. Stage of fibrous tissue.
2. Stage of extending bone formation.
3. Stage of bone remodelling.
4. Stage of mature bone.

Vectors of DO—Vertical; horizontal and oblique.

Types of distractors—Extra-oral; intra-oral; subcutaneous; hybrid; monodirectional; bidirectional and multidirectional.

BIORESORBABLE OSTEOSYNTHESIS

- Polyglycolic acid (PGA), polylactic acid (PLA) and PGA–PLA copolymer are bioresorbable materials used for fractures fixation.
- No 2nd surgery required, as is required with metallic implant.
- Maintain their strength till 4–6 weeks and then degrade.
- Eliminate STRESS-SHIELDING PHENOMENON, and hence maintain bone density.
- Metallic implants in children cause growth restrictions, so PGA/PLA should be used.
    - Indicated for Re of comminuted fractures of naso ethmoidal area, lacrimal and frontal sinus bone, infra-orbital margin, paediatric patient, etc.
    - Self reinforced (SR) technique has improved mechanical properties by 5 times.
    - Sterile abscess may develop in vicinity of bioresorbable plates placed subcutaneously.

5

Local Anaesthesia

Pain impulses

Through myelinated, fast conducting, **A-delta fibres** = are strong localised pain, are the first alert to tissue injury.

Through unmyelinated slow conducting **C-fibres** = poorly localised, burning and aching pain.

Components of local anaesthesia

2% lignocaine – HCl:	21.3 mg	Main component.
Adrenaline	0.005 mg	vasoconstrictor
Sodium chloride	6.0 mg	isotonicity of solution
Sodium metabisulphite	0.5 mg	preservative of adrenaline.
Methyl paraben	1.0 mg	preservative/fungicide
Water to make	1.0 ml	vehicle

BASIC CONCEPTS ABOUT NERVE CONDUCTIONS

1. **Action potential**: brief increase in the permeability of membrane to sodium, delayed increase in the permeability of membrane to potassium.
2. **Primary effect** of local anaesthesia occurs during depolarisation phase.

3. **Primary site of local anaesthesia action** is nerve membrane, its outer bimolecular lipoprotein layer.
4. **Primary effect of local anaesthesia** is to decrease permeability of nerve membrane to sodium ions.
5. Action of local anaesthesia is to stabilise the nerve membrane in polarised state, i.e. non-depolarising block, so blocking the nerve conduction.
6. Nerve block by local anaesthesia is called as **non-depolarisation nerve block.**
7. Local anaesthesia lengthens the refractory period, decreases the amplitude of action potential and increases the firing threshold.
8. Solution is absorbed in lipoid tissues of the nerve and prevents depolarisation of the nerve membrane.
9. For maximum benefit the local anaesthesia must come **in contact with at least 8–10 mm** of the nerve to block 2–3 adj. Nodes of Ranvier.
10. Local anaesthesia contacts nerve membrane at nodes of Ranvier only, rest is absorbed by myelin sheath.
11. So higher concentration of local anaesthesia is required to block myelinated nerve fibres.
12. Impulse transmission in myelinated nerve fibres is **saltatory conduction,** i.e impulse jumps from one node to other, so faster rate of conduction.
13. Intraligamentary injection for securing anaesthesia of a single tooth, is best for the children, as to avoid the injuries after the block.

Local anaesthesia action = **specific receptor theory is the nost popular theory.**

Release of calcium ions from sites within the nerve membrane is the step in nerve membrane depolarisation, and sudden increase of permeability to sodium.

Local anaesthesia may act by **competitive antagonism / inhibition with calcium** ions for same receptors, thus displacing the calcium and binding the receptor, so it prevents initiation of depolarisation and stabilises the nerve membrane.

DIFFERENT TECHNIQUES

Infraorbital block: mesiobuccal root of maxillary first molar is also anaesthetised, the needle is below quadratus labii superioris and above he caninus muscles.

Post superior alveolar block, the needle pierces post fibres of buccinator, does not anaesthetise mesiobuccal root of maxillary first molar,

Inferior alveolar block, the needle passes through buccinator.

CHEMISTRY OF LOCAL ANAESTHESIA

All synthetic local anaesthesia are weak bases and poorly soluble in water, but their HCl salts are water soluble and acidic, With balanced lipophilic and hydrophilic properties.

If **hydrophilic** is more, diffusion in lipid rich, nerve is reduced. If **lipophilic** is more, diffusion through the soft tissues is reduced, as it is insoluble in water.

pH = pka, the compound is half ionised and half unionised,
pH = pka – log (RNH+ - RN)

High pka = few molecules as **free base,** lipid soluble, poor anaesthetic quality, poor penetration,

Low pka = large no. of free base, but **lesser no. of cationic form,** good penetration but poor blockade of nerve conduction.

Low pH = **pus** prevents deprotonization and liberation of free base—poor anaesthesia.

RN is free base, fat soluble.

Alkalies increase concentration of unionised free base which is soluble in lipids

RNH+ ⇔ RN + H^+, this reaction depends on pH and pka of solution.

As pH decreases, the H^+ increase, the equilibrium shifts to charged cationic form, i.e. water soluble.

As pH increases, the H^+ decrease, the equilibrium shifts to uncharged free base form, i.e. fat soluble.

Deprotonation is brought about by alkalinity of tissues, pH = 7.3–7.4, which liberates free base and penetrate the nerve membrane,

Uncharged fat soluble form is required to diffuse through nerve sheath and cell membrane

Charged cation binds the receptor site which is responsible for suppressing the nerve conduction.

Higher the lipid solubility and % of protein binding, more rapid and long lasting effects.

Local anaesthesia produces a **loss of function in following order**, i.e. Pain, temp, touch, pressure and skeletal muscle tone and return of sensation in the reverse order (PTTPM).

Degree of anaesthesia depends not on the concentration of local anaesthesia but on the **molar concentration** of local anaesthesia in contact with nerve fibres.

Motor nerve require a higher concentration for depression of their action than sensory nerve.

Perineurium is the **major barrier** to diffusion of local anaesthesia into nerve fibres.

Perillema / innermost layer of perineurium is the major diffusion barrier within the nerve trunk.

Concentration of local anaesthesia required to block conduction in a peripheral nerve is about six times greater than that required for CNS.

All local anaesthesia are **amphipathic.**

PH of normal tissue = 7.4

PH of infected/inflammed tissue = 5–6

PH of solution without adrenaline. = 5.5

PH of solution with adrenaline = 3.3

It is the **extracellular pH** which determines the ease of local anaesthesia to move from site of injection to nerves.

Periodontal ligament inj of local anaesthesia is not recommended in primary teeth.

Primary effect of local anaesthesia on BP is hypotension

Local anaesthesia also **causes nm blockade** due to inhibition of sodium diffusion through a blockage of sodium channel in cell membrane.

Drugs like **barbiturates** induce the production of hepatic microsomal enzymes, which increase the rate of metabolism of local anaesthesia.

Biotransformation of local anaesthesia—

Once absorbed the **skeletal muscles have the highest %** of local anaesthesia.

Local anaesthesia salts are hydrolysed by plasma cholinesterase or biotransformation in liver.

CLASSIFICATION OF LA

I. According to duration of action :

- ultra-short acting = (< 30 min.), e.g. procaine, 2-chloroprocaine, 2 % lidocaine, 4% lidocaine
- short-acting = (45 – 75 min), e.g. 2 % lidocaine with 1 : 1 lac adr, 4 % prilocaine, etc.
- medium acting = (90 – 150 min), e.g. 4 % prilocaine with 1 : 2 lac adr; 2 % lidocaine with vasoconstrictor.
- Long acting (> 180 min), e.g. 0.5 % bupivacaine, etidocaine.

II. According to chemical nature =

- Ester group =
  - a. Benzoic acid = cocaine; benzocaine (topical only)
  - b. PABA esters = procaine, tetracaine, propoxycaine, 2–chloro-procaine.
- Non- ester/amide =
  - a. Anilide type = bupiva-; etido-; lido-; mepiva-; prilo-caines.

Important

Ester group	Mainly metabolised by plasma cholinesterase; some in liver
Amide group	Metabolised only in liver
Prilocaine	Metabolised in lungs also
Procaine	Metabolised in kidneys also
Chloroprocaine	Least toxic; safest; used in children; short acting
Tetracaine	Most toxic; compatible with sulfonamides; only topical use
Cocaine	Only LA with vasoconstrictor property; excreted unaltered by kidneys so C/I in kidneys disease; used only topical
Procaine	First synthetic LA; greatest vasodilating property of all LAs
Propoxycaine	Always combined with 2 % procaine; useful in absolute C/I of amide type LAs
Propoxycaine/ rovacaine	Effective in inflammed tissues
Lidocaine	First non- ester type of LA; suitable in inflammed tissues; agent of choice in patients with abnormal amounts of plasma cholinesterase enzyme
Mepivacaine	Longer duration; can be used in patients where Adr is not recommended
Priolocaine	May cause methemoglobulinemia
Prilocaine + 1: 2 lac Adr	Safest amide LA; longest duration effect
Bupivacaine	Long acting; no need of post–op. Analgesics should not be given in children

Important (*Contd.*)

Articaine	Metabolised by saponification/ hydrolysis in liver; only LA C/I in patients allergic to Sulphur containing compounds
Etidocaine	Not given in children due to longer duration; rapid redistribution
Amide LA	C/I in patients with malignant hyperthermia
Benzocaine	Topical; inhibits sulfonamides
Dyclonine HCl	Given in patients with known sensitivity to LAs
Centbucridine	No CNS/ CVS effects
Allergy	Common with ester type LAs; due to PABA, methyl paraben
Toxicity of LA	First S/S is CNS effects as TALKATIVENESS
EMLA	Lignocaine + Prilocaine

- **Ester group** local anaesthesia is metabolised by **plasma cholinesterase** and some in liver; **amide type** local anaesthesia **in liver only** by microsomal enzymes.
- **Prilocaine** in small % is metabolised **in lungs** also.
- **Procaine** also undergoes some biotransformation in **kidney.**
- **Ester type local anaesthesia should not be given in the patients with cholinesterase deficiency, but amide type can be used.**

1. Choloroprocaine: most rapidly hydrolysed, least toxic.

Safest local anaesthesia due to its extremely high rate of hydrolysis by plasma cholinesterase.

Indicated in patient with allergy to amide type local anaesthesia.

Short duration and short-acting – so used in **children**

2. **Tetracaine: most slowly hydrolysed, most toxic.**

3. Cocaine is the **only local anaesthesia** with **vasoconstrictor properties**, by inhibiting the uptake of adrenaline in tissue binding sites.

Cocaine is excreted almost completely in an unaltered form by the kidneys. So it should be precluded in patients with severe kidney dysfunction or on dialysis.

4. Procaine is the **first synthetic injectable** local anaesthesia drug.

Has greatest vasodilating properties of all local anaesthesia.

It is the **drug of choice** in immediate m/m of accidental I/A inj, of the drug, as its vasodilating property aids in breaking the arteriospasm.

It can **decrease the effectiveness of sulfonamides** due to excessive PABA, which can reverse the action of this antibiotic. Mechanism of Action of sulfonamides is through competitive antagonism with PABA, which is an essential bacterial nutrient.

Metabolism is by plasma cholinesterase, so no toxicity in patients of liver dysfunction and 90% metabolite is PABA. **Allergic** reactions of procaine are due to **DEAE** (diethylaminoethanol). Readily crosses the blood brain barrier. Its effect on heart is **quinidine like**.

5. Propoxycaine: always combined with 2% procaine, due to its high toxicity, useful if absolute C/I of amide local anaesthesia exists.

6. Tetracaine (pontocaine): Compatible with sulfonamides.

Available for **topical use only**, not for injection, Rapidly absorbed systemically so should not be sprayed on mucous membrane, but placed in a cotton pledget.

7. Propoxycaine/ravocaine: *Effective in the inflammed tissues,*

Anilide/non-ester derivatives

1. **Lidocaine** is the first non-ester type local anaesthetic used, developed by Lofgren 1943,

   More suitable than ester type in inflammed tissues due to its low pka.

   An analogue of lidocaine which is **effective orally = tocainide –HCl,** it is also an oral anti- dysrhythmic agent.

It is **derivative of xylidine** which is antiarrhythmic,

Cardiac lidocaine = lidocaine + sod. chloride.

Respiratory arrest is the most common cause of death with its overdose.

Not affected by plasma cholinesterase, so is the agent of choice in patients with abnormal amount of this enzyme.

Maximum acceptable dose = **4.4 mg/kg (300 mg) without vasoconstrictor** and 7 mg/kg (500 mg) with vasoconstrictor

2. **Mepivacaine/carbocaine:** longer duration effects, **3% can be given to patient where adrenaline is not recommended.**

   Most commonly used in pediatric and geriatric dentistry

3. **Prilocaine**: derivative of **toluidine**, slow reabsorption from injection site, metabolised in liver and lungs. Its one metabolite is **orthotoluidine** which may cause **methemoglobinemia** , it can be reversed with **1–2 mg/kg of 1% methylene blue** solution i/v over a 5-minute period.

   Prilocaine with adrenaline 1: 2. lac is **safest of all amide local anaesthesia,** as it provides long effect (3–8 hrs), with least concentration of adrenaline, so can be recommended in adrenaline sensitive patients.

   It is C/I in congenital or idiopathic methemoglobinemia cases.

4. **Citanest forte** = 4% citanest and 1:2 lac adrenaline.

5. **Bupivacaine** long acting.

   There remains a period of analgesia which persists after all other senses have returned, so post op. need of analgesics is decreased.

   Should **not be given to children** due to its long effects.

   Biotransformed in liver by conjugation with glucuronic acid,

6. ***Articaine: metabolism is initiated by saponification / hydrolysis in liver.***

   Only local anaesthesia with thiophene ring. It is the only local anaesthesia C/I in the patients allergic to sulphur containing drugs.

7. **Etidocaine/duranest**: should not be given in children,

   Because of high tissue solubility, it redistributes rapidly,

   No post op analgesia required.

Amide local anaesthesia are C/I in patients with malignant hyperpyrexia.

Use of vasoconstrictors is to be avoided in patients on MAO inhibitors.

Topical local anaesthesia: are poorly soluble in water as they **lack hydrophilic** substituted amine group, do not form soluble acid salts,

Most common exceptions are lidocaine and tetracaine whose higher concentration are required for diffusion through mucous membrane

Cocaine is used exclusively topical, inj is C/I

Benzocaine is the most popular topical, poor soluble in water, so minimum absorption and rare systemic toxicity. It inhibits antibacterial action of sulfonamides.

Water soluble topical local anaesthesia should not be sprayed on mucous membrane, e.g. benzyl alcohol, tetracaine HCl/ pontacaine 2% — its onset of action is slow but of longer duration,

Dyclonine HCl: unique as it **has a ketone**, no cross sensitivity so it can be given to patients with known sensitivity to other local anaesthesia.

Centbucridine–does not effect CNS/CVS.

Renal diseases are relative c/i to local anaesthesia esp. Cocaine.

VASOCONSTRICTORS

Decrease the toxicity of local anaesthesia,

Sodium bisulfite is added to preserve the vasoconstrictor against the oxidation, then sodium bisulfite gets changed in sodium bisulfate thus sparing the vasoconstrictor.

Phenylephrine is the weakest of all.

All vasoconstrictors used with local anaesthesia are directly acting agents.

Receptors

Adrenaline stimulates alpha-receptors at higher doses (vasoconstrictor)

And stimulates beta-receptors at lower doses (vasodilator).

Nor-adrenaline stimulates mainly alpha-receptors (vasoconstrictor).

1. Adrenaline: Vasoconstriction effect is by arteriolar and on precapillary sphincters, so only local hemostasis is possible. Causes glycogenolysis in liver and muscles and increase blood sugar level.

Hyperthyroidism patients are sensitive to adrenaline, so adrenaline should be sparingly used in these patients.

Safe maximum dose = 0.2 mg. In healthy patients and 0.04 mg in patients with organic cardiac problems.

If 1: 1 lac adrenaline = then 1 gm in 100,000 ml = 0.01 mg/ml

So approx. 20 ml solution of local anaesthesia (0.2 mg) can be given.

2. Nor-adrenaline: Acts mainly on alpha receptors,

It has no beta 2 effects, so respiratory effects are nil.

Not effective in management of bronchospasm.

Dose; is used in twice the concentration of adrenaline and total dose should not exceed 0.34 mg, And 0.14 mg in CVS patients.

It has **local ischemic effect** due to local vasoconstriction by alpha receptors, causing **tissue necrosis**, so not more than 4 ml local anaesthesia should be injected at one time in one area to avoid ischemia and sloughing.

3. Levonordefrin acts on **alpha receptors exclusively**, arteriolar constriction is the only action, causes no CNS stimulation, causes tissue ischemia and necrosis.

<u>Total dose</u> = 1 mg only and 0.4 mg in CVS patients.

4. Phenylephrine: most stable and **weakest** vasoconstrictor, Used in the concentration of 1: 2500, **pure alpha receptor agonist**, no beta action, post-op phase passes with less bleeding.

Maximum dose: 4 mg for normal patients and 1.6 mg for heart patients

Termination of action

By **reuptake** of the sympathomimetic amines by the nerve terminal and storage in its original locations. It causes the action on beta-receptors and so vasodilation and rebound activity occurs causing increased bleeding.

Tricyclic antidepressants prolong its action and increase its toxic actions.

COMT enzymes also can inactivate these, i.e Adrenaline to metanephrine, and nor-adrenaline to nor metanephrine.

Intraneuronal enzymatic destruction is by MAO enzyme. It prevents excessive intracellular accumulation of naturally occurring amines. Vasoconstrictors are C/I in presence of MAO-I drugs.

Absolute c/i to vasoconstrictor is—thyrotoxicosis.

In **diabetes mellitus**, adrenaline may result in local ischemia and tissue sloughing due to blockage of microcirculation and impaired blood flow.

It can be given with GA agents, i.e. halothane, enflurane.

Fellypresin: is a synthetic analogue of ADH (vasopressin).

Is **non-dysrhythmogenic**, minimum CVS stimulation,

No effect on adrenergic nerve transmission—so **safer in hyperthyroid** and in patients on MAO-I and tricyclic antidepressant.

Has both diuretic and **oxytocic** action –so **C/I in pregnant** patients

Not recommended for hemostasis, as they effect venous return rather than arterial muscles.

Can be given with halogenated GA compounds (adrenaline can not be given).

SIDE-EFFECTS

1. Allergy

To ester is common, due to PABA, but rarest with amide type.

If allergy to both ester and amide type local anaesthesia exist then **an injectable antihistamine,** e.g. Diphenhydramine can be used as anaesthetic = in 1.5–2.0 ml or 15–20 mg to give 30 min of action.

Involves antigen-antibody reaction, with release of histamine.

Methyl paraben is the cause of allergy.

2. Malignant hyperthermia: non-ester type of local anaesthesia/ GA are provoking agents. Calcium ions are released from sarcoplasmic reticulum of muscles, which leads to metabolic acidosis, etc.

Ester type local anaesthesia are useful in the treatment of certain aspects of malignant hyperthermia and so they are **local anaesthesia of choice** in them.

Treatment: Dantrolene sodium 350 mg i/v

Rate of administration of local anaesthesia = 1 ml/min

3. Toxicity of I/V local anaesthesia is 16 times and of I/A local anaesthesia is 4 times than normal.

4. Effect on CNS is **biphasic**, i.e. stimulation is followed by depression.

CNS stimulation: occurs due to depression of certain inhibitory centers, which allow the excitatory actions to occur unopposed.

Primary site of action is amygdala.

a. *At 0.5–4.0 microgm/ml* ***of blood levels = procaine and lidocaine have anti-convulsant effects.***

b. At **4.0–7.0 microgm/ml** of blood levels = procaine and lidocaine have CNS **stimulation**, generalised cortical sensitivity, effects. **Talkativeness is the first sign.**

First toxic s/s of all synthetic local anaesthesia is CNS stimulation, i.e. talkativeness.

Generalised numbness of oral cavity is the pathognomonic sign of toxicity of local anaesthesia, which is due to direct effect of high blood level of local anaesthesia rather than effects on CNS.

c. At **7.5–10.0 microgm/ml** of blood levels = **generalised tonic clonic seizures** occur, which are short lived and self limiting, 30 sec.

CNS depression /sedation can be the first s/s rather than CNS excitement with = **lidocaine**

5. Toxic effects on CVS = only depression, quinidine like effects

Local anaesthesia has **anti arrhythmic action** in low doses.

Most popular being lidocaine 1.5–5.0 microgm/ml.

Dose required is 1.0–1.5 mg/kg

At 5.0 microgm/ml, severe CVS depression

At > 10.0 microgm/ml, severe CVS collapse due to intensive vasodilatation and asystole.

LOCAL COMPLICATIONS

Post injection pain is the most common local complication of local anaesthesia.

Paresthesia is most common with lingual n block.

Trismus = the most common cause is trauma to muscles in the infratemporal fossa.

Trauma to nerve sheath: sensation of an electric shock through out the distribution of the nerve.

Syncope: most common dental complication,

Is a form of **neurogenic shock,** also known as vasovagal attack or fainting fit.

Prolonged anaesthesia: due to hemorrhage in neural sheath.

Haematoma: most common with post superior alveolar, block (produce largest size) and infraorbital nerve block, Rarest with palatal injection due to dense hard palatal tissue.

Facial paralysis: due to injection of local anaesthesia in parotid gland capsule.

Post injection infection: mostly due to infected local anaesthesia solution.

Idiosyncracy: due to underlying genetic cause.

Sterile abscess: in palatal tissue only,

Overdose: mostly with amide local anaesthesia., Allergy mostly with esters local anaesthesia.

Oxygen is given with overdose to prevent acidosis.

RESUSCITATION

Lung inflation = once every 5 sec (12/min)

Maximum carotid artery flow which can be achieved with CPR = 25 33% of the normal.

One rescuer =

Artificial ventilation: circulation = 2: 15, i.e. 2 very quick lung inflation (within 4–5 sec), followed by 15 chest compressions.

Two rescuers =

Chest compressions = 60/min.

Lung inflation = on the upstroke of each 5th compression.

6

MCQs in Oral Surgery and Anaesthesia

1. From the choices listed below, what are the two most important steps in the initial management of a laryngospasm?
A. Administering epinephrine
B. Applying oxygen under positive pressure
C. Administering succinylcholine
D. Placing the patient in the Trendelenburg position

2. The optimal bone grafting material should be of what origin?
A. Foreign
B. Synthetic
C. Autogenous
D. Mixed

3. Which of the following are requirements for successful implant placement?
A. Mucosal seal
B. Adequate transfer of force
C. Biocompatibility
D. All of the above

4. Which of the following can be used for removing bone?
A. Rongeur forceps
B. Chisel and mallet
C. Bone file

D. Bur and hand piece
E. All of the above

5. **Ultrashort-acting barbiturates produce loss of consciousness by depression of the:**
A. Medulla oblongata
B. Ascending portion of the reticular activating system
C. Substantia nigra
D. Descending portion of the reticular activating system

6. **The facial nerve, the retromandibular vein, and the external carotid artery lie within which salivary gland listed below?**
A. Submandibular gland
B. Parotid gland
C. Sublingual gland
D. None of the above

7. **All of the following may prevent a patient from developing a vasovagal syncopal reaction after the uses of a local anesthetic except:**
A. Slowly injecting the anesthetic solution
B. Watching the patient's color change during the injection
C. Using a topical anesthetic prior to administration of the local anesthetic
D. Injecting the anesthetic solution as quickly as possible
E. Using a low concentration of vasoconstrictor
F. Premedicating extremely anxious patients
G. Sympathetic, but confident handling of the patient

8. **How will a larger than normal functional residual capacity affect nitrous oxide sedation?**
A. Nitrous oxide sedation will happen much quicker
B. Nitrous oxide sedation will take longer
C. Functional residual capacity does not effect nitrous oxide sedation
D. All of the above.

9. **A serious condition in which the quantity of blood pumped by the heart each minute (cardiac output) is insufficient to meet the body's normal requirements for oxygen and nutrients is called:**
A. Heart block

B. Ventricular tachycardia
C. Congestive heart failure
D. Atrial fibrillation

10. All of the following are contraindication to implant placement except one. Which is the exception:
A. The presence of pathology within the bone
B. The presence of limiting anatomic structures such as the inferior alveolar nerve or maxillary sinus
C. Unrealistic expectations of the patient
D. The patient has a pronounced gag reflex
E. Acute illness or uncontrolled metabolic disease

11. A mandibular fracture that extends only through the cortical portion of the bone without complete fracture of the bone is called a:
A. Simple fracture
B. Greenstick fracture
C. Compound fracture
D. Comminuted fracture

12. Acetaminophen and propoxyphene are used together to treat moderate to severe pain due to:
A. Dental procedures
B. Headache
C. Arthralgias
D. Myalgias
E. All of the above

13. Major oral surgery includes all of the following procedures except:
A. The treatment of maxillary and mandibular fractures
B. Exodontia
C. Pre-prosthetic surgery
D. Reconstructive surgery
E. Traumatology

14. Which drug listed below is most commonly used to attain general anaesthesia?
A. Valium
B. Chloral hydrate

C. Phenergan
D. Brevital

15. If the fracture line results in a muscle pull displacing the fractured segment, it is termed a (an):
A. Favorable fracture
B. Unfavorable fracture
C. Complex fracture
D. Complicated fracture

16. Which of the following is the process by which the total removal of a cystic lesion is achieved?
A. Marsupialization
B. Decompression
C. Enucleation
D. The Partsch operation

17. Which of the following is the primary direction of luxation for extracting maxillary deciduous molars?
A. Buccal
B. Palatal
C. Mesial
D. Distal

18. Which of the following are the most common causes of dehydration?
A. Fever
B. Vomiting
C. Diarrhoea
D. Heat exhaustion
E. All of the above

19. Which of the following can contribute to the non-healing (non-union) of a fracture?
A. Ischemia
B. Excessive mobility
C. Interposition of soft tissue
D. Infection
E. All of the above

20. Local anesthetics depress small, nonmyelinated nerve fibers:

A. First
B. Last
C. At the same time as large, myelinated nerve fibers
D. After the large, myelinated nerve fibers

21. Dead space in a wound usually fills with

A. Pus
B. Water
C. Blood
D. Tissue

22. All of the following are considered to be inhalational anaesthetics except?

A. Nitrous Oxide
B. Cyclopropane
C. Halothane
D. Isoflurane
E. Lidocaine

23. Which surgical approach listed below is the best to expose the TMJ?

A. Preauricular
B. Submandibular
C. Both are the same
D. None of the above

24. The internal jugular vein descends through the neck within the:

A. Arachnoid sheath
B. Carotid sheath
C. Spiral sheath
D. Dural sheath

25. All of the following statements concerning the articular eminence are true except:

A. It is also called the articular tubercle
B. It is convex
C. It is ridge that extends mediolaterally just in front of the mandibular fossa

D. It is considered to be the non-functioning portion of the temporomandibular joint
E. It is lined with a thick layer of fibrous connective tissue (fibrocartilage).

26. The universal sign of laryngeal obstruction is:
A. Mydriasis
B. Stridor (crowing sounds)
C. Sweating
D. Tachycardia

27. Squamous cell carcinoma is most easily managed when found where?
A. Floor of the mouth
B. Palate
C. Lower lip
D. Side of the tongue

28. What is the best way to palpate the posterior aspect of the mandibular condyle?
A. Intraorally
B. Lateral to the external auditory meatus
C. Through the external auditory meatus
D. Any of the above

29. Rheumatic fever is:
A. Inflammation of joints (arthritis) and the spleen (splenomegaly) resulting from a streptococcal infection, usually of the throat.
B. Inflammation of joints (arthritis) and the parotid glands (parotitis) resulting from a staphylococcal infection, usually of the middle ear.
C. Inflammation of the joints (arthritis) and the heart (carditis) resulting form a streptococcal infection, usually of the throat.
D. Inflammation of the joints (arthritis) and the thyroid gland (goiter) resulting from a staphylococcal infection, usually of the blood.

30. Which of the following is that phase of anaesthesia that begins with the administration of anesthetic and continues until the desired level of patient unresponsiveness is reached?
A. Amnesia

B. Induction
C. Maintenance
D. Recovery

31. Which of the following is not an indication for excisional biopsy?
A. A small lesion (less than 1 cm in diameter)
B. A lesion that can be removed completely without traumatizing the tissue
C. When there is a suspicion of malignancy
D. A pigmented or small vascular lesion

32. Strong apical pressure with a small straight elevator may displace root tips of maxillary premolars and molars into the:
A. Submandibular space
B. Maxillary sinus
C. Mandibular canal
D. Infratemporal fossa

33. Which size suture listed below has the least strength and the smallest diameter?
A. 9-0
B. 3-0
C. 2
D. 5

34. All of the following drugs can potentiate a patient's bleeding following an extraction except:
A. Aspirin
B. Anticoagulants
C. Antianxiety drugs
D. Anticancer drugs

35. Which of the following delay healing process of an extraction site?
A. A patient that has a protein deficiency
B. A patient on glucocorticoid therapy
C. An older patient
D. Local infections
E. All of the above

36. All of the following statements concerning hemophilia are true, except:

A. Hemophilia A and B are inherited as a sex-linked recessive trait by which males are affected and females are carriers.
B. Bleeding time is abnormally prolonged.
C. The majority of people affected with manifestations include Type A and are under the age of 25.
D. The signs, symptoms and clinical manifestations include excessive bleeding from minor cuts, epistaxis, hematomas, and hemarthroses.
E. Chronic complications include impaired renal function and osteoarthritis.

37. What is the proper rate of rescue breathing in an adult?

A. 15 times per minute
B. 12 times per minute
C. 20 times per minute
D. 25 times per minute

38. Which vein listed below is the optimum site for I / V sedation for an outpatient?

A. Median basilic vein
B. Median cephalic vein
C. Median antebrachial vein
D. Angular vein

39. Which of the following is the most common pathognomonic sign of a mandibular fracture?

A. Nasal bleeding
B. Exophthalmos
C. Malocclusion
D. Numbness in the infraorbital nerve distribution

40. Which artery listed below supplies the mucosa of the hard palate posterior to the maxillary canine?

A. Sphenopalatine artery
B. Greater palatine artery
C. Posterior superior alveolar artery
D. Nasopalatine artery

41. Which of the following is the fixative of choice used for a routine biopsy specimen?

A. Hydrogen peroxide
B. Sodium hypochlorite
C. 10% formalin
D. Saline

42. The mandibular left second molar of a 14 year-old boy is unerupted. Radiographs show a small dentigerous cyst surrounding the crown. What is the treatment of choice?

A. Surgically extract the unerupted second molar
B. Uncover the crown and keep it exposed
C. Prescribe an anti-inflammatory medication and schedule a follow-up appointment in six months
D. No treatment is necessary at this time

43. All of the following drugs can reduce salivary flow during dental treatment. Which one, however, works by reducing anxiety and sensitivity during the procedure?

A. Scopolamine
B. Atropine
C. Local anaesthesia
D. Benztropine

44. Therapeutic anticoagulation is administered to patients with all of the following except:

A. Post-myocardial infarction
B. Cerebrovascular thrombosis
C. Asthma
D. Pulmonary thrombosis

45. Body temperature can be measured in several different ways, which one is the least accurate?

A. Orally
B. Axillary
C. Rectally
D. Aurally

46. Serum calcium will be increased in all of the following conditions except:
A. Hyperparathyroidism
B. Chronic glomerulonephritis
C. Diabetes mellitus
D. Hypervitaminosis D
E. Malignant diseases of the skeleton (i.e., multiple myeloma)

47. Minor oral surgery includes all of the following procedures except:
A. Exodontia
B. The treatment of maxillary and mandibular fractures
C. The treatment of dental infections
D. The treatment of hard tissue pathologies
E. The treatment of soft tissue pathologies

48. Which of the following narcotics is contained in the analgesics Percodan and Percoset?
A. Codeine
B. Oxycodone
C. Hydrocodone
D. Morphine

49. Which form of the reduction listed below is best used to reduce a fracture when teeth are missing in one or more of the fractured segments?
A. Open reduction
B. Closed reduction

50. Which cranial nerve listed below provides motor innervation that allows for movements of the mandible?
A. Trigeminal (CN V)
B. Olfactory (CN I)
C. Facial (CN VII)
D. Vagus (CN X)

51. What is the only direction in which the TMJ can be dislocated?
A. Laterally
B. Medially
C. Anteriorly
D. Posteriorly

52. Which of the following are physiological symptoms of a patient taking barbiturates?

A. Slurred speech & Shallow breathing
B. Sluggishness & Fatigue
C. Disorientation & Lack of coordination
D. Dilated pupils (mydriasis)
E. All of the above

53. The mesioangular impaction is generally acknowledged as:

A. The most difficult impaction to remove
B. The least difficult impaction to remove
C. Neither of the above
D. Cannot be said.

54. The following signs i.e. a) Nausea b) Pallor and cold perspiration c) Widely dilated pupils d) Eyes rolled up e) Brief convulsions are indicative of a patient having which type of reaction?

A. Somatogenic reaction
B. Psychogenic reaction

55. Which of the following is considered to be the most common cause of TMJ pain?

A. Internal derangement
B. Degenerative joint disease (DJD)
C. Myofascial pain dysfunction (MPD) syndrome
D. None of the above

56. Which of the following statements are true concerning ecchymosis?

A. Ecchymosis is an area of hemorrhage into the skin and subcutaneous tissue >1 cm in diameter.
B. An ecchymosis is often the result of injury; clotting and bleeding disorders can predispose to the formation of an ecchymosis
C. Grossly, an ecchymosis presents as a bluish lesion at the earliest stages of onset.
D. As the red blood cells in the lesion undergo progressive degeneration and the hemoglobin becomes converted through bilirubin into hemosiderin, the lesion progressively changes

color from blue through green through purple to finally a brownish discoloration.

E. All of the above statements concerning ecchymosis are true

57. Alloplastic grafts are:

A. Those where the bone to be grafted to jaw is taken or harvested from one's own body

B. Taken from human donors

C. Inert, man made synthetic materials

D. Harvested from animals

58. Which of the following is a peculiar thermal alteration that occurs during surgery in susceptible persons?

A. Malignant hypothermia

B. Heat stroke

C. Malignant hyperthermia

D. Hyperreflexia

59. Ketamine is most commonly used to obtain:

A. Neurolept anaesthesia

B. Local anaesthesia

C. Dissociative anaesthesia

D. Regional anaesthesia

60. The American Society of Anesthesiologists would give what ASA classification to a healthy young patient with an unremarkable medical history and no systemic disease?

A. ASA-O

B. ASA-I

C. ASA-II

D. ASA-V

61. Which scalpel below is universally used for oral surgical procedures?

A. No. 2 blade

B. No. 6 blade

C. No. 10 blade

D. No. 15 blade

62. Chronic bronchitis is primarily a disease of:
A. Alcoholics
B. Cigarette smokers
C. Miners
D. Patients with a family history of allergy

63. What is the first step when initiating CPR?
A. Administer oxygen
B. Establish unresponsiveness
C. Administer epinephrine
D. Place a cool towel on the person's forehead

64. The most commonly used allogenic bone is:
A. Freeze-dried
B. Artificial
C. Both of the above
D. Neither of the above

65. Which of the following teeth could be removed without pain after administration of an inferior alveolar and lingual nerve block?
A. All anterior teeth on the side of the injection
B. Canine and first premolar on the side of the injection
C. Both premolars and first molar on the side of the injection
D. All the mandibular teeth

66. When a patient attempts protrusion, the mandible deviates markedly to the left which muscle listed below is unable to contract?
A. Buccinator muscle
B. Temporalis muscle
C. Right lateral pterygoid muscle
D. Left lateral pterygoid muscle

67. Incision for drainage (I&D) in an area of acute infection should only be performed after which of the following has occurred?
A. A culture for antibiotic sensitivity has been performed
B. Localization of the infection
C. A sinus tract is formed
D. All of the above

68. Which of the following is the maximum allowable dose for 2% lidocaine with 1:100,000 epinephrine?

A. 3.0 mg lidocaine/per lb.
B. 3.5 mg lidocaine/per lb.
C. 6.0 mg lidocaine/per lb.
D. 7.0 mg lidocaine/per lb.

69. The stylomandibular ligament of the TMJ is a band of cervical fascia that runs from the styloid process of the sphenoid bone to the:

A. Mandibular condyle
B. Ramus of the mandible
C. Angle of the mandible
D. Lingula of the mandible

70. The ideal time to remove impacted third molars is :

A. When the root is fully formed
B. When the root is approximately two-third formed
C. Makes no differences how much of the root is formed
D. When the root is approximately one-third formed

71. Which of the following will produce neurolept anaesthesia?

A. Neuroleptic agent + narcotic analgesic
B. Neuroleptic agent + nitrous oxide
C. Neuroleptic agent + narcotic analgesic + nitrous oxide
D. Narcotic analgesic + nitrous oxide

72. When would you place a suture over a single extraction socket?

A. Routinely
B. Never
C. If the patient requests it
D. When there is severe bleeding form the gingiva or if the gingival cuff is torn or loose.

73. A patient with dry socket develops severe dull throbbing pain:

A. Two to three hours following a tooth extraction
B. One day following a tooth extraction
C. Two to four days following a tooth extraction
D. Immediately following a tooth extraction

74. A patient with a paralyzed left lateral pterygoid muscle is instructed to open his mouth wide. Which direction will the mandible take upon opening?
A. To the right
B. To the left
C. Straight
D. Is not able to open the mouth.

75. When performing CPR, if there is a pulse but the victim is not breathing, you should give rescue - breathing at a rate of:
A. 2 breaths every 20 seconds
B. 1 breath every 15 seconds
C. 1 breath every 5 seconds
D. 2 breaths every 30 seconds

76. Which suture pattern (or method) listed below is most commonly used in oral surgery?
A. Continuous pattern
B. Interrupted pattern
C. Mattress pattern
D. Sling suture pattern

77. Atelectasis can result from which of the following after a patient has undergone oral surgery?
A. Inactivity after surgery
B. Post operative narcotic analgesics
C. An endotracheal tube which has misplaced during the oral surgery procedure
D. All of the above

78. How long should one wait before obtaining a biopsy of an oral ulcer?
A. 4 days
B. 7 days
C. 14 days
D. 30 days

79. During an inferior alveolar nerve block injection, the needle passes through the mucous membrane and the buccinator muscle and lies lateral to the:
A. Masseter muscle

B. Temporalis muscle
C. Medial pterygoid muscle
D. Lateral pterygoid muscle

80. Nitrous oxide works on the:
A. Peripheral Nervous System (PNS)
B. Central Nervous System (CNS)
C. Autonomic Nervous System (ANS)
D. All of the above

81. Stage I of anaesthesia describes which level of sedation?
A. Unconscious sedation
B. Conscious sedation
C. None of the above

82. Allogenic grafts (also called allografts) are composed of tissue taken from:
A. Another species
B. An individual of the same species who is not genetically related to the recipient
C. An individual of the same species who is genetically related to the recipient
D. The same individual

83. Which of the following is the most common indication for tooth transplantation?
A. Severe decay of a central incisor
B. Severe decay of a first molar
C. Severe decay of a third molar
D. Severe decay of a canine

84. All of the following are systemic contraindication to elective surgery except:
A. Blood dyscrasias (i.e., hemophilia, leukemia)
B. Controlled diabetes mellitus
C. Addison's disease or any steroid deficiency
D. Nephritis
E. Any debilitating disease
F. Cardiac disease

85. Management of an acute asthmatic episode occurring during oral surgery includes all of the following except:

A. Terminate all dental treatment
B. Position the patient in an erect or semierect position
C. Patient should administer their own bronchodilator using an inhaler
D. Administer nitroglycerin
E. Administer oxygen
F. Monitor vital signs

86. A 52-year-old woman requests removal of a painful mandibular second molar. She tells you that she has not rested for two days and nights because of the pain. Her medical history is unremarkable, except that she takes 20 mg of Prednisone daily for erythema multiforme . How do you treat this patient?

A. Have patient discontinue the Prednisone for two days prior to the extraction
B. Give steroid supplementation and remove the tooth with local anaesthesia and sedation
C. Instruct the patient to take 3 grams of amoxicillin one hour prior to extraction
D. No special treatment is necessary prior to extraction

87. Wharton's duct is associated with the:

A. Parotid gland
B. Submandibular gland
C. Sublingual gland
D. von Ebner's glands

88. All of the following are reasons that vasoconstrictors are included in local anesthetics except:

A. They prolong the duration of action of the local anesthetic
B. They reduce the chance of an allergic reaction to the local anesthetic
C. They reduce the toxicity because less local anesthetic is necessary
D. They reduce the rate of vascular absorption by causing vasoconstriction

E. They help to make the anaesthesia more profound by increasing the concentrations of the local anesthetic at the nerve membrane.

89. How many milligrams of epinephrine are in each cartridge (1.8 cc) of 2% lidocaine with 1:100,000 epinephrine?
A. 0.018 mg
B. 18 mg
C. 0.036 mg
D. 36 mg

90. The maxillary first molar is innervated by the:
A. Anterior superior alveolar and middle superior alveolar nerves
B. Middle superior alveolar and posterior superior alveolar nerves
C. Posterior superior alveolar and inferior alveolar nerves
D. Middle superior alveolar and palatine nerves

91. A surgical procedure for recontouring alveolar structures, usually in preparation for a prosthesis is called a (an):
A. Closed reduction
B. Operculectomy
C. Alveoloplasty
D. Gingivoplasty

92. Muscle fibers covered by a mucous membrane that attaches the cheek, lips and / or tongue to the associated dental mucosa is called:
A. Gingiva
B. Frenum
C. Operculum
D. Abutment

93. Cavernous sinus thrombosis can be caused by:
A. An infection of the central face or para-nasal sinuses
B. Bacteremia
C. Trauma
D. Infections of the ear or maxillary teeth
E. All of the above

94. Clinically scopolamine is used to:
A. Prevent nausea and vomiting associated with motion sickness
B. Reduce salivation and excess bronchial secretions prior to surgery
C. Reduce spastic states in parkinsonism
D. Produce sedation and as a preanesthetic medication
E. All of the above

95. In the head and neck, all the lymph ultimately drains into the:
A. Submental lymph nodes
B. Submandibular lymph nodes
C. Deep cervical lymph nodes
D. Retropharyngeal lymph nodes

96. Which local anesthetic listed below may possibly manifest its toxicity clinically by initial depression and drowsiness rather than stimulation and convulsion?
A. Lidocaine
B. Procaine
C. Benzocaine
D. Tetracaine

97. All of the following are contraindications to the use of nitrous oxide except:
A. Hypoxemia
B. Respiratory disease
C. Children
D. Emotional instability
E. Contagious diseases

98. All of the following are causes of metabolic alkalosis except:
A. Use of diuretics (thiazides, furosemide, ethacrynic acid)
B. Vomiting
C. Chronic renal failure
D. Overactive adrenal gland (Cushing's syndrome or use of corticosteroids)

99. Implants that are surgically inserted into the jawbone are called:
A. Endosseous implants

B. Subperiosteal implants
C. Transosscous implants
D. Supra-periosteal implants
E. None of the above

100. The treatment of a mandibular fracture using only intermaxillary fixation (IMF) is called:
A. Open reduction
B. Closed reduction
C. Fixation
D. Approximation

101. A complete blood count (CBC) includes:
A. Hematocrit
B. Hemoglobin
C. White blood cell count
D. Red blood cell count
E. All of the above

102. Zygomatic arch fractures can be nicely demonstrated by which radiograph?
A. Water's view
B. Lateral skull view
C. Posteroanterior skull view
D. Submento vertex view

103. Which artery listed below supplies the tongue?
A. Palatine artery
B. Inferior alveolar artery
C. Lingual artery
D. Vertebral artery

104. Which two of the following are useful for sedation and analgesia only?
A. Halothane
B. Methoxyflurane
C. Cyclopropane
D. Nitrous oxide
E. Ethylene

105. On physical examination, painless induration of soft tissue is suggestive of:

A. Normal tissue
B. Infection
C. Invasive malignant lesions
D. Benign lesions

106. Which division of the trigeminal nerve below passes through the foramen ovale and supplies motor innervation to the tensor veli palatini, tensor tympani, muscles of mastication (temporalis, masseter, lateral and medial pterygoids), and the anterior belly of digastric and mylohyoid muscles?

A. Ophthalmic division (V-1)
B. Maxillary division (V-2)
C. Mandibular division (V-3)
D. None of the above

107. All of the following drugs are anticholinergic except:

A. Atropine
B. Benztropine & Scopolamine
C. Fenfluramine
D. Trihexyphenidy
E. Ipratropium & Probanthine

108. By far and away the most commonly performed mandibular procedure for the correction of mandibular retrognathia is the:

A. Segmental osteotomy
B. Sagittal split osteotomy
C. Vertical ramus ostcotomy
D. Body osteotomy

109. While attempting to remove a grossly decayed mandibular molar, the crown fractures. What is recommended next step in order to facilitate the removal of this tooth?

A. Use a larger forceps and luxate remaining portion of tooth to the lingual
B. Separate the roots
C. Irrigate the area and proceed to remove the rest of the tooth
D. Place a sedative filling and reschedule patient

110. All of the following are elements of general anaesthesia except:
A. Analgesia
B. Relaxation
C. Hyperpyrexia
D. Hyporeflexia
E. Narcosis

111. Arrange the following five phases of healing of an extraction site in their correct order
1 Replacement of the connective tissue by fibrillar bone
2. Hemorrhage and clot formation
3. Replacement of granulation tissue by connective tissue and epithelialization of the site
4. Recontouring of the alveolar bone and maturation
5. Organization of the clot by granulation tissue
A. 4,1,3,5,2
B. 1,2,3,4,5
C. 3,4,2,1,5
D. 4,2,3,1,5

112. While extracting a mandibular third molar, you notice that the distal root tip is missing. Where is it most likely to be found?
A. In the infratemporal fossa
B. In the submandibular space
C. In the mandibular canal
D. In the pterygopalatine fossa

113. Which of the following is the most common error in recording blood pressure?
A. Applying the blood pressure cuff too tightly
B. Applying the blood pressure cuff too loosely
C. Overinflating the blood pressure cuff
D. Under-inflating the blood pressure cuff
E. Use of the wrong size cuff

114. A prothrombin time (PT) of:
A. 5-7 seconds is considered normal
B. 6-9 seconds is considered normal

C. 12-14 seconds is considered normal
D. 20-25 seconds is considered normal

115. All of following are weak points in the mandible where fractures are most common except:
A. The angle
B. The coronoid process
C. The condylar neck
D. The symphysis area

116. Which two diseases below cause more than 60% of all cases of end-stage renal disease in the United States?
A. Diabetes
B. Leukemia
C. High blood pressure (hypertension)
D. Pernicious anemia
E. Tuberculosis

117. All of the following local anesthetics are amides except:
A. Prilocaine
B. Bupivacaine
C. Lidocaine
D. Procaine

118. Which nerve below supplies motor function to the buccinator muscle?
A. Trigeminal nerve (CN V)
B. Facial nerve (CN VII)
C. Vagus nerve (CN X)
D. Glossopharyngeal nerve (CN IX)

119. Which of the following tests should be routinely performed in the preoperative work up for a patient that is being admitted to a hospital for surgery
A. A complete blood count (CBC)
B. A total white blood cell count
C. An assessment of the circulating platelets
D. A urinalysis
E. All of the above

120. Before dental treatment prophylactic antibiotic coverage is indicated for patient with each of the following conditions except:

A. Previous coronary artery bypass graft surgery
B. Rheumatic heart disease
C. Prosthetic aortic valve
D. Kidney damage needing hemodialysis
E. Total joint prosthesis

121. Inadvertent intravascular injection of a local anesthetic with a vasoconstrictor may cause which of the following clinical signs?

A. Nervousness
B. Dizziness
C. Blurred vision
D. Excitation and/or depression of the CNS
E. All of the above

122. Which of the following can result in masticator space infections?

A. Infections of the mandibular molar, especially the third molar
B. Non-aseptic technique in local anaesthesia of the inferior alveolar nerve
C. Trauma to the mandibular (either external or fracture into the socket of a diseased third molar)
D. All of the above

123. Diazepam (Valium) can be used for

A. Candida albicans infections
B. Sedation induction
C. Hypothyroidism diagnosis
D. Myasthenia gravis

124. Which of the following are local contraindications for tooth extractions?

A. ANUG
B. Irradiated jaws
C. Malignant disease
D. All of the above

125. Chronic obstructive pulmonary disease (COPD) is a group of disorders characterized by airflow obstruction during respiration. Which one of those disorders listed below is marked by dyspnea and wheezing expiration caused by episodic narrowing of the airways?

A. Bronchial asthma
B. Chronic bronchitis
C. Emphysema
D. Bronchiectasis

126. Alloplastic materials used for augmentation genioplasty generally have a tendency to do what?

A. Produce an immunologic response
B. Be replaced by the host bone
C. Migrate from the position in which they were placed at the time of surgery
D. Be rejected

127. The most frequent location for a maxillary torus is:

A. The right sides of the hard palate
B. The left side of the hard palate
C. The midline of the hard palate
D. On the soft palate

128. Which teeth listed below are the most frequently impacted?

A. Maxillary canines
B. Maxillary third molars
C. Mandibular third molar
D. Mandibular premolars

129. Of the following drugs, which is most likely to cause seizures as an adverse reaction?

A. Aspirin
B. Morphine
C. Meperidine
D. Acetaminophen

130. The normal serum concentration of glucose is:

A. 20-40 mg/dl
B. 50-70 mg/dl

C. 80-120 mg/dl
D. 130-150 mg/dl

131. Which of the following are indications for biopsy?

A. A lesion that persists for more than two weeks with no apparent etiologic basis
B. Persistent hyperkeratotic changes in surface tissues
C. A lesion that has the characteristics of malignancy
D. An inflammatory lesion that does not respond to local treatment after 14 days (such as removing local irritant)
E. A persistent swelling, either visible or palpable, beneath relatively normal tissue
F. All of the above are indications for biopsy

132. A posterior superior alveolar nerve block (tuberosity injection) will provide anaesthesias for:

A. The second and third molar along with the mucoperiosteum of he palate
B. The first, second molars along with the mucoperiosteum of the palate
C. The first, second, and third molar but not the mucoperiosteum of the palate
D. The first, and third molars along with the mucoperiosteum of the palate

133. The unpleasant sensation of difficulty in breathing is called:

A. Hypercapnea
B. Dyspnoea
C. Hypocapnea
D. Apnea

134. Phlebitis of a vein after administration of IV valium is usually attributed to the presence of which of the following in the mixture?

A. Hydroquinone
B. Water
C. Alcohol
D. Propylene glycol

135. In preparing the edentulous mandible for dentures, each of the following may be safely excised except:
A. A labial frenum
B. A lingual frenum
C. The mylohyoid ridge
D. The genial tubercles
E. An exostosis

136. During extraction of a maxillary third molar, you realize the tuberosity has also been extracted. What is the proper treatment in this case?
A. Remove the tuberosity from the tooth and reimplant the tuberosity
B. Smooth the sharp edges of the remaining bone and replace and suture the remaining soft tissue
C. No special treatment is necessary
D. None of the above

137. Diabetes Mellitus Type 2 is associated with all of the following characteristic except:
A. Normal or increased insulin synthesis
B. Onset in adulthood
C. Autoimmune origin
D. Associated with obesity
E. Rare ketoacidosis

138. Which muscle below is responsible for the forward displacement of the condylar head when the neck of the condyle is fractured?
A. Masseter muscle
B. Mylohyoid muscle
C. Lateral pterygoid muscle
D. Medial pterygoid muscle

139. Which paranasal sinuses are the largest?
A. Frontal
B. Ethmoidal
C. Maxillary
D. Sphenoidal

140. How much hydrocortisone is secreted by the adrenal cortex daily?

A. About 1 mg
B. About 100 mg
C. About 20 mg
D. About 200 mg

141. Osteomyelitis is an infection of the bone and marrow. It is most often caused by:

A. Streptococcus pyogenes
B. Staphylococcus aureus
C. Mycobacterium tuberculosis
D. Neisseria meningitidis

142. Which of the following are important points to remember in the management of a diabetic patient?

A. Defer surgery until diabetes is well-controlled; consult physician
B. Schedule an early morning appointment and avoid lengthy appointments
C. Watch for signs of hypoglycemia
D. Treat infections aggressively
E. All of the above

143. The TMJ is the articulation between the condyle of the mandible and the squamous portion of the:

A. Sphenoid bone
B. Temporal bone
C. Ethmoid bone
D. Zygomatic bone

144. Which of the following arteries does not accompany the corresponding nerve throughout its course

A. Infraorbital artery
B. Inferior alveolar artery
C. Lingual artery
D. Posterior superior alveolar artery

145. The pterygopalatine fossa communicates laterally with the infratemporal fossa by way of:

A. The sphenopalatine foramen

B. The pterygoid canal
C. The foramen rotundum
D. The petrotympanic fissure
E. The pterygomaxillary fissure

146. The nerve to the mylohyoid muscle is a branch of the:
A. Ophthalmic nerve (CN V-1)
B. Maxillary nerve (CN V-2)
C. Mandibular nerve (CNV-3)
D. Facial nerve (CN VIII)

147. Which type of shock listed below is most often associated with severe trauma and reactive peripheral vasodilation?
A. Hypovolemic shock
B. Cardiogenic shock
C. Septic shock
D. Neurogenic shock
E. Anaphylactic shock

148. Which nerve listed below innervates the facial muscles with motor fibers, the lacrimal gland and salivary gland with parasympathetic fibers, and the anterior tongue with sensory fibers?
A. Trigeminal
B. Vagus
C. Facial
D. Glossopharyngeal

149. Which type of maxillary third molar impaction is most likely to be displaced into the antrum (maxillary sinus) and infratemporal space if correct extraction technique are not employed?
A. Vertical impaction
B. Distoangular impaction
C. Mesioangular impaction
D. Horizontal impaction

150. All of the following are advantages of using nitrous oxide analgesia except:
A. Rapid onset and recovery
B. Pleasant induction

C. It is a complete pain reliever
D. Nonirritating to the GI tract

151. Which of the following are likely signs and symptoms of a zygomatic fracture?
A. Nasal bleeding
B. Pain over zygomatic region
C. Numbness in the infratemporal nerve distribution
D. Exophthalmos
E. Diplopia
F. All of the above

152. When removing maxillary teeth, the upper jaw of the patient should be where in relation to the dentists's shoulder?
A. Below
B. Above
C. At the same height
D. It makes no difference where the patients's upper jaw is in relation to the dentist's shoulder

153. Local anesthetics are most effective in tissues that have what pH?
A. Below 7
B. Above 7
C. Below 4
D. Makes no difference what the pH of the tissue is.

154. What is usually the first clinical sign of mild lidocaine toxicity?
A. Itching
B. Nervousness
C. Vomiting
D. Sleepiness

155. Which type of bone healing involves both endosteal and periosteal proliferation?
A. Primary (bone- to bone)
B. Secondary (space fills in with callus)
C. Gap healing
D. None of the above

156. If a small communication is made with the maxillary sinus during extraction of a maxillary second molar, what treatment is recommended?

A. The sinus communication should be closed with a flap procedure

B. No additional surgical treatment is necessary

C. A figure- of - eight suture should be placed over the tooth socket

D. None of the above

157. Branches of which artery listed below supply the maxillary and mandibular teeth?

A. Vertebral

B. Occipital

C. Maxillary

D. Subclavian

158. Which of the following is a mandibular disorder caused by a chronic excess of glucocorticoids?

A. Cushing syndrome

B. Addison's disease

C. Cretinism

D. Grave's disease

159. How do local anesthetics affect the nerve membrane?

A. They increase potassium influx

B. They increase the membrane excitability by increasing the membrane's permeability to sodium ions

C. They decrease the membrane's permeability to sodium ions and reduce the membrane excitability

D. They increase the calcium and chloride flux

160. Which salivary gland listed below is the smallest and contains both serous and mucous acini?

A. Submandibular gland

B. Parotid gland

C. Subingual gland

D. Minor salivary glands

161. Which of the arteries listed below supply blood to the TMJ?

A. Facial artery
B. Lingual artery
C. Superficial temporal artery
D. Vertebral artery

162. The most common site of a pericoronal infection (pericoronitis) is

A. Around the site of a recent extraction
B. Around a newly erupted primary tooth
C. Around periodontally involved mandibular incisors
D. Around mandibular third molars

163. Which of the following is the most common cause of bleeding disorders?

A. Polycythemia vera
B. Thrombocytopenia
C. Myelofibrosis
D. Chronic myelocytic leukemia

164. Which of the following statement concerning the hypoglossal nerve are true?

A. It is a motor nerve supplying all of the intrinsic and extrinsic muscles of the tongue, except the palatoglossus, which is supplied by the vagus nerve.
B. It leaves the skull through the hypoglossal canal medial to the carotid canal and jugular foramen
C. It passes above the hyoid bone on the lateral surface of the hyoglossus muscle deep to mylohyoid muscle
D. It loops around the occipital artery and passes between the external carotid artery and internal jugular vein.
E. In the upper part of its course, it is joined by C1 fibers from the cervical plexus
F. All of the above statements are true concerning the hypoglossal nerve

165. Which nerve listed below is the largest of the 12 cranial nerves and is the principal general sensory nerve to the head, particularly the face?

A. Vagus (CN X)

B. Glossopharyngeal (CN IX)
C. Facial (CN VII)
D. Trigeminal (CN V)

166. Which of the following is the main reason to use water irrigation when cutting bone
A. It helps to wash away debris
B. Because heat generated by the drill affects bone vitality
C. To decrease the smell of freshly cut bone
D. It helps to flush out the high speed suction

167. The most severe tissue reaction is seen with which type of suture material?
A. Plain catgut
B. Chromic catgut
C. Polyglycolic acid
D. Polyglactin 910

168. Postoperative hypotension may be due to the effect of
A. Transfusion reaction
B. The anesthetic or analgesics on the myocardium
C. Liver failure
D. Anaphylaxis
E. All of the above

169. In patients having a Le Fort II fracture, a common finding is parasthesia over the distribution of the :
A. Infraorbital nerve
B. Inferior alveolar nerve
C. Mylohyoid nerve
D. Hypoglossal nerve

170. A person who has been on suppressive doses of steroid will
A. Never regain full adrenal cortical function
B. Take as much as a year to regain full adrenal cortical function
C. Take as little as a week to regain full adrenal cortical function
D. Take usually a couple of days to regain full adrenal cortical function

171. The initial event in a vasovagal syncope episode is the stress-induced release of increased amounts of catecholamines that cause all of the following except:
A. A decrease in peripheral vascular resistance
B. Tachycardia
C. Sweating
D. Bradycardia

Answer Key to MCQs in Oral Surgery and Anaesthesia

1	B, C	2	C	3	D	4	E
5	B	6	B	7	D	8	B
9	C	10	D	11	B	12	E
13	B	14	D	15	B	16	C
17	B	18	E	19	E	20	A
21	C	22	E	23	A	24	B
25	D	26	B	27	C	28	C
29	C	30	B	31	C	32	B
33	A	34	C	35	E	36	B
37	B	38	B	39	C	40	B
41	C	42	B	43	C	44	C
45	B	46	C	47	B	48	B
49	A	50	A	51	C	52	E
53	B	54	B	55	C	56	E
57	C	58	C	59	C	60	B
61	D	62	B	63	B	64	A
65	B	66	D	67	B	68	B
69	C	70	B	71	C	72	D
73	C	74	B	75	C	76	B
77	D	78	C	79	C	80	B
81	B	82	B	83	B	84	B
85	D	86	B	87	B	88	B
89	A	90	B	91	C	92	B
93	E	94	E	95	C	96	A
97	C	98	C	99	A	100	B
101	E	102	D	103	C	104	D, E
105	C	106	C	107	C	108	B

109 B	110 C	111 A	112 B
113 B	114 C	115 B	116 A, C
117 D	118 B	119 E	120 A
121 E	122 D	123 B	124 D
125 A	126 C	127 C	128 C
129 C	130 C	131 F	132 C
133 B	134 D	135 D	136 B
137 C	138 C	139 C	140 C
141 B	142 E	143 B	144 C
145 E	146 C	147 D	148 C
149 B	150 C	151 F	152 C
153 B	154 B	155 A	156 B
157 C	158 A	159 C	160 C
161 C	162 D	163 B	164 F
165 D	166 B	167 A	168 E
169 A	170 B	171 D	

7

Orthodontics

GROWTH

⇒ **Cephalocaudal gradient** of growth = mandible grows more and up to later age than maxilla.

⇒ Helps **decrease the overjet** which is especially marked during first 6 months of life.

⇒ General direction of growth of face with respect to skull and cranial base = D and F

Growth in maxillary length by = apposition at maxillary tuberosity

⇒ Different tissues grow at different rates at different times, i.e. **differential growth pattern, Scammon's growth curves.**

⇒ Nearly all tissues of face and neck originate from ECTODERM (including muscles and bone also, which elsewhere in the body originate from the MESODERM).

⇒ Most of these tissues develop from neural crest cells (NCC).

⇒ Most of the problems which results in craniofacial anomalies arise in 3rd stage of development, i.e. 19–28 days (4th week).

Most of facial structures arise from NCC-interference with their movement leads to deformities, e.g. hemifacial microsomia, mandibulofacial dysostosis, i.e. Treacher Collins synd–both U/L jaws involved, esp. lateral face is involved due to excessive cell death in trigeminal ganglion which affects NCCs.

⇒ Most common congenital defect of face = CLP

⇒ Most common congenital defect = Club foot

⇒ Formation of organ system **(primary palate)** in 28–38 days

⇒ **Secondary palate** in 42–55 days.

⇒ **Clefts arise during 4th developmental stage.**

⇒ Maturation of oral functions follows **a gradient from anterior to posterior, e.g.**

Speech	1st sounds = bilabial	m, p, b
(A→P)	Tongue tip consonants	t, d
	Sibilants	s, z
	Posterior tongue positioning	r

PALATE: Fusion progresses from A to P and reaches soft palate

MANDIBLE: **Mandible recognisable in** shape at 8th week.

CRANIUM

⇒ Cranial base (neurocranium) = growth esp. at synchondroses

⇒ Cranial vault (desmocranium) – sutural growth

⇒ Cartilage grows both by INTERSTITIAL and APPOSITIONAL GROWTH

⇒ Epiphyseal C (if transplanted) can grow independently – so it is a primary cartilage with genetic potential. But **condylar cartilage is secondary cartilage** and cannot grow after transplantation.

⇒ Bone grows by additive or apposition only (it cannot grow by interstitial or expansile activity).

⇒ **In newborn = cranium is 8–9 × larger than face (cephalo-caudal gradient of growth).**

⇒ Original pattern of skeleton is constant and **stationary biologic center lies in the body of sphenoid bone.**

UP to 5th year = Neurocranial dominance

After 5 year = Orofacial dominance of growth.

⇒ **Epigenetic factors**: are genetically determined but influence in an indirect way by intermediary action on associated structures (eye, brain, etc.).

⇒ **Nasal septum** = more important in anteroposterior growth than vertical growth of maxilla.

CRANIAL BASE: Endochondral esp. of midline structures.

⇒ By synchondroses = i.e. cartilaginous growth.
⇒ Sphenoethmoidal = close at 5–25 year (exactly unknown)
⇒ Intersphenoidal = Birth
⇒ Sphenooccipital = 20th year = main synchondroses and **most important**
⇒ Interoccipital = 3–5 years

⇒ Metcpic suture = between frontal bones.

BASIC CONCEPTS

- **Development** = growth + differentiation + translocation
- **Growth** = is an increase in size.
- **Development** = is progress towards maturity.
- **Differentiation** = is a change from generalised cell to a specialised kind, i.e. a change in quality.
- **Translocation** = i.e. passive growth. It is a change in the position of whole bone. It depends on capsular matrix and is ka displacement of the bone.
- **Primary growth** = Actual **translation** (passive growth) and remodelling of bones.
- **Transformation** = is active growth. It is the apposition and resorption in a bone. It is a local change and occurs under the influence of periosteal matrix, and is aka the apposition and resorption in a bone.
- **Secondary growth** = **transformation** (periosteal) + sutural growth.
- **Maturation** = it expresses the qualitative changes which occur with age.

Mechanisms of bone growth

- Bone deposition and resorption = aka **bone remodelling.**
- **Cortical drift** = combination of bone deposition ad resorption resulting in a growth movement towards the depository surface.

- **Displacement** = is the movement of whole bone as a unit. It is due to pull or push of different soft and bone tissues as they all continue to enlarge.
- **Primary or active displacement** = i.e. if bone gets displaced due to its own growth, e.g. growth at maxillary tuberosity pushes maxilla anteriorly.
- **Secondary or passive displacement** = i.e. if the bone gets displaced due to growth and enlargement of an adjacent bone.
- Sutural growth.
- **Enlow's expanding V – principle** = many bones/parts of the bone have V-shape pattern of the growth, which occurs towards wider ends of the V due to selective apposition and resorption.
- **Enlow's counterpart principle** = states that the growth of any given facial or cranial part relates specifically to other structural and geometric counterparts in face and cranium.
- **Neurotrophism** = is a non-impulse transmitting neural function which involves axoplasmic transport and provides for long term interaction b/w neurons and innervated tissues, which homeostatically regulates the morphological, compositional and functional integrity of these tissues.

⇒ Midsagittal suture does not close until the middle of 3rd decade of life.

⇒ **CRANIAL BASE GROWTH:**	**Size of face: Size of body**
⇒ At Birth = 55–60% of adult size	50%
⇒ 4–7 years = 94% of adult size	33%
⇒ 8–13 years = 98% of adult size	12%

⇒ Neurocranium = follows neural growth pattern

⇒ Splanchnocranium (lower face) = follows general / bodily growth pattern

⇒ Desmocranium = has neurocranial capsule and orofacial capsule

⇒ According to Scammon's growth =Lymphoid > Neural > General > Genital growth

Pure intramembranous	Frontal, zygomatic, parietal, palatal, maxilla, vomer, nasal, lacrimal
Pure endochondral	Ethmoid, inferior nasal concha
Mixed	Mandible, occipital, sphenoid, temporal

Direction of growth

⇒ Basal cranium = U/F

⇒ Maxilla = D/F

⇒ Mandible condyle = U/B

GROWTH OF MAXILLA

Maxilla is mainly **INTRAMEMBRANOUS** except

- Paranasal processes of nasal capsule
- Alveolar border of zygomatic process

2 areas: (1) Neural and alveolar areas

⇒ (2) Frontal, zygomatic, palatal processes.

⇒ A passive/**secondary displacement** of nasomaxillary complex is D and F due to cranial base growth.

⇒ **Primary displacement** of nasomaxillary complex occurs by growth of maxillary tuberosity in posterior direction.

3 primary ossification centers = one above canine fossa for maxilla proper and two for premaxilla.

⇒ **Sutures** = all are oblique and parallel to each other - growth moves maxilla D/F or cranium U/B – But sutural growth is secondary.

⇒ **Basic maxillary skeletal unit** = INFRAORBITAL NEUROVASCULAR TRIAD

⇒ Maxillary width is completed quite at early age (i.e. follows neural growth curve – as it is attached to cranial base.

⇒ Elongation of dental arches occurs at free (distal) ends only.

⇒ Actual changes which occur in maxilla are controlled by EPIGENETIC FACTORS.

Growth completion in dimensions with age = WDH (width earliest completed).

⇒ In late stages = vertical growth dominates the horizontal growth in maxilla.

⇒ Mainly sutural and remodelling – Translation and transformation;

⇒ Midpalatal suture: does not start closing till 8–10 yrs of age.

⇒ Nasal septum shows endochondral growth.

MANDIBLE

⇒ It starts developing prenatally and is recognisable in shape by 8th week IU.

⇒ **Meckel's cartilage** acts only as a template for **intramembranous** growth of mandible and does not contribute to mandible bone, develops lateral to Meckel's cartilage.

It ossifies by **2 ossification centres,** one each in the area of future mental foramen, (appear in 6 week IU) lateral to Meckel's cartilage, **ossification stops at a point which later becomes Lingula.**

⇒ **Remanants of Meckel's cartilage** are malleus, incus, spine of sphenoid, sphenomandibular, ligament, etc.

⇒ Lower jaw is the first to develop in the facial skeleton.

Its growth **follows General Tissue growth curve**, while that of vault follows neural growth curve

⇒ At birth = Size of mandible arch is sufficient to accommodate all primary teeth if erupted.

⇒ 2 halves of mandible fuse by 16–18 months age.

⇒ Main growth of mandible after birth occurs at condyle, Ramus, Alveolar bone

CONDYLE

⇒ **Condyle** is the major growth Centre of mandible, it has **fibrocartilage** which is a secondary cartilage, grows by proliferation of cartilage. **Condyle is the only bone in body** which shows **both interstitial and appositional growth .**

Condyle grows in U and B direction – so mandible moves in D and F direction, along the arch which runs from foramen ovale to mandibular foramen to mental foramen (**unloaded nerve concept**).

⇒ **Basal tubular part** = protects mandibular nerve (**unloaded nerve concept)** and follows a logarithmic spiral in its D/F growth.

⇒ Most constant portion of mandible is the =ARC from **F. ovale to mandibular f. to mental f.**

⇒ D/F movement of mandible is primarily passive translation.

⇒ **Active transformation** = minor D/F changes but mainly U/B compensatory growth of ramus.

⇒ Condyles are not primary site of mandibular growth, but are loci with secondary, compensatory growth potential.

CHIN

⇒ Only human and elephant have got chin.

Area of chin just above symphysis menti is resorptive, which gives the chin its prominence.

⇒ Mandibular growth is more sustained in boys than in girls (i.e. up to 25 years age).

RAMAL GROWTH

⇒ In infancy = the ramus is located at approx. primary first molar area.

Growth occurs along the **V-principle**. Anterior border is resorptive to provide space for eruption of permanent molars. After 6 years age, greatest increase in size of mandible occurs distal to first molars. Posterior surface is depository.

Ramal growth **provides space vertically** in which both U/L alveolar bones grow, the teeth being their functional matrices.

LATE MANDIBULAR GROWTH occurs in horizontal direction and is mainly responsible for lower anterior crowding, rather than mandibular third molars, which appears, develops or increases in the adult age/ postpubertal age (20–30 years age).

⇒ (L) incisors tend to upright under the terminal horizontal growth increments, which occurs due to U and F rotation of mandible, leading to lingual movement of lower incisors.

⇒ **ALVEOLAR GROWTH**

Distance between mental foramina = changes little after 6 years age (i.e. width of mandible).

Mental foramen level changes with growth, from near mandibular border (infants) to middle of the body (in adults) to at alveolar crest (in edentulous patient).

Level of mandibular foramen lies below OP in children and at the level of OP in adults.

CRANIUM: DW (H) (i.e. growth in D is most rapid, with growth in W and H in that order).

FACE: HD (W)

H shows greatest incremental changes with age.

W shows least incremental change with age.

⇒ So **at birth, height of cranium and width of face are closest to adult size.**

⇒ Growth is generally completed first in head, then in W of face and last in L (D) of face.

⇒ female pubertal spurt occurs 2–3 yrs ahead of that of male.

THEORIES OF GROWTH

The most important is **functional matrix theory by Moss.**

FCC

Functional matrix

- Periosteal matrix
- Capsular matrix
  1. neurocranial capsule
  2. orofacial capsule

Skeletal unit

1. Macroskeletal unit
2. Microskeletal unit

⇒ Major difference in the theories is the Location at which genetic control is expressed.

⇒ Indirect genetic control is known as Epigenetic.

⇒ **SITE** = is a location where growth occurs

⇒ **CENTER** = is a location **at which independent, genetically controlled growth occurs,** i.e. independent of environment.

⇒ 2 capsular matrices —neurocranial and orofacial

GROWTH SPURTS

	Female	**Male**
1st peak (Childhood)	3 years	3 years
2nd peak (Juvenile)	6–7 years	7–9 years
3rd peak (Prepubertal)	11–12 years	14–15 years

⇒ More boys to have 2–3 peaks

⇒ Girls show only 2 peaks

⇒ Very few girls show MDP growth spurt, but all show pubertal growth spurt.

⇒ So MDP jaw changes (with FJO) is more successful in boys.

⇒ Female mature earlier (2–3 years) than males, so early treatment is more critical in girls than in boys.

⇒ During pubertal growth period = there is directional change from vertical to horizontal.

CLINICAL IMPLICATIONS

1. Intercanine width-increases upto:

Sex	Maxilla	Mandibular
M	18 years	9–10 years
F	12 years	9–10 years

2. Maxillary intercanine width is a **Safety Valve** – when the final horizontal growth of mandible esp in males, causes a forward movement of mandibular base with teeth.

⇒ In both M, F = Maxillary intercanine dimension serves as a safety valve for pubertal growth spurt, where basal horizontal mandibular growth partly unmatched by maxilla, as mandible grows D and F.

⇒ Onset of menstruation = growth spurt is all but complete.

3. Growth modulation therapy is better and results are stable, if given during the spurts period.

GROWTH COMPLETION SEQUENCE

1. W = Both jaws + arches = before adolescent growth spurt, esp. on canine regions, but in M2/M3 region, width increases due to jaws growth in length posteriorly.
2. D (length) = continues through period of puberty

   F = 14–15 years (2–3 years after menstruation)

   M = approx. 18 years (4 years after sexual maturity)
3. H in F = 17–18 years and in M = early 20's

DEVELOPMENT OF DENTITION

A. Gum pads

Dental arches till no teeth erupted are ka gum pads.

Touch in future primary first molar region only.

Anterior open bite is present which helps in tongue positioning during suckling.

Anterior overjet due to smaller lower jaw.

Posterior overjet due to wider upper arch than lower.

Intercuspation of occlusal height in primary dentition establishes for the first time = at eruption of primary first molars only.

Deep bite in primary dentition is due to more upright incisors.

B. Baume's classification of occlusion

Flush terminal plane 76% (to be observed most critically)

Mesial step 14%

Distal step 10%

- Distal step = a. to Class II, if minimum growth differential is there.
  b. change in end – on, by loss of leeway space and forward mandibular growth.
- FTP = a. end – on if minimum growth differential is there.
  b. in Class I due to loss of leeway space of mandibular E.
  c. in Class II if maxillary E is lost before mandibular E.
- Mesial step = a. to Class I if minimum growth differential is there.
  b. to Class III, due to loss of leeway space and forward mandibular growth.

Spacing in deciduous dentition – if present, it is known as **open dentition.** If absent, it is known as **closed dentition.**

Class	In deciduous teeth	Crowding chances in permanent teeth
I	Crowded	10 in 10
II	No spaces	7 in 10
III	≤ 3 mm spacing	5 in 10
IV	3 – 6 mm spacing	2 in 10
V	> 6 mm spacing	None

Primary spacing/ physiological /developmental spacing—occurs due to growth, helps in proper alignment of bigger size permanent teeth, 70% in maxilla and 63% in mandible.

Primate/simian/anthropoid spaces are found mesial to primary maxillary canines and distal to primary mandibular canines, named as it is found in primates, i.e. between BC/CD.

C. MIXED DENTITION PERIOD

Begins with the eruption of first permanent molars at 6 yeas of age, generally in end–on relationship, marks the Stage I of natural bite opening.

First transitional period/ early MDP—eruption of 6, 1, 2, mostly lower erupt first, 6–8 years age.

Correction of FTP/end on relation to class I occurs by utilisation of physiologic space, leeway space and differential forward growth of the mandible.

Early mesial shift occurs in **open dentition at 6–7 years**, due to closure of primate spaces by pressure of erupting molars.

Late mesial shift occurs **in closed dentition at 10–11 years**, due to closure of leeway spaces after shedding of primary second molars.

Incisal liability—difference between sizes of primary and permanent incisors, 7 mm in upper and 5 mm in lower arch, overcome by – utilisation of interdental spacing, incisor inclination labially, increased intercanine width **(Warren Mayne's 4 principles).**

Method	Maxilla	Mandible
I/D spacing	0 –10 mm, av. = 4 mm	0 – 6 mm, av. = 3 mm
Increase in intercanine width	4.5 mm	3 mm
Incisor position	2.2 mm	1.3 mm

⇒ **Incisor liability**: Diff. in size of permanent and primary teeth, space comes from 3 sources:

1. <u>Increase intercanine width</u> = 2 mm, M > F, U > L

   Girls have greater liability to incisor crowding
2. <u>Labial positioning</u> of permanent incisors = 1–2 mm
3. <u>Repositioning</u> of mandibular canines distally in primate spaces when mandibular. LIs erupt = 1 mm space. (But not in U arch, as primate space is between B and C.)

⇒ In primary dentition – An equivalent of Class III is never seen, due to growth pattern of mandible which lags behind the maxilla.

⇒ **Also C2 D2 is not seen in primary dentition.**

⇒ If a child has FTP in MDP, then approx. 3.5 mm of movement of mandibular first molar forward with respect to maxillary first molar is required for smooth, transition to class I relation in permanent DP (i.e. a one half cusp transition in molar relation).

Inter-transitional period is a quite period, 8–10 years of age, no change in dentition occurs.

Late mixed dentition/second transitional period — eruption of 3, 4, 5 : leeway space of Nance is the difference between MD sizes of CDE and 345; 1.8 mm in maxilla and 3.4 mm in mandible; mostly due to primary mandibular second molar ka E–space (2–3 mm), helps in late mesial shift to achieve class I molars.

Space age = is MDP.

Pronounced attrition in MDP is observed to help in–decrease in deep bite, prevent interlocking and thus paving way to unhindered forward growth of mandible.

Deep bite decreases by eruption of permanent molars, attrition of incisors and forward movement of mandible due to growth.

Intercanine width increases more in spaced dentition, more in maxilla, up to a later age in maxilla.

Secondary spacing occurs in closed dentition, with eruption of lower incisors which pushes primary mandibular canine laterally. It creates space for proper eruption of maxillary lateral incisors. It helps to increase the intercanine width in both arches and increase in arch circumference in maxilla.

Ugly duckling stage of Broadbent: in maxilla, 8–9 years age, canines pressing roots of laterals, root crowding, crowns move distally, spaces develop, should not be disturbed till eruption of canines, is a self correcting anomaly.

Arch length decreases by 2–3 mm when MDP changes to PDP, both from anterior and posterior sides. Also posterior teeth move mesially throughout life due to attrition and anterior component of force.

Largest arch length = is before eruption of first permanent molar.

Signs of incipient malocclusion are lack of interdental spacing in primary dentition, crowding in permanent incisors in MDP and premature loss of primary canines esp. mandibular.

Transition in chewing pattern develops in conjunction with eruption of permanent canines at age 12 years.

Self-correcting anomalies

GUM PADS STAGE	PRIMARY D P	MIXED D P
Open bite	Deep bite	End-on molars
Increased overjet	FTP	Ugly-duckling stage
Tongue in between gum pads	Primary spacing	< 2 mm of lower incisors crowding
Primate spacing Small mandible More upright incisors		

⇒ Owen says = Space loss (due to caries) is most likely in mandibular deciduous second molar area.

⇒ **Chewing pattern of child Vs adult** – adult opens straight and then lateral/child moves laterally.

<u>**Natural bite opening**</u> –at 6, 12, 18 years of age, with eruption of permanent molars.

⇒ 3 periods of bite opening (Schwarz)

⇒ 6 years =when Ist molar erupts; 12 years = 2nd molar erupts; 18 years – 3rd molar erupts.

⇒ U/L permanent incisors erupt lingual to primary teeth and move forward under the tongue pressure as they erupt.

⇒ 7–8 years age = critical period

⇒ sudden change during the eruption of the CI and LI is shown by = **1.5 mm. Crowding** in both M and F. Average female recovers slightly better than males.

⇒ No great relief of crowding in incisor region is expected after full eruption of LI.

⇒ Maxillary CI seem to erupt from LABIAL
⇒ Mandibular CI, LI seem to erupt from LINGUAL
⇒ Maxillary LI = no labial gingival bulge.
⇒ maxillary second molar erupts D and F
⇒ maxillary third molar erupts D and B and outward

⇒ Axial inclination of maxillary teeth tend to converge apicaly esp. at the end of the arch and mandibular axes tend to diverge following the CO Spee.

MISCELLANEOUS POINTS

⇒ Most crowding = (L) anterior segments

⇒ Occlusal contact is only 2–6% in 24 hrs period.

⇒ Primary incisors are more vertical and interincisal angle is more greater causing deep bite.

⇒ Normal overbite = 33% of crowns of lower incisors.

⇒ **Key ridge** = corresponds to MB root of maxillary first molar and is lowermost point on contour of anterior wall of infratemporal fossa.

⇒ **Ortho treatment is C/I in = MARFAN'S syndrome**

⇒ Catalans appliance should not be worn for > 6 weeks.

⇒ Palatal cribs should be worn for at least 6 mos.

⇒ OTM in pulpless teeth compared to vital teeth is = same

⇒ Basic difference in facial growth during puberty is greater vertical development in males.

⇒ Distance between x-ray source and mid sagittal plane of patient = 5 feet while taking a lateral cephalogram.

⇒ Lateral nasal process = does not contribute to (U) lip.

⇒ Philtrum = line of fusion of MNP and maxillary process.

⇒ At 8th week: Nasolacrimal groove = between LNP and maxillary, process = forms nasolacrimal duct.

⇒ Primary palate forms :

– Premaxilla, alveolar process underlying it and part of inside of (U) lip

⇒ Mandible takes shape during 8th week.

⇒ Bones in skull at birth = 45

Bones in skull of adults = 22, i.e. 14 face and 8 cranium.

First primary teeth to erupt are mandibular central incisors = at 6–8 months of age.

Sequence of primary teeth eruption = ABDCE

By 3 years of age, roots of all deciduous, teeth completed, crown of permanent first molars completed.

Sequence of permanent teeth eruption = 61245378 in maxilla, 61234578 in mandible.

At 5-6 years of age, just before the shedding of primary incisors, there are **maximum number** (52) of teeth in jaws than at any other time.

STOMATOGNATHOLOGY

⇒ Trabecular alignment is due primarily to functional forces (according to Wolff) = known as **Law of Orthogonality.**

⇒ **Law of Transformation** of bone, i.e. stresses of tension or pressure on bone stimulates bone formation.

⇒ **Buccinator mechanism** involves Orbicularis oris m., Buccinator m, Superior constrictor m of pharynx attached at pterygomandibular raphe.

⇒ **Chondrocranium** is a continuous plate of cartilage, extends from nasal capsule to foramen magnum.

⇒ Major center of growth of long bones = epiphyseal plate cartilage which has uncalcified cartilage.

⇒ Most anterior part of chondrocranium = Nasal capsule.

PRE-EMERGENT ERUPTION

⇒ Eruptive movements begin soon after the root begins to form – because metabolic activity in PDL is a major part of eruption.

POST-EMERGENT ERUPTION: till the teeth come in occlusion; and also to keep pace with occlusal attrition.

⇒ Eruption occurs mainly at night.

JUVENILE OCCLUSAL EQUILIBRIUM

⇒ Teeth which are in function erupt at a rate which parallels the rate of VERTICAL GROWTH of mandibulr.r ramus.

ETIOLOGY

SYNDROMES

Class II	**Class III**
• Pierre Robin Synd	• Klienfelter syndrome
	• CLP, osteogenesis imperfecta
• Mouth breathing	• Cleidocranial dysostosis
• Ankylosis of condyles	• Achondroplasia
• Millwaukee brace	• Down's syndrome
• Mandibulofacial dysostosis (Treacher Collin syndrome)	• Bilateral condylar hyperplasia
• Still's disease	• Marfan Synd
• Goldenhar synd	• Hyperpituitarism
	• Craniofacial dystosis (Crouzon's dis)
• Mobius syndrome	• Gorlin syndrome

1. Class III, Class II = hereditary; skeletal growth pattern

⇒ In majority of C2 D1= maxillary second molar tends to erupt earlier than mandibular second molar (which may be due to space problem in the mandibular arch).

⇒ Eruption of maxillary canine before maxillary first premolar leads to labial displacement of maxillary canine (and hence crowding) due to lack of space.

⇒ maxillary 2 are displaced generally LINGUALLY.
⇒ maxillary 3 are displaced generally LABIALLY
⇒ maxillary 5 are displaced generally PALATALLY.

2. Most common local cause = premature fall of primary-teeth due to high caries
3. Deep bite– Hereditary
4. As growth pattern predetermines the occurrence of class II m.o. = so it cannot be prevented as such.
5. Growth cannot be prevented but only can be redirected.
6. Major etiology of Cl II m.o.= growth discrepancy
7. **Adenoid facies** = Dolichofacial, vertical growth

⇒ Thumb sucking habit = considered normal up to 3–4 years age.

⇒ Infantile swallow seen normally up to = 1½ – 2 years

⇒ **Pseudo class III** = deviated forward path (anteriorly) of closure due to occlusal prematurities; Skeletal class I, but may change to true class III if not treated in time.

⇒ **True class III** – is Skeletal class III

⇒ C2, D2= Backward path of closure
= Horizontal growth pattern
= Increased freeway space
= Closed / deep bite

⇒ **Sunday bite** = Bite achieved by patient by bringing his mandible forward in C2, D1

⇒ C2, D1= hypotonic (U) lip, hyperactive mentalis

DIAGNOSIS

Soft tissue examinations

1. VERTICALLY, face can be divided in 3 parts in 1: 1 ratio as
   a. upper third = from hair line to root of the nose/glabella
   b. middle third = from root of the nose/glabella to subnasale
   c. lower third = from subnasale to lowermost point on chin.
2. Transversely, face can be divided in 5 equal parts.
3. Width of the nose is equal to medial intercanthal distance.
4. Width of the mouth = distance b/w medial limbus of one eye to other.

5. Subnasale to vermillion border of lower lip = vermillion border of lower lip to lowermost point on chin.
6. Ratio of the distance of "Subnasale to the junction of upper and lower lips" to the distance from the junction of upper and lower lips to lowermost point on chin = 1:2

♦ **Angle's classification**

Angle's Class I = 60%
II = 25%
III = 5%

♦ **Simon's Law of Canines**: Orbital plane (i.e. perpendicular to FHP under the pupil) passes through distal third of upper canines. In class I canine relation, mesial incisal ridge of maxillary canine overlaps the distal incisal ridge of mandibular canine. Also, the tip of upper canine falls in the embrasure between lower canine and first premolar.

♦ **Dewey's modification**

TYPE I	CROWDING
TYPE II	SPACING
TYPE III	ANTERIOR CROSS BITE
TYPE IV	POSTERIOR CROSS BITE
TYPE V	DISTURBED MOLAR RELATION DUE TO EARLY LOSS OF PRIMARY SECOND MOLARS.

Ackermann–Proffit classification

1. Alignment
2. Profile
3. Type, transverse dimension
4. Class, sagittal dimension
5. Bite, vertical dimension

♦ <u>**Cephalic Index**</u> : Breadth × 100/ Width

1. Dolichocephalic: 75 or less
2. Mesocephalic: 75–80
3. Brachycephalic: 80 or more

CAST ANALYSIS

1. Ashley Howe's analysis

If PMBAW

≤ 37%	Extraction
37–44%	Border Line
> 44%	Non-Extraction

2. Bolton's Analysis

⇒ Anterior Ratio = 77.2%

⇒ Overall Ratio = 91.3%

3. Peck and Peck Ratio

(L)	CI	=	88–92%
(L)	LI	=	90–95%

4. Proffit's space analysis

If TSALD is 0–5 mm = Non-extraction case

5–9 mm = Borderline case

> 9 mm = Extraction case

5. Carey's analysis

If crowding is 0–2.5 mm = non extraction case

2.5–4 mm = second premolar extraction case

more than 4 mm = first premolar extraction case

Ideal cases for serial extraction are:

– 8½ – 9½ year age (growing period)

TSALD≥ 10 mm

– Skeletal Class I relations

– but it causes lingual tipping of lower incisors and deep bite development.

CEPHALOMETRICS

1. Main reference plane used in Downs analysis = FHP
2. Reference plane used in Steiners analysis = SN plane

3. Reference plane used in Ricketts an analysis is = Anatomic FHP
4. FHP = Po – Or
5. ANB > 8° = Sk Class II
   ANB < 0° = Sk Class III
6. FMA > 30° = Vertical growth pattern
   SN-MP>35° = Vertical growth pattern
   Bjork's Sum > 400° = Vertical growth pattern
   Jarabak ratio < 60% = Vertical growth pattern
7. FMA < 20° = Horizontal growth pattern
   SN-MP<25° = Horizontal growth pattern
   Bjork's Sum > 390° = Horizontal growth pattern
   Jarabak ratio > 65% = Horizontal growth pattern
8. Rickett's E-Line joins = soft tissue chin with tip of nose
9. Acceptable magnification on ceph its 5–7% (80 KV/8mA/ 0.8 sec.)
10. Distance of film from midsagittal plane in ceph = 18 cm
11. Distance of x-ray source to midsagittal plane = 5 Feet
12. Mainly LHS of ceph in taken
12. Jarabak ratio = PFH/AFH % = 62–65%
13. Ratio of AUFH to ALFH is = 45 : 55 or 1 : 1.2
14. Bjork's sum = NSAr + SArGo + arGoMe = 396° ± 6°
15. An increased SNA denotes maxillary prognathism
16. An decreased SNA denotes maxillary retrognathism
17. An increased SNB denotes mandibular prognathism
18. An decreased SNB denotes mandibular retrognathism
19. Facial angle is the angle between FHP and facial plane (N-Pog)
20. Tweed's triangle includes FMA, FMIA and IMPA.
21. By Ballard's method = relation between lower incisor inclination with MP and maxillary–mandibular plane angle is inversely proportional
22. Angle of convexity is the angle between NA and A-pog planes.

23. Ratio of UAFH to LAFH = 45 : 55, i.e. 1.2
24. Normal nasolabial angle = 110°
25. Normal interincisal distance = 40–45 mm

Various soft tissue lines are = (MRSH)

1. Merrifield's line = line passing from soft tissue pogonion to the most prominent lip, whether upper or lower.
2. Rickett's line = line passing from soft tissue pogonion to the tip of the nose.
3. Steiner's line = line passing from soft tissue pogonion to the centre of the S-shaped curve formed by passing from nose to the upper lip.
4. Holdaway's line = line passing from soft tissue pogonion to the most prominent point on upper lip.

Cervical vertebra maturation index

Stage	Growth status	Shape	Inferior border
Initiation	80 – 100 %	Wedge	Flat
Acceleration	65 – 85 %	Rectangular	Slight concavity
Transition	25 – 65 %	Rectangular	Slight concave
Deceleration	10 – 25%	Square	Distinct concave
Maturation	5 – 10 %	Square	Accentuated concavity
Completion	0 – little	Vert. Dim > horizontal	Deep concavities

Hand Wrist R/G

1. Absence of sesamoid bone at average onset of puberty in a female implies retardation of pubertal development.
2. Initiation ossification of pisiform and hook of hamate = preceded peak growth in most males and females.
3. Initial ossification of thumb and advanced ossification of hook of hamate coincided with peak growth in most M and that was true in only about half of the F.

METHODS OF GAINING SPACE

1. Expansion = 1 mm / mm of space from expansion can be gained in intercanine region.
2. Reproximation = 0.5 mm per interdental area, i.e. 0.25 mm per tooth surface.
3. Distalisation of molars = up to 5–6 mm space can be gained on each side of the upper arch. It is not possible in lower arch, where only distal tipping is achieved.
4. Protrusion of incisors = 1 mm / mm of space by protrusion can be gained, i.e. 0.5 mm / side of the arch.
5. Derotation of molars / PMs = rotated posteriors occupy more space.
6. Uprighting of incisors = MD inclined anteriors occupy more space.
7. Uprighting of molars
8. Extraction = 7 mm / side of space can be gained by removal of first premolars.

Stripping indicated if TSALD = 0–2.5 mm

- Not > 50% enamel thickness should be reduced, i.e. 0.25 mm/ surface
- Immediate fluoride application is recommended to replenish the surface layer of enamel with fluoride.
- ARS, i.e. air rotor stripping is better than the hand strips.

FORCES

Types of forces

1. **Continuous** – e.g. light wire appliance;
   - Very light force
   - Direct resorption
   - No rest period
   - Decrease little in magnitude

2. **Intermittent** – e.g. removable appliance
   - Become zero with time
   - High forces
3. **Interrupted forces** – e.g. Headgears, FA
   - Heavy forces (200–300 gm)
   - Used for 12–14 hrs/day
   - Become zero abruptly when appliances are removed

Orthodontic forces	**Orthopaedic forces**
Light, 50–100 gm	Heavy > 400 gm/side
Continuous	Interrupted 12–14 hrs.
Dentoalveolar effects	Skeletal effects

⇒ Main fibers affected during OTM and most abundant are OBLIQUE FIBRES.

Squeeze film effect (by Bien) — When very heavy forces are applied, the interstitial fluid of PDL gets squeezed out and moves towards apex and cervical margins and results in decreased OTM.

⇒ **PHASES OF OTM**
Very rapid OTM = In Initial phase, by compressed PDL.
Little / no OTM = In lag phase, DUE TO HYALINISATION
Rapid OTM = In post-lag phase, due to removal of hyalinised areas

Theories of OTM

1. Pressure – tension theory
2. Fluid dynamic theory
3. Peizoelectric theory

⇒ **First messengers** in OTM = PTH, PG, Subs P, VIP

⇒ **2nd messengers** in OTM= CAMP, CGMP, Ca^{2+}

⇒ **step child of dentition =** third molars

⇒ **corner stone of the dentition** = first molars

⇒ **corner tooth** = canines

⇒ **servient of the tooth** = alveolar process

⇒ **bed of OTM** = PDL

Forces required for tooth movements

1. Tipping	-	50–75 gm
2. Bodily movement	-	100–150 gm
3. Intrusion	-	15–25 gm
4. Extrusion	-	50–75 gm
5. Torquing	-	50–75 gm
6. Uprighting	-	75–125 gm
7. Rotation	-	50–75 gm
8. Head Gears	-	350–450 gm on each side for a minimum of 12–14 hrs/day
9. Face mask	-	1 pound (450 gm) per side, (12–14 hr),
10. Chin cup	-	Initially 150–300 gm /side next two months force in 450–700 gm per side (for 12–14 hrs.)

11. **Optimal force** = 20–26 gm/cm^2 RSA. It is the force which moves the teeth most rapidly and causes no damage to tooth and associated tissues; and with minimum patient discomfort.
12. Forces in expansion - SME = 2–4 lbs
    - RME = 10–20 lbs
13. Minimum force to be applied to cause tooth movement = 7 gm/cm^2
14. Minimum time for which force is to be applied to cause tooth movement = 6 hours

⇒ D and F pull of headgear force (15–20° to OP) is applied (450 gm/side for 12–14 hrs/day by reverse face mask.

⇒ Orthodontic force should be light and gentle for rapid OTM and should be 1–2 Oz.

⇒ Light continuous forces are better and preferred and cause **frontal resorption.**

⇒ Heavy forces cause **rear resorption, undermining resorption**.

⇒ PGE1 plays role in OTM (arachidonic acid metabolites)

⇒ NSAIDS, i.e. Brufen, etc. inhibit OTM as they interfere with production of prostaglandins.

⇒ Nimesulide does not interfere with PG production and so can be safely given during OTM.

CHARACTERISTICS OF WIRES: Longer/thinner wires decrease the load-deflection rate and provide a more gentle force system.

STRENGTH = STIFFNESS × RANGE.

$$\frac{D^3}{L} = \frac{D^4}{L^3} \times \frac{L^2}{D}$$

SPRIGINESS = 1/ STIFFNESS

⇒ Loops / Helices given in wire – to increase wire length and so to decrease the forces applied (lighter) and decrease LDR, increase the range of action.

⇒ Force is directly proportional to D^4 / L^3, long lever arm

ANCHORAGE

Simple	- Resistance to tipping
Stationary	- Resistance to bodily OTM
Reciprocal	- Tooth move equal and opposite
Minimum	- > 1/2 space can be lost by mesial movement of the anchor teeth.
Moderate	- 1/4 to 1/2 space can be lost by mesial movement of the anchor teeth.
Maximum	- < 1/4 space can be lost by mesial movement of the anchor teeth.
Hammock	- By PDL

Muscular - By lower lip, e.g. lip bumper, etc.

Cortical - By mandibular cortex (Rickett's)

Extraoral Anchorage = HG

Intra oral Anchorage = Elastics, TPA, LHA, NPA, More number of teeth involved

Baker's Anchorage = Class II, III elastics

Single/primary anchorage = only one tooth acts as anchorage

Compound anchorage = more than one tooth acts as anchorage

Reinforced/multiple anchorage = where more than one type of resistance unit is used.

Anchorage loss is more in maxilla than mandible, due to more cancellous bone in maxilla.

Mandibular teeth provide better anchorage than maxillary teeth due to dense bone and direction of trabeculae.

Anchorage savers = HG, TPA, LHA, NPA, etc.

EXPANSION

Pitch of screw = 360°, i.e. 0.8 mm

Expansion schedule: SME = 90° / 3 days

RME = 90° / BD

Fixed Expansion by - Coffin, Haas, Hyrex, quad helix, w-arch, bihelix, NPE

RME Vs SME

1 Opening	0.5–1 mm /day (3.5–7 mm / week	1 mm/week
	90° BD	90° / 2–3 days
2 Force generated	10–20 lbs	2–4 lbs
3 Tissue damage	More	Less
4 Skeletal: dental expansion.	8:2	5:5
5 After 4 months of retention	5:5	5:5

EXTRACTION

⇒ **Wilkinson's extraction** = Removal of all first permanent molars, at 8½ – 9½ years age

⇒ **Stowbiz extraction** = Removal of ADJACENT premolars at one time.

⇒ **Therapeutic extraction** = Removal of teeth for treatment purpose.

⇒ **Balancing** = Removal of teeth from both sides in same arch

⇒ **Compensating** = Removal of teeth from same side in both arches.

⇒ **Serial extraction** = removal of CD4

⇒ Serial extraction procedures are usually related to the eruption pattern of permanent mandibular 3, 4.

⇒ Serial extraction causes **deepening of bite**, due to lingual inclination and uprighting of lower incisors. It always requires a second phase of orthodontic treatment by fixed orthodontic appliance.

⇒ Maxillary deciduous canine during serial extraction should not be extracted until 11–12 yrs age, otherwise proper intercanine width cannot be achieved.

APPLIANCES

Coffin Spring	Expansion
quad helix	Expansion
Jack screw	Expansion
Porter (W-arch)	Expansion
Bihelix	Expansion
Schwarz Appliance	Expansion
NPE I, II	Expansion
TPA, LHA, NPA	Space maintenance, anchorage savers

APPLIANCES (*Contd.*)

Distal shoe appliance	For guiding mandibular, permanent first molar to erupt after premature loss of primary mandibular first molar
Anterior bite plate	Bite opening
Posterior bite plate with z-spring	Treatment of Anterior cross bite
Reverse bite plate	Bite opening and mandibular forward displacement
Catalan's/(L) inclined plane	Treatment of Anterior cross bite
Bionater, Twin-block	Myofunctional
Activator, FR, etc.	Myofunctional
Herbst, Jasper Jumper	Myofunctional, fixed
Chin cup, Petit's/and Hickham appliance, Delaire's face mask	For treatment of Skeletal Class III
Oral screen	For treatment of protruded incisors with spacing, and for expansion of arches
Cetlin appliance, pendulum app., distal jet	Molar distalisation
Lip bumper/plumber	For hyperactive mentalis, lip sucking habit
Tongue blade	Treatment of anterior cross bite
M-spring	Closure of midline diastema
Hewley's appliance	For retention (also known as DENTAL CRUTCH)
Clip on retainer	For retention
Kesling tooth positioner	For retention
Nakamura's	Treatment of class III

APPLIANCES (*Contd.*)

Jackson's Clasp	U-shaped
3/4 circumferential	C-shaped
Southend Clasp	M-shaped (anterior region)
Triangular clasp	
Ball-end clasp	
Schwarz clasp	Also known as Arrow Head Clasp with a number of arrow heads
Crozat Pin head	U-shaped with wire soldered

⇒ Finger spring for MD OTM

⇒ Z spring for labial OTM

⇒ T- spring, paddle/ flapper for labial OTM

⇒ M spring = closure of midline diastema

ANTERIOR BITE PLATE

⇒ For opening of deep bite, best in average/horizontal growth patterns; C/I in vertical growth cases.

⇒ 2–3 mm inter occlusal gap at one time for supra eruption of molars. The plane is kept parallel to the OP.

⇒ If gap is > 4–5 mm = Tongue interferes with molar eruption and bite does not correct

⇒ Causes anterior force on (U) incisors, good for C2D2 m.o.

REVERSE BITE PLATE

⇒ Opens the bite, shift mandible forward; plane is at 45–60 degrees to OP.

⇒ Causes anterior force on (L) incisors and their flaring

POSTERIOR BITE PLATE

⇒ To create gap between incisal edges of U/L teeth, i.e. incisal clearance, for treatment of anterior cross bite

⇒ To treat the anterior open bite by causing intrusive forces on molars.

⇒ All the posterior teeth should be touching the acrylic ramp evenly on both the sides for efficient mastication.

Oral screen

⇒ Best age = early MDP, 8–9 years, time of palatal width increase.

⇒ Helps = Expansion of arches

⇒ Retraction of upper anteriors

⇒ Treatment of mouth breathing, tongue thrusting

⇒ Ring = Kept at junction of middle and incisal 3rd of upper CI, Used for lip exercises

⇒ Spacer = Provides space for expansion of arches by tongue pressure

⇒ Modified with holes, cribs, lingual screen, etc. for specific purposes.

FIXED APPLIANCES

Plastic brackets are made of	Polycarbonate
Nitinol wires contain	Ni, Ti in 55 : 45, i.e. 1:1 stoichiometric ratio
β- titanium (TMA) contain	Ti, Mo
elgiloy contains	Co, Cr, Ni
18:8 S.S. contains	18 Cr, 8 Ni

Elastics are made of latex rubber

Class I Elastics	Intra arch, close space and retract the teeth
Class II Elastics	Inter arch, class II molar correction, retraction of (U) anterior
Class III Elastics	Inter arch, class III molar correction, retraction of (L) anterior

(Class II, Class III also known as Baker's anchorage)

Box elastics	for treatment open bite
Cross elastics	for treatment posterior cross bite
Triangular and check patterns	For occlusal settling

FIXED ORTHO APPLIANCE

1. Band material:
   - ⇒ 0.180 × 0.005" – 0.006" – for molars
   - ⇒ 0.150 × 0.004" – for PMs, canines
   - ⇒ 0.125 × 0.003" – for incisors
2. Brackets:
   a. Edgewise = 022 × 028", 018 × 025" slot size
   - ⇒ Rectangular wire = Two point contact, help torquing.
   - ⇒ Bodily tooth movement
   - ⇒ High forces required, more time required
3. Begg's Buccal tube = 030"
   - ⇒ Only tipping movement, light forces required
   - ⇒ Round wire, single point contact

FUNCTIONAL APPLIANCES

⇒ Best age for treatment with FA = 10 years to pubertal growth phase

- M =12–14 years ± 1 year
- F =10–12 years ± 1 year,

2–3 years earlier in girls than boys.

⇒ Best in horizontal growth pattern cases with normal sized but retrognathic mandible

⇒ **Pterygoid response** = Lat pterygoid m. (inferior head) is affected. Checked at 6–8 weeks after start of FA therapy.

⇒ **Head gear effect** = U/B force on maxilla

⇒ Class II elastic effect on lower anteriors → flowing

⇒ With construction bite, bite is opened 2–3 mm beyond free way space.

⇒ Bionator is based on philosophy of tongue.

⇒ Main function of coffin spring in bionator is to stimulate the tongue and to bring in effect FM theory concept of growth.

⇒ FR appliance functions in vestibule of oral cavity, stretches the periosteum and causes bone growth and adaptation.

⇒ Twin block is better because it is a two piece appliance comfortable, allows mandibular movement and speech and worn for 24 hrs.

⇒ Appliance therapy to control oral habits is not recommended for children < 8 years age.

C Res of single rooted tooth	In midroot region, 2/3rd the distance from apex of the root.
C Res of molar	Bifurcation, midroot region
C Res of maxillary	Zygomatic maxillary suture
Crot. for bodily OTM	at infinity
Cervical Hg	Extrusion of Maxillary molars
	Increase LFH
HPHG and Kloehn HG	Intrusion of Maxillary molars and restricts maxillary growth

CLEFT

Epidemiology

1:800 patients, incidence increases with mother's age,

CLP more in males than females.

CL is 3 times more on left side than on right.

Isolated CP is more common in females.

Appears between lateral incisor and canines, generally LI are missing.

CL = MNP – LNP not fused = during 6th wk IU.

CP = Palatal shelves not fused = during 8th wk IU.

Lip repair = **Millard's rule of 10**

i.e. 10 wks age so as to assist suckling

10 lbs wt

10 gm% Hb

10,000 WBCs.

Palate repair = 12–24 mos age, i.e. before speech development starts

Ortho treatment during MDP is most important treatment phase for control of growth and dentition.

No ortho treatment is required during DDP except correction of cross bite.

SURGICAL PROCEDURES

1. **Frenectomy:** High labial frenum causes midline diastema, frenum should be clipped only after orthodontic diastema closure.
   - IF done earlier than diastema closure, then scar elastic tissue leads to relapse.
2. **Pericision (CSF) :** Circumferential supracrestal fibrotomy by Edwards
   - to prevent rotational relapse,
   - min. retention period required to avoid the rotation relapse = 232 days, which are required for readaptation of transseptal fibers + Alveolar crest groups of gingival fibers.
3. BSSO = Bilateral sagittal split osteotomy and

TOVRO = Transoral vertical ramal osteotomy are for treatment of mandibular sagittal discrepancy.

4. Reduction genioplasty = for treatment of mandibular prognathism, Augmentation genioplasty for Mandibular retognathism.
5. Lefort I osteotomy with advancement: for Maxillary retrognathism

RELAPSE

⇒ It is the loss of any correction achieved by orthodontic treatment.

⇒ Its **causes** are the following:

1. **PDL traction** = mainly supracrestal fibres, transeptal fibres of gingival fibers ≃ 232 days for readaptation, e.g. rotations. To avoid relapse either circumferential supracrestal fibrotomy is done OR a prolonged retention is given.

   - PDL fibers require 4–5 months only for reorganisation.
2. Due to **muscular forces and occlusal imbalances.**
3. Due to **growth changes** - Prolonged retention is given until active growth is complete to avoid relapse of skeletal problems (e.g. Class II, III), e.g. head gear, chin cup are used. It is known as **DYNAMIC RETENTION**
4. Treated anterior cross bites with sufficient overbite are self-retentive.
5. Relapse of lower anterior crowding after growth has ceased is mainly by **LATE MANDIBULAR GROWTH** (18–25–30 years) in which mandible rotates U/F pushing the mandibular arch against the upper anterior teeth. Also 3rd molars have been implicated for it, which has been proved a wrong contention.
6. Minimum time for which retention is given for a mild malocclusion = 9–12 months
7. **Midline diastema** closure, expansion in CLP cases, large tongue size with tongue thrusting and severe rotations require PROLONGED RETENTION.
8. Anterior bite plate should be incorporated in retainer in case of horizontal growth pattern.

SOLDERING:

It is defined as a process of joining metals by the use of a filler metal which has a substantially lower fusion temperature than that of the metals being joined.

The filler metals having fusion temperature less than 450 C are used for soldering

If the fusion temperature of filler metals exceeds than 450 C then the procedure is ka brazing.

It involves the flow of the molten filler metal due to capillary action between the metallic parts to be joined.

Ideal requisites of Dental solders:

It should exhibit excellent tarnish and corrosion resistance in the oral environment.

The fusion temperature of the solder should be lower than that of the parts being joined. It should 50 – 100 C lesser.

It should be free – flowing and should adequately wet the metal parts.

The strength of the solder should be similar to that of the metal being joined.

The color of the solder should match with that of the parts being joined.

Most dental solders are composed of gold, silver, copper, zinc, tin and nickel.

Flux:

- It helps in flow of the solder.
- It aids in removal of oxide coating so as to increase the flow of the molten solder.
- It also dissolves any surface impurities.
- It prevents oxidation of the metals and also reduces the melting point of the dental solder.
- Flux contains borax glass and boric acid and silica : as 55: 35: 10%.

- Fluoride fluxes contain boric acid and potassium fluoride in 1: 1 ratio; and produce excellent solder joints.

Antiflux:

It is defined as a material that is used to confine the flow of the molten solder over the meals being joined.

Eg lead pencil markings; graphite lines and iron rouge.

Types of soldering:

- **Investment soldering** – it has gap of approx 0.13 mm.
- **Free hand soldeing.**

  Reducing flame is used during soldering.

TYPES OF SOLDERS:

- Hard solders: they have high melting temperature and have greater strength and hardness.
- Soft solders: they have low melting range of about 260 C ; but lack corrosion resistance.

COMPOSITION:

Composition	Gold solder	Silver solder
Gold	45–81%	—
Silver	8–30	10–80
Copper	7–20	15–50
Tin	2–4	
Zinc	2–4	4–35

Cadmium or phosphorous may be present in small amounts.

Fusion temperature	690–870 C	620–700 C

WELDING:

It involves the joining of 2 or more metal parts directly under pressure without the introduction of an intermediary filler metal.

Types:

- **Cold welding**: done by hammerng or pressue eg gold foil fillings
- **Hot welding** : uses heat of sufficient intensity to melt the metals being joined.
- **Spot welding**: used to join orthodontic components; heat sources is usually a high amperage electric machine called as spot welder. It employs the electrode technique.

8

Pedodontics

- A child's behavior problem can be handled by familiarization if the basis of problem is = fear.
- The greatest period of growth of cranium occurs b/w = birth and 5 years of age.
- A broad understanding of the development of human behavior requires a knowledge of basic concepts of = maturation and learning.
- Acute herpetic gingivo-stomatitis is main cause of generalized acute gingival inflammation in a preschool child.
- Small, irregular bright red spots on child's buccal mucosa with bluish white specks in the centre is of = rubeola.

Mile stones

Age	Milestone
1 month	Holds head up
2 months	Smile with recognition
3 months	Reaches for objects but misses
4 months	Sits up with support
5 months	Sits on lap grasp with support
6 months	Sits in chair with back rest
7 months	Sits unaided
8 months	Stands with aid
9 months	Stands holding into furniture
10 months	Crawls
11 months	Walk with support

Mile stones (*Contd.*)

12 months	Pulls to standing position using furniture
13 months	Crawls up steps
14 months	Stands unaided
15 months	Walks unaided

Development of different tissues of the body

Age of IUL	Tissues
4 weeks	Thyroid gland
6 week	Parotid and submandibular glands
6–7 weeks	Cleft lip
6–8 weeks	Human face
7 weeks	Muscles of mastication
8 weeks	Sublingual gland
8 weeks	Premaxilla/maxilla
4–8 weeks	Tongue
14 weeks	Bony palate established
32 weeks	Infantile swallowing established
12–15 months of age	Adult swallowing is established.

GROWTH

- RATIO b/w skull and face at birth = 8:1.
- Neurocranium = desmocranium + chondrocranium.
- Desmocranium = cranial vault; formed by intra- membranous ossification.
- Chondrocranium = base of skull; formed by endochondral ossification.
- Viscerocranium = i.e. bones of facial skeleton; formed by intramembranous ossification.

FONTANELLES: 6 in no.

1 Frontal/ anterior	b/w 2 parietal and frontal bones	Close at 8–12 months
1 Occipital/ posterior	b/w 2 parietal and occipital bones	Close by 2 months
2 Sphenoid/ antero-lateral	paired; b/w frontal, parietal; temporal and sphenoid bones	Close by 3 months
2 Mastoid/ postero-lateral	paired; b/w parietal; occipital and temporal bones	Close by 12 months

- Cephalo-caudal gradient of growth.

Head circumference at birth = 35 cm approx.

Head size

At birth	22 % of the total body length.
10 yrs	95 % of total head growth completed.
15 yrs	98 % of total head growth completed.
3 yrs	Width of head completed.
17–18 yrs	Length of head is completed.

Mandibular foramen

- Lies below OP = in very young child.
- At OP level = during primary dentition phase.
- Above OP approx 7 mm = in adults.

Height and weight predictions

	Boys	**Girls**
Adult height Adult weight	2 × height at 8 yrs 5 × weight at 2 yrs	2 × height at 7.6 yrs 5 × the weight at 1.6 yrs

Height and weight charts

Age	Increment	Height
Birth	–	20 inches
0–6 months	1 inch/month	26 inches
6–12 months	0.5 inch/month	32 inches
1–7 yrs	3 inch/year	50 inches
8–15 yrs	1 inch/year	62 inches

Weight chart

Age	Increment	Weight
Birth	–	7–8 lbs
0–4 months	2 lbs/month	15–16 lbs
4–12 months	2 lbs/month	23–24 lbs
1–2 yrs	1/2 lbs/yr	29–30 lbs
2–10 yrs	5 lbs/yr	69–70 lbs

Changes from birth to adulthood

Head	2 × that of birth size
Trunk	3 × that of birth size
Arms	4 × that of birth size
Legs	5 × that of birth size

Tonsils/adenoids

At birth	Very small; may regress after few days
First few months.	Growth occurs
6 mos–2 yrs	Maximum growth occurs know as primary physiological enlargement
6 yrs	Hypertrophy occurs know as secondary physiological enlargement
Puberty	Regression and atrophy occurs

According to **Scammon's growth curve**

Growth of lymphatic tissues > neural > somatic > genital tissues.

Later on, lymphatic tissues start regressing.

PHYSIOLOGY OF GROWTH (Also refer to orthodontics in Vol 1.)

Effect of hormones

- GH, thyroxine, corticosteroids and insulin = bring changes in growth rate.
- PTH, vitamin D, calcitonin = affect skeletal maturation and pubertal growth.
- GH and insulin = stimulate stomatomedin release and cause cartilage growth.
- Pubertal growth spurt is enhanced by steroids and GH and helps in accelerated bone maturation.
- PTH = osteoclastic activity.
- Calcitonin = bone deposition enhancer.

Methods of growth assessment

- **Biometrics** = i.e. a science of statistical biology in which collection and statistical analysis of data regarding a living being is considered, e.g. cross-sectional study; longitudinal study; semi-longitudinal study.
- **Craniometry** = is the measurement of cranial dimensions in dry skulls.
- **Somatometry** = is the measurement of facial dimensions on a living person. Only soft tissues measurement can be done.
- **Cephalometry** = measurements of cranio-facial complex made on a standardized x-ray plate. It is a 2 D picture of a 3 D figure.
- **Implant metals indicators** = by Bjork; metal acts as a reference point and so growth of bone is studied on x-ray.
- **Superimposition** = of a series of x-rays on some reference points and comparing.
- **Stereo-pair images** = 3 D computer analysis is done by digital imaging method.
- **EMG.**
- **Animal experiments.**

- **Vital staining = alizarine dye** is found in **madder plants**; which gets deposited in the areas of active growth. But animal has to killed for studying.
- **Radio-isotopes** = get collected in the areas of growth. Growth is measured with Geiger-Muller counter by studying the emission of radiations. Mainly **99 m Tc** is used.
- **Natural markers** = certain developmental features of bone act as reference markers.
- **Anthropometry** = certain landmarks on soft tissues corresponding to bony landmarks are studied and measured, e.g. data by Farkas.

AGES AS THE GROWTH DETERMINANTS

1. **Chronologic age** = is calculated from child's Date of birth. It is not a good predictor of growth.
2. **Somatotypic age** = 3 somatotypes exist according to Sheldon. Ectomorphics are late maturers, i.e. growth in them continues for longer time. Endomorphs are early maturers. It is also not a good predictor of growth.
3. **Height and weight ages** = height and weight are affected by genetic and environmental factors and cannot be used as a sole predictor of developmental age of child.
4. **Dental age** = is calculated by observing the state of dental development and teeth eruptions. It is simplest but least accurate method. Calcification of a tooth is also an indicator of somatic maturation, e.g. mandibular canine calcification stages.
5. **Sexual age** = pubertal changes are observed in males and females due to hormonal changes. Peak height velocity PHV occurs early in females than in males. Maturation occurs early 2–3 yrs in females than the males. Onset of menstruation indicates completion of pubertal growth spurt.
6. **Facial age**
7. **Skeletal age** = most reliable method; many methods can be used, e.g. hand wrist x-ray; CVMI; (cervical vertebra maturation indicator); SMI (skeletal maturation indicators), etc.

Influence of deciduous tooth morphology on cavity design and restoration placement

Anatomy of deciduous teeth	Implication for cavity design and tooth restoration
Enamel thinner than in permanent teeth	Dentin involved more rapidly
Crowns more bulbous than permanent teeth	Influences placement of floor of i/d box in class II cavities
Primary molars are narrower occlusally, esp Ds	Adaptation of matrices is more difficult Cusp strength is influenced by width of occlusal restoration
Broad contact points in molars	In proximal caries diagnosis; so bitewing r/gs are required for detection
Pulp chambers are larger; pulphorns are more pointed; pulpal outline follows DEJ	Cavity size must be restricted. Limited space for sufficient bulk bulk of restorative material to resist fracture.

Atraumatic caries treatment ART = here, caries is removed using the hand instruments and restored with GI cements.

Non-mechanical caries removal/chemical caries removal = carious dentin is removed by using ***N–mono-chloro-amino-butyric acid NMAB.***

Traumatic injuries

1. Concussion = tooth traumatised but not loosened.
2. Subluxation = tooth is dislocated in the socket but not displaced.
3. Extrusion = tooth displaced in occlusal direction.
4. Intrusion = tooth displaced in apical direction in the socket.
5. Lateral displacement = tooth pushed laterally, buccally, or palatally.
6. Avulsion = tooth totally displaced from socket.

CLASSIFICATION OF TOOTH DISCOLORATION

(I) Intrinsic Discoloration: Occurs following a change in the structural composition of hard dental tissues, e.g.

1. Aging
2. Alkaptonuria
3. Amelogenesis imperfecta
4. Congenital erythropoietic porphyria
5. Congenital hyperbilirubenenaemia
6. Dentinogenesis imperfecta
7. Enamel hypoplasia
8. Fluorosis
9. Pulpal haemorrhage products
10. Root resorption
11. Tetracyline staining

(II) Extrinsic Discoloration

1. Metallic
2. Non metallic

(III) Internalised Discoloration: Is due to incorporation of extrinsic stains within the tooth substance following dental development. It occurs in enamel defects and in the porous surface of exposed dentine, e.g. in acquired defects like:

(a) Tooth wear and gingival recession.

(b) Dental caries.

(c) Restorative materials.

- Bitewing r/g is good for the detection of proximal caries lesions.
- Caries lesions always appear smaller on the r/g than it actually is, because the r/g is a 2 D picture of a 3 D object.
- Proximal caries if not restored timely leads to the loss of arch length due to mesial migration of the adjacent tooth.
- Child's first dental visit and oral examination should be at least at 9–12 months of age or as soon as the first tooth erupts in the oral cavity.

- Cleaning of the gum pads of the child should be done regularly by a soft moist cloth.

INFECTION CONTROL PROCEDURES IN A DENTAL CLINIC: As approved by ADA and CDC PHS in US dept of health.

1. Obtain a thorough medical history.
2. Clean instruments in an ultrasonic cleaner or soap and water solutions. Wear heavy rubber gloves during cleaning. Adhering blood or tissues do not allow proper penetration of heat and sterilisation.
3. Sterilize all reusable instruments.
4. Monitor the use and functions of sterilizer by using spores test routinely. **Spores of actinobacillus stereothermophillus** bacteria are used.
5. Use gloves during all treatment procedures.
6. Wear surgical masks and protective eyewears to avoid aerosols and splatter.
7. Wear protective gowns and uniforms during Rx.
8. Protect operatory surfaces by protective covers, e.g. plastic wrap, aluminium foils, etc.
9. Use rubber dam and high speed suctions.
10. Require vaccinations vs Hep B, etc.
11. Hand wash between the patients contacts by antimicrobial surgical hand scrubs, e.g. STERILLIUM.
12. Perform waste-disposal properly.
13. Use disposables syringes, etc. where ever possible. Destroy syringes/needles, etc. after use before rejection.
14. Incineration of soiled items should be done at a proper place.
15. Place biopsy specimen in sturdy containers with a tight lid to prevent leakage (10% formalin).
16. Disinfect all contaminated operatory surfaces in b/w the patients, e.g. 1:10 diluted solution of household bleach for non-metallic surfaces or with Iodophore.
17. Clean and sterilize all handpieces.

18. Clean and disinfect impressions and intra-oral appliances before handling, e.g. glutraldehyde; surgi-scrub; iodophore solutions, etc.

CHILD ABUSE AND NEGLECT

First documented and reported case of child abuse occurred in 1874.

Battered child syndrome term was coined by Henry Kempe in 1962. Its S/S are:

- Fractures of any long bones
- Subdural hematoma
- Failure to thrive
- Soft tissue swelling
- Skin bruising

Types of child abuse

1. Physical abuse/non-accidental trauma
2. Child sexual abuse/exploitation
3. Failure to thrive
4. Health care neglect
5. Dental neglect
6. Safety neglect
7. Emotional neglect
8. Emotional abuse
9. Physical neglect
10. Educational abuse
11. Intentional drugging or poisoning.
12. **Munchausen syndrome by proxy** = i.e. children who are victims of parentally fabricated or induced illness.

Physical abuse = is most important type of abuse; it is the injury inflicted on a person below 18 yrs of age.

Soft tissues injuries esp bruises are most common injury sustained in child abusc.

DATING THE BRUISES

Time elapsed	Characteristics
0–2 days	Swollen, tender
0–5 days	Red, blue, purple
5–7 days	Green
7–10 days	Yellow
10–14 days	Brown
2–4 weeks	Cleared

CHILD PSYCHOLOGY

Pedodontic treatment triangle

- Rx of a child is a one-to-one relationship.
- Triangle consists of the CHILD-DENTIST-FAMILY esp mother.
- Child is at the apex of the triangle and focus of attention of family and dentist.

Developmental milestones = are the physical changes appearing at the specific chronologic ages during the development of the child.

Intelligent quotient IQ by **Binet:**

IQ = mental age × 100/chronologic age.

IQ classification guide.

American association of mental deficiency classification

52–68	Mild	140 and up	Very superior
36–51	Moderate	120–139	Superior
20–35	Severe	110–119	High average
19 and below	Profound	90–109 80–89 70–79 69 and below	Average Low average Borderlinedefective Mentally retarded

How does the maternal anxiety affects the child's behavior in the dental clinic? The highly anxious parents tend to affect their child's behavior NEGATIVELY.

FRANKL BEHAVIOR RATING SCALE

- Rating 1 = definitely negative
- Rating 2 = negative
- Rating 3 = positive
- Rating 4 = definitely positive

Types of PARENTS

1. **Over-protective parents** = their behavior often prevents the natural development of the child towards independence.
2. **Manipulative parents** = have excessively demanding attitude.
3. **Hostile parents** = they question the necessity of the Rx. The question is posed in a distrusting manner.
4. **Neglectful parents** = failure of co-operation; miss the appointment, etc.

DEVELOPMENT OF DENTITION (Also refer to the section of orthodontics.)

- Mandibular D = no resemblance to any tooth-primary or permanent.
- Max. D = resembles max 5.
- Max E = resembles max 6.
- Mandibular E = resembles mandibular 6.
- Mandibular D = buccal cervical ridge is MOST prominent; and oblique.
- Mandibular E = MB pulp horn is the HIGHEST.

Eruption sequence = ABDCE.

Calcification sequence of primary teeth = ADBCE.

Evolution of dentition

3 stages of tooth evolution:

- Reptilian stage/haplodont = simplest; single cone type.
- Early mammalian stage = triconodont.
- Triangular stage = tritubercular molars.
- Quadri-tubercular molars.

Characteristics of dentition

Acrodont	Teeth attached to jaws by a connective tissue.
Pleurodont	Teeth are set inside the jaws.
Thecodont	Teeth are inserted in bony socket.
Polyphyodont	Teeth replaced through out the life.
Diphyodont	2 sets of teeth, e.g. human teeth.
Monophyodont	Single set of teeth.
Homodont	Single type of the teeth.
Heterodont	Many types of teeth, e.g. human teeth.
Human teeth are	Heterodont; diphyodont and continuously invested teeth.

Origin of teeth

- Theory of concrescence.
- Theory of trituberculy = widely accepted.
- Theory of multi-tuberculy.

Types of eruption

- Continuously growing teeth.
- Continuously extruding teeth.
- Continuously invested teeth = e.g. human teeth.
- Clinical eruption = i.e. movement of tooth from its position in the socket to the functional position in an occlusal plane.

Stages of tooth eruption

Pre-emergence eruption = occurs when crown formation is completed and root development starts post-emergent eruption.

Theories of eruption

- Root growth theory
- Constriction of pulp
- Pulp growth
- Bone growth
- Tissue fluid pressure
- Shrinkage of collagen

Eruption rhythm = mean daily eruption velocity is approx 71 microns/day.

Accelerated eruption	Retarded eruption
Hyperthyroidism Hyper-pituitarism Turner's syndrome	Hypothyroidism Hypopituitarism Cleidocranial dysostosis Downs syndrome Achondroplasia Hypovitaminosis A, D Amelogenesis imperfecta Osteopetrosis

Special points wrt morphology of primary teeth (Also refer to the section of dental anatomy.)

- **Max CI** = its MD diameter of crown is more than the cervico-incisal length (opposite of permanent max CI).
- **Max LI** = its cervico-incisal dimension is more than the MD width.
- **Max C** = root is more than the twice the length of the crown.
- **Mandibular LI** = is similar to the mandibular CI but is somewhat larger in all dimensions except labio-lingually. Its incisal edge slopes towards the distal aspect of the tooth.
- **Max D** = ML cusp is largest and sharpest. MD dim is greatest and then converges cervically.

- **Max E** = it resembles max 6. Its root bifurcation on buccal side is close to the CEJ. Cusp of Carabelli is on ML cusp. Oblique ridge joins ML cusp to DB cusp.

Mandibular D

- Does not resemble any permanent tooth.
- Distal area of tooth is shorter than mesial area.
- Has prominent buccal ridge.
- Pronounced lingual convergence of the crown on the mesial aspect.
- MMR is so well developed that it appears as another small cusp lingually.
- Cervical line slants upward from the buccal to the lingual surface because crown length is more in MB area than the ML area.

Mandibular E = it resembles mandibular 6.

- 3 buccal cusps are of equal size but in mandibular 6, the distal cusp is smaller than the other 2 buccal cusps.

RADIOGRAPHY

(Also refer to section on radiography in volume I and operative dentistry in Vol. III.)

Primary **biologic effects** of low level radiations are: carcinogenesis; teratogenesis; mutagenesis.

Younger the tissue and more actively it is dividing, the more sensitive it is to the radiations.

Which **stage of mitosis** is affected most by the radiations?

Critical organs = which should be shielded from radiations are:

- Skin
- Red bone marrow
- Gonads
- Eyes
- Thyroid
- Pregnancy
- Breasts

1. Lead apron and thyroid collar should be used to protect from stray radiations.
2. Annual maximum permissible dose/MPD = 5 rem for occupationally exposed person.
3. Cumulative MPD = 5 (N–18) rem, where N = age of the person.
4. Non-occupational exposure = 10% of that for radiation workers = 0.5 rem.

Size of the x-ray films

For a young child = 2.2 × 3.5 cm IOPA.

For an older child = 3.1 × 4.1 cm IOPA.

Occlusal film = 5.7 × 7.6 cm.

Sizes of the film

No. 1	22 × 35 mm	Pediatric film
No. 2	24 × 40 mm	Adult anterior
No. 3	32 × 41 mm	Standard adult
No. 4	27 × 54 mm	Bite wing
No. 5	57 × 76 mm	Occlusal film
Screen films	4 × 5 inches 5 × 12 inches 8 × 10 inches	

- **ALARA rule** = also known as reasonably achievable.
- **Bite wing** r/g is used to detect the proximal caries lesions when the teeth are in tight contacts.
- **15 IOPA films** are used for full all-around intra-oral examination, i.e. 8 in upper arch and 7 in lower arch. An additional IOPA is required in max incisor region because the teeth are larger in size.
- **SLOB rule** (same lingual, opposite buccal)= as known as **buccal object/CLARK'S rule**, i.e. if the cone of the rays is displaced

while shooting the r/g, the lingual object moves in the same direction and the buccal object moves in the opposite direction.

- Films are available as A to E speed films from lowest to highest speed, the **E-speed films should be used**. These films help in reducing the radiation exposure to the patient.

Suggested R/G protocols for a child patient

Age	R/G survey	Views
3–5 yrs	4 film survey	2 = U and L anterior occlusals 2 = R and L posterior bitewings
6–7 yrs	8 film survey	2 = U and L anterior occlusals/ IOPA. 2 = R and L max posterior occlusals. 2 = R and L mandibular posterior IOPA. 2 = R and L posterior bitewings.
8–9 yrs	12 film survey	4 = U and L, R and L posterior IOPA. 4 = U and L, R and L canine IOPAs. 2 = U and L anterior IOPAs2 = R and L posterior bitewings.
10–12 yrs	16 film survey	12 film survey + 4 = U and L; R and L permanent molars IOPAs.

Positioning the patient

- Sagittal plane must be vertical and perpendicular to the floor.
- **Ala-tragus line** should be parallel to the floor for the maxillary teeth.
- **Angle of mouth-tragal line** should be parallel to the floor for the mandibular teeth.

Tooth	Centering point	Vertical angle
Lower molar region	3 cm anterior to angle of mandible, 1 cm above the lower border.	0–10 degrees
Unerupted 3rd molar	2 cm anterior to angle, 1 cm above the lower border.	0
Lower PMs	Line down from angle of mouth when open, 1 cm above the lower border.	–10–15
Lower	Along the line of tooth.	–20–30
Canine	1 cm above the lower border.	
Lower incisors	1 cm above the lower border in the midline.	–20–30
Max molars	At the intersection of a line perpendicular 1 cm behind the outer canthus of eye crosses the ala-tragus line.	20–30
Max 3rd molar		5–10
Max PMs	At the intersection point, where the perpendicular from the midpoint of infraorbital margin crosses ala-tragus line or above the corner of mouth.	35–40
Max canine	Ala of nose along the inter-dental space b/w canine and first PM	45–50
Upper incisors	Along the I/D area b/w CI and LI. Centering point is along the vertical axis of tooth through the nose to extension of ala-tragus line in incisor region.	50–55

- Proclined teeth require more degree of angulation than the normal.
- If high dome of palate/deep palate is there = the small angle between tooth and film is taken.
- Angle of incidence increases, when alveolar processes get resorbed.
- Mostly, D and E speed films are used.
- High kVp helps = decreasing patient's exposure; decreases contrast; decreases exposure time.
- Anode to film distance is kept = 10–20 cm.
- Slightly more angle is required for max LI than CI.

GENETIC ASPECTS OF DENTAL ANOMALIES

- **Differentiation of cells** = is a progressive specialization and hence limitation of cell functions.
- Protein synthesis is the critical element which determines cell functions and the cell type.
- DNA is the genetic material which controls the functions and differentiation and protein synthesis.
- **Gene** = the genetic material DNA controls the production of a single protein/polypeptide chain.
- **Cytogenetics** = is the study of human chromosomes.
- **Karyotyping** = is the technique of chromosome analysis.

By karyotyping, the human chromosomal set has been divided in 8 groups as:

Group	Chromosomes	Group	Chromosomes
A	1–3	E	16–18
B	4–5	F	19–20
C	6–12	G	21–22
D	13–15	Sex	XX/XY

- **Deletion** = is the absence of a piece of chromosome.
- **Duplication** = the insertion of an extra fragment into a chromosome from its now deficient homolog.
- **Inversion** = breaking of a chromosome in 2 places and subsequent rejoining with middle piece inverted.
- **Translocation** = attachment of a broken piece from one chromosome to another but non-homologous chromosome.
- **Denver nomenclature** = is the most commonly accepted system for chromosomal identification. It is based on chromosomal morphology.
- **Monogenic trait** = it is produced and regulated by a single gene. It follows simple Mandelian principles.
- **Polygenic trait** = controlled by many genes at different loci, e.g. skin colour, height, etc.
- **Multifactorial inheritence** = i.e. determined by a combination of genetic and environmental factors.
- **Proband/propositus** = is the first affected person in the family who brings that family to attention.
- **Siblings** = i.e. brothers and sisters in a family.
- **Phenotype** = i.e. the clinical appearance of a given trait for an individual.
- **Genotype** = i.e. the specific genetic make up which controls that phenotype.
- **Alleles** = genes at the same locus on a pair of homologous chromosomes.
- **Homozygous** = when both members of a pair of alleles are identical.
- **Heterozygous** = i.e. when the 2 alleles at a given locus are different.
- **Dominant gene** = i.e. a gene which expresses a particular phenotype in single dose.
- **Recessive gene** = i.e. a gene required in double dose to express a phenotype.

CHROMOSOMAL ABNORMALITIES

- **Trisomy** = i.e. when an extra chromosome is present, e.g.
  - Trisomy 21 = as known as Down syndrome.
  - Trisomy 18 = Edwards syndrome.
  - Trisomy 13 = Patau syndrome.
- **Monosomy** = i.e. one chromosome is missing.

SOME INHERITANCE-LINKED DISORDERS

Autosomal dominant inheritance	Autosomal recessive inheritance
• e.g. dentinogenesis imperfecta. • **50 % offsprings** affected. • **Both sexes** are equally affected. • Mostly, **heterozygous** individuals.	• i.e. expressed by the individual who has both altered recessive alleles and **Homozygous.** • **25% siblings** are affected. • e.g. **acatalasia,** i.e. absence of enz. Catalase. • So H_2O_2 is not metabolized to H_2O and O_2, leading to gangrenous stomatitis in the absence of O_2 and nutrition. • Incidence = 1:10,000. • Heterozygous parents are **carriers** and unaffected. • Higher frequency of **parental consanguinity.** Other examples are = albinism; juvenil periodontitis; Papillon-Lefevre syndrome; hypophosphatasia; Phenyl ketonuria; sickle cell anemia; fibromatosis gingiva; ectodermal dysplasia.

- **Turner syndrome** = monosomy of X-chromosome, i.e. XO.
  - Missing one X-chromosome.
  - Phenotypic FEMALES.
  - 1:10,000 live births.
- **Deletion** = e.g. short arm of chr. No. 5 = cri-du-chat syndrome
- **Translocation = philadelphia chromosome** = T 22, 9. It is related to the etiology of CHRONIC GRANULOCYTIC LEUKEMIA.

Polygenic traits = are susceptible to environmental modifications, i.e. a multi-factorial course, e.g. CLP.

Sex linked recessive inheritance, SLRI	**Sex linked dominant inheritance, SLRI**
Males are hemizygous for all X-linked genes, i.e. they have XY pair.	Gene is dominant, so seen **more in females.**
So in males, even a recessive gene on X-chromosome can express itself.	**All daughters** of an affected father get affected. because of X-chromosome.
So rare SLRI are **practically restricted to males.**	**Affected males do not transfer the trait** to their sons (as seen in SLRI).
Affected father passes genes to all his daughters, who are now carriers and not to the sons. It is know as **criss-cross inheritance**.	It appears about **TWICE in females** than males.
e.g. hypohidrotic ectodermal dysplasia; hemophilia.	Its transmission is indistinguishable from ADI and can be differentiated only by observation of offspring of affected males, not the affected females, e.g. hypoplastic amelogenesis imperfecta.

Environment = is defined as those non-genetic circumstances which render an individual more or less susceptible to a disease state.

Disease **risk to offsprings** of an affected person

Monogenic dominant trait = 50%

Monogenic recessive trait = 25%

Polygenic trait = < 10%

Genetic aspects of dental caries

- **Vipeholm study** = done by Gustafson and associates.
- Because of genetic differences certain environmental factors are more cariogenic for some people than for others.
- Children especially daughters show remarkable similarity in caries to their parents caries' susceptibility esp to mothers.
- **Proline-rich proteins PRP** in saliva have been linked to early plaque/pellicle formation. They bond tightly to hydroxyapatite. They are inherited as ADI trait. Coded by a block of genes know as **salivary protein complex,** which is located on **short arm of Chr 12.**
- Patients with high resistance to dental caries have a specific immunoglobulin in saliva, which lyses the cariogenic bacteria. It is transmitted as ADI trait.
- Caries a **polygenic trait,** i.e. a multi-factorial disease.
- Genetic modifications of caries concept, i.e. food, vaccine, etc.
- **BRAX–I gene** is responsible for enamel growth in teeth.

DEVELOPMENTAL/INFECTIONS DISORDERS OF TEETH (Also refer to sec. on oral pathology in volume I.)

Condition	**Features**
Alveolar abscess	Caused by Strept. Viridans. Localized by fibrous capsule bacteria are not susceptible to TETRA-CYCLINE R/g shows thickened PDL. A gum boil/fistula can be seen in chronic cases.

Condition	Features
Cellulitis	Diffuse and massive swelling of soft tissues, a serious infections may lead to cavernous sinus thrombosis CST. Ka as Ludwig's angina if it involves submandibular, sublingual and submental spaces bilaterally. Caused by streptococci, which produce Enz. hyaluronidase, i.e. spreading factor and fibrinolysins, which help in spread of infections. Some staphylococci may also be present.
Fusion of teeth	It is the union of 2 independent teeth. Have separate pulp chambers and root canals. Mostly involve the **anterior teeth.** May be seen in both deciduous/permanent teeth.
Gemination	It is an incomplete division of a single tooth germ by invagination occurring during proliferation stage. Bifid crown on a single root is present seen in both deciduous/permanent teeth but mostly in deciduous teeth.
Dens in dente	i.e. tooth with in a tooth/pregnant tooth. Mostly seen in permanent max LI. Is a lingual invagination of enamel. Invagination is lined with enamel and the presence of foramen cecum/lingual pit, which may lead to caries and a very early pulp involvement. The enamel is very thin in the depth of pit.

EARLY EXFOLIATION OF TEETH

A variation of 18 months in the exfoliation time of primary teeth is considered normal.

A delay of 6 months in the eruption time of primary teeth is considered normal.

Main **causes** are:

1. Periodontosis
2. Cherubism

3. Acrodynia
4. Hypophosphatasia
5. Pseudohypophosphatasia

Cherubism	As known as familial fibrous dysplasia. Multi-locular areas of bone destruction and thinning of cortical plates esp. mandible. Premature exfoliation of primary teeth due to loss of support and root resorption. Premature loss of permanent teeth due to interference in root development. Conservative approach is taken as they are self-limiting lesions and tend to resolve with maturity.
Acrodynia	As known as pink disease. Due to mercury poisoning.
Hypophosphatasia	Absence of severe gingivitis, but still loss of alveolar bone and teeth; limited to ANTERIOR region only. Low alkaline Pase levels = 7 King-Armstrong units (normal is 13–17 KA units) Hypocementosis of affected teeth.
Pseudo-hypophosphatasia Anomalous dental development	Serum alk. Pase levels are normal. Patients exhibit osteopathy of long bones/skull. Defective root development in dentinal Dysplasia and shell teeth. Absence of cementum from root surface and so loss of PDL support.
Cyclic neutropenia	Decreased no. of PMN neutrophils. Occurs after every 3 weeks cycle. Severe gingivitis and ulceration. Prepubertal periodontitis = due to repeated infections and considerable loss of supporting bones.

6. Anomalous dental development
7. Cyclic neutropenia
8. Acatalasia
9. Hyperpituitarism
10. Juvenile diabetes
11. Progeria
12. Histocytosis X
13. Leukemia, etc.

ENAMEL HYPOPLASIA

- Interference in normal enamel matrix formation and so surface defects appear.
- **Prenatal disturbance** is seen as an accentuated neonatal ring in the primary teeth.
- **Postnatal amelogenesis** is confined to the part of crown located cervically from the enamel are present at birth.
- Lead poisoning as known as **plumbism;** lead can cross placenta. It delays the development and eruption of primary teeth.
- **Turner's tooth** = i.e. due to local infection or trauma.
- Radiations = ameloblasts are resistant to rays, but **dentin is severely affected**; root formation is stunted; development of tooth arrested.
- **Fluoride** = lead to mottled enamel; pigmentation is **limited to outer 3rd of enamel;** nitrogen content of enamel is higher than normal.
- Other causes = rubella/german measles; deficiency of vitamin A, C, D, Ca, P, etc.

DENTINOGENESIS IMPERFECTA

- Its is an ADI trait. It is a MESODERMAL DEFECT.
- Seen with osteogenesis imperfecta.
- Type I = DI + OI.
- Type II – DI only. It is as known as hereditary opalescent dentin.

- Enamel gets chipped off due to **lack of scalloping at DEJ;** exposed dentin gets abraded.
- Pulp chambers are **small or entirely absent.**
- Pulp canals are very small.
- Extraction of affected teeth is difficult due to brittleness of dentin.

AMELOGENESIS IMPERFECTA

- 1:14,000 to 1:16,000 incidence.
- 3 types, i.e. hypocalcified type; hypomaturation type and hypoplastic type.
- Hypoplastic type.
  - Enamel matrix is imperfectly formed.
  - Calcification occurs and enamel is hard.
  - But enamel is defective in amount and has a rough and pitted surface.
- **Hypocalcified type**
  - Matrix formation is of normal thickness.
  - But calcification is defective, enamel is soft and rough.
- **Odontogenesis imperfecta**
  - It is the combination of amelogenesis and dentinogenesis imperfecta.
  - It is as known as enamel and dentin dysplasia.
- **Very large pulp chambers** and root canals
  - Teeth are devoid of enamel.
  - Cementum is normal and acellular.
  - DEJ lacks scalloping.

SHELL TEETH

- **Very large pulp chambers** and root canals.
- Roots are short and early exfoliation of teeth occurs.
- Very small amount of enamel and dentin formed.

Taurodontism = as known as bull teeth:

- Crowns enlarge at the expense of roots.
- **Pulp chambers are elongated** and extend deeply in the areas of roots.
- It is a familial trait.

Conditions having large pulp chambers of teeth

1. Odontogenesis imperfecta
2. Shell teeth
3. Taurodontism

Ankylosed tooth = i.e. lack of PDL in some areas of tooth; mandibular deciduous teeth esp D/E are most common; a solid sound is heard on percussion. Tooth not able to erupt.

Submerged tooth = teeth adjacent to ankylosed tooth are free to erupt and carry the alveolar bone with them, so the occlusal level of ankylosed tooth is at a lower level than the adj. teeth.

Impacted tooth = tooth is not able to erupt due to interference in its path of eruption.

Inostosis of enamel may lead to ankylosis of a permanent tooth. It occurs due to a chronic infection of deciduous tooth, which irritates the follicle of permanent tooth. So the enamel epithelium disintegrates and coronal cementum or bone gets deposited leading to ankylosis.

Anodontia

- Complete failure of teeth to develop is very rare.
- Partial anodontia, i.e. congenital absence of a few teeth is a common condition, e.g. in ectodermal dysplasia.
- Partial anodontia has SLRI pattern and criss–cross inheritance occurs.
- Partial anodontia is as known as oligodontia or hypodontia.
- There is lack of alveolar growth as the teeth act as the functional matrix for its growth.
- But skeletal structures/jaw bases are normal.
- Lack of sweat glands and so no sweating.
- Pt is uncomfortable in hot weathers.

- **Induced anodontia** = is due to extraction of teeth.
- Every distal tooth of a group is missing, e.g. 2nd premolars; 3rd molars and max LI, except in lower incisor region, where central incisors are congenitally are missing.

DOWN SYNDROME: Also known as mongolism/trisomy 21.

- Delayed tooth eruption.
- Prolonged retention of primary teeth.
- Defect gets initiated b/w 6–8 weeks IU.
- It is linked to **increased age of mother.**
- Depressed nasal bridge; maxillary growth deficiency; skeletal class III relation.
- Increased periodontal diseases; high prevalance of bacteroides melaninogenicus.
- Low susceptibility to dental caries = due to increased salivation.
- Large fissured tongue; protruded.

Hypothyroidism

- Delayed eruption of teeth.
- Cretinism = congenital hypothyroidism; it is present at birth; short arms and legs; dwarf; head is disproportionately large.
- Delayed primary/permanent dentition.
- **Macroglossia** = so anterior open bite.

Hypopituitarism

- Decreased/retarded growth.
- Delayed dentition and eruption; prolonged retention of deciduous teeth.
- Is due to decreased growth hormones.
- Usually does not appear before 4 yrs of age.

Achondroplasia: Autosomal dominant

- Growth of limbs is limited due to lack of calcification in cartilages of long bones.
- Head size is large.

- Nasal bridge and maxilla is deficient.
- Skeletal Class III relation; due to early closure of synchondroses in the base of skull and so limited growth of maxilla.

Delayed dentition is also seen in following:

1. Fibromatosis gingiva.
2. Rickets.
3. Gardener syndrome.
4. Chondro-ectodermal dyslplasia/Ellis-Van Creveld synd.

INTRINSIC PIGMENTATION OF TEETH

Erythroblatosis fetalis

- Dentin is affected; it is due to excessive destruction of RBCs.
- Colour of teeth is blue-green due to deposition of bilirubin and biliverdin in dentin which are the products of Hb.
- Mother's blood is Rh –ve with a Rh +ve baby.

Porphyria

- It is due to increased production of porphyrin pigments in the body.
- Patient is **hypersensitive** to light.
- Red colour urine.
- Porphyrins get deposited in the teeth giving them purplish brown colour.

Cystic fibrosis

- Teeth are yellowish gray to dark brown.
- Patients are given TETRACYCLINE during childhood for its Rx, which causes discoloration of teeth.
- Mouth breathing and open bite due to nasal obstruction.
- Delayed dental development and erup.
- Seat the patient in an upright posture during treatment as in asthma.
- Low dental caries.

- Abnormal water and electrolyte transport across the epithelial cells.
- Involvement of multiple systems, e.g. pancreas, sweat glands, liver, GIT, respiratory system, etc.

Tetracycline Rx

- Teeth are yellow to brown in colour.
- Dentin is affected more as compared to enamel (9:1).
- Tetracycline forms chelate-complexes in the calcifying tissues which get deposited.
- Exposure of teeth to light causes oxidation and so colour changes from yellow to brown.
- Fluorescence occurs under UV light.
- Tetracycline can cross placenta and can affect the developing teeth.
- **Most critical period** = 4 to 9 months of age for the primary anterior; and 3–5 months to 7 yrs of age for permanent anteriors.
- Rx = is by vital bleaching; done by 35% H_2O_2 + ethyl ether solution (5:1) at 120°F for 30–40 sec. It decreases the oxidation process and so discoloration of teeth under light.

CONDITIONS OF TONGUE

Circumvallate papillae	Are 10–15 in no. Largest size, have taste buds, are vascularized.
Fungiform/mushroom shaped papillae	Present on the dorsum of the tongue esp. tip and lateral margins vascularized.
Filiform	Most numerous thin and hair like evenly present on dorsal surface of tongue no. vascularization.

CONDITIONS OF TONGUE (*Contd.*)

Foliate	Arranged in folds along the lateral margins of tongue taste sensation is associated with them.
Macroglossia	Is over-development of lingual ms, e.g. in cretinism/hyperthyroidism in infants in Downs syndrome. Abnormal growth of jaws with class III m.o. and flared lower incisors and generalized spacing tongue is fissured and crenated due to continuous pressure of teeth on the lateral border of tongue.
Ankyloglossia	i.e. tongue tie due to forward attachment of the lingual frenum on the ventral surface of tongue. Speech problems due to restricted tongue movement. Stripping of lingual tissues may occur in anterior region. Nursing problems in infants. Partial ankyloglossia is more common. Rx = lingual frenectomy.
Fissured tongue	e.g. seen in cretinism, Downs syndrome. Vitamin B deficiency.
White straw berry tongue	Enlargement of FUNGIFORM PAPILLAE, e.g. in scarlet fever.
Black hairy tongue	Enlargement of FILIFORM PAPILLAE in middle 3rd of tongue due to prolonged antibiotics Rx.
Geographic tongue	Also known as benign migratory glossitis due to lack of FILIFORM PAPILLAE.

CONDITIONS OF TONGUE (*Contd.*)

	H/E = desquamation of keratin layers of papillae and inflammation of corium.
Medial rhomboid glossitis	Seen immediately anterior to circumvallate papillae. No FILIFORM PAPILLAE, due to *Candida albicans* infections.

ABNORMAL LABIAL FRENUM

- Labial frenum has 2 layers of **epithelium** enclosing **loose vascular connective tissue**. **Muscles fibers are absent**, but if present, the fibers are from orbicualris oris m.
- Arises at the midline on the inner surface of lip and inserted in the midline in the outer layer of periosteum and in the connective tissue of internal maxillary suture and alveolar process.
- It is attached to palatine papilla at birth and **receds with the growth** of alveolar process.
- Diagnosis = by BLANCH TEST.
- It causes midline diastema if remains attached to palatine papilla, as it does not allow the approximation of max CIs after eruption of permanent canines.
- Orthodontic closure of midline diastema = **wait till eruption of permanent canines**. Then close the spaces. Frenectomy/ **Wanton's clipping** is to be done only after orthodontic closure.
- If frenectomy is done before ortho Rx = the **elastic scar tissue** formed will not allow the closure of space and will lead to relapse.

ERUPTION OF TEETH (See ortho section and oral path section also in Vol. I)

1. Max teeth are ahead of mandibular teeth in the development.
2. Teeth of females erupt earlier than males.
3. Mandibular teeth erupt earlier than max teeth.

4. First clinical sign of tooth eruption in a child is increased salivation and a habit of poking finger in the mouth.
5. A variation of 6 months of the usual eruption time is considered normal for primary teeth.
6. Teeth start moving in the bone when 1/2–2/3rd root has been formed and erupt in the oral cavity when 3/4th root has been formed.
7. Teeth move 1 mm in 3–4 months period in bone during eruption under normal eruptive forces.
8. Enamel calcification requires 2 more yrs to be completed after eruption in p.o. saliva.
9. Development of tooth starts at 11 weeks, i.e.
10. No tooth erupts in oral cavity during 9 yrs of age, i.e. a period of quiescence.
11. Hammock–ligament theory is the most important theory for eruption. Changes occur in the intermediate layer of PDL.
12. Interval between crown completion and until the tooth is in full occlusion is approx 5 yrs for the permanent teeth.
13. Mandibular 6 is often the first permanent tooth to erupt in oral cavity.
14. Sequence of eruption in mandibular arch is 6 1 2 3 4 5 7 8; in max arch is 6 1 2 4 5 3 7 8 or 6 1 2 4 3 5 7 8.
15. It is desirable that mandibular 3 erupts before 4, 5. It helps in maintaining adequate arch length and prevents lingual tipping of incisors.
16. If 7 erupts before 5 in any arch, it may lead to loss of arch length as it may push 6 mesially and loss of E-space occurs.
17. If lower incisors erupt lingually and slightly crowded (< 2 mm), before 7½ yrs age—then no intervention should be done, as it may resolve itself by tongue forces, alveolar and basal growth of jaws.
18. **Natal teeth** = i.e. which are present at birth.
19. **Neonatal teeth** = erupt during first 30 days of life.
20. 85% of natal/neonatal teeth are lower deciduous incisors. They should not be removed if not supernumerary.

21. **Epstein's pearls** = along the midpalatine raphe. It is the remnants of epithelial tissue trapped along the raphe.
22. **Bohn's nodules** = present along the buccal and lingual aspects of dental ridges. These are remnants of mucous glands tissues.
23. **Dental lamina cysts** = present on the crest of U/L ridges. Arise from remnants of dental lamina.
24. **Eruption cysts** = bluish purple fluid filled area; esp. in E and 6 regions.

DEVELOPMENT OF DENTITION

A. Gum pads: Dental arches till no teeth erupted are known as gum pads.

- Touch in future primary first molar region only.
- Anterior open bite is present which helps in tongue positioning during suckling.
- Anter or overjet due to smaller lower jaw.

Gum pads

Transverse groove	Divides the pads in 10 segments.	Correspond to the deciduous teeth.
Lateral sulcus	Lies b/w C and D.	
Gingival groove	Separates the gum pad from palate.	
Dental groove	Starts in incisive papilla region; extends backwards to touch gingival groove in canine region and then laterally to end in molar region.	
U and L gum pads contact	In D region only.	Overjet all around.
Shape	U = horse-shoe shaped. L = U-shaped.	

- ♦ Posterior overjet due to wider upper arch than lower.
- ♦ Intercuspation of occlusal height in primary dentition establishes for the first time = at eruption of primary first molars only.
- ♦ Tongue lies in b/w the gum pads and helps in suckling.
- ♦ Upper gum pad is horse-shoe shaped and lower is U-shaped.

B. Baume's classification of PRIMARY MOLARS occlusion.

- Flush terminal plane 76% (to be observed most critically).
- Mesial step 14%.
- Distal step 10%.

- ♦ **Distal step** = (a) changes to Class II, if minimum growth differential is there. (b) changes in end-on, by loss of leeway space and forward mandibular growth.
- ♦ **FTP** = (a) end-on if minimum growth differential is there.
  (b) in Class I, due to loss of leeway space of mandibular E.
  (c) in Class II, if maxillary E is lost before mandibular E.
- ♦ **Mesial step** = (a) to Class I, if minimum growth differential is there.
  (b) to Class III, due to loss of leeway space and forward mandibular growth.

Spacing in deciduous dentition = if present, it is known as **open dentition.** If absent, it is known as **closed dentition.**

Class	If deciduous teeth	Crowding chances in permanent teeth
I	Crowded	10 in 10
II	No spaces	7 in 10
III	< = 3 mm spacing	5 in 10
IV	3–6 mm spacing	2 in 10
V	> 6 mm spacing	None

Primary spacing/physiological/developmental spacing = occurs due to growth, helps in proper alignment of bigger size permanent teeth, 70% in maxilla and 63% in mandible.

Primate/simian/anthropoid spaces are found mesial to primary maxillary canines and distal to primary mandibular canines, named as it is found in primates, i.e. between BC/CD.

C. Mixed dentition period

- Begins with the eruption of first permanent molars at 6 years of age, generally in end-on relationship, marks the Stage I of natural bite opening.
- **First transitional period/early MDP** = eruption of 6, 1, 2, mostly lower erupt first, 6–8 years age.
- Correction of FTP/end on relation to Class I occurs by utilisation of physiologic space, leeway space and differential forward growth of the mandible.
- **Early mesial shift** occurs in **open dentition at 6–7 years**, due to closure of primate spaces by pressure of erupting molars.
- **Late mesial shift** occurs **in closed dentition at 10–11 years**, due to closure of leeway spaces after shedding of primary second molars.
- **Incisal liability** = difference between sizes of primary and permanent incisors, 7 mm in upper and 5 mm in lower arch; overcome by—utilisation of inter-dental spacing, incisor inclination labially, increased intercanine width.

(Warren Mayne's principles)

Method	Maxilla	Mandible
I/D spacing	0–10 mm, av = 4 mm	0–6 mm, av = 3 mm
Increase in intercanine width	4.5 mm	3 mm
Incisor position	2.2 mm	1.3 mm

- **Incisor liability** = difference in sizes of permanent and primary teeth, space comes from 3 sources.
  1. Increase intercanine width = 2 mm, M > F, U > L.
     Girls have greater liability to incisor crowding.
  2. Labial positioning of permanent incisors = 1–2 mm.
  3. Repositioning of mandibular, canines distally in primate spaces when mandibular LIs erupt = 1 mm space. (But not in (U) Arch, as primate space is between B and C.
- If a child has FTP in MDP, then approx 3.5 mm of movement of mandibular first molar forward with respect to maxillary first molar is required for smooth, transition to Class I relation in permanent DP (i.e. a one half cusp transition in molar relation).
- **Inter-transitional period** = is a quite period, 8–10 years of age, no change in dentition occurs.
- **Late mixed dentition/second transitional period** = eruption of 3, 4, 5, leeway space of Nance is the difference between MD sizes of CDE and 345; 1.8 mm in maxilla and 3.4 mm in mandible; mostly due to primary mandibular second molar known as **E-space** (2–3 mm), helps in late mesial shift to achieve Class I molars.
- **Significance of pronounced attrition** in MDP is observed to help in—decrease in deep bite, prevent interlocking and thus, paving way to unhindered forward growth of mandible.
- **Deep bite decreases** by—eruption of permanent molars, attrition of incisors, and forward movement of mandible due to growth.
- **Intercanine width** increases more in spaced dentition, more in maxilla, up to a later age in maxilla.
- **Secondary spacing** occurs in closed dentition, with eruption of lower incisors, which pushes primary mandibular canine laterally. It creates space for proper eruption of maxillary lateral incisors. It helps to increase the intercanine width in both arches and increase in arch circumference in maxilla.

- **Ugly duckling stage of broadbent** = in maxillary, 8–9 years age, canines pressing roots of laterals, root crowding, crowns move distally, spaces develop should not be disturbed till eruption of canines, is a self correcting anomaly.
- Arch length decreases by 2–3 mm when MDP changes to PDP, both from anterior and posterior sides. Also posterior teeth move mesially throughout life due to attrition and anterior component of force.
- **Largest arch length = is before eruption of first permanent molar.**
- **Signs of incipient malocclusion** are = lack of inter-dental spacing in primary dentition, crowding in permanent incisors in MDP and premature loss of primary canines esp mandibular.
- Transition in chewing pattern develops in conjunction with eruption of permanent canines at age 12 years.

Self-correcting anomalies

Gum pads Stage	Primary D P	Mixed DP
Open bite	Deep bite	End–on molars
Increased overjet	FTP	Ugly–duckling stage
Tongue in between gum pads	Primary spacing Primate spacing Small mandible More upright incisors	< 2 mm of lower incisors crowding

- According to Owen, the Space loss (due to caries) is most likely in mandibular deciduous second molar area.
- Arch length decreases during change from the mixed dentition to permanent dentition. It is mainly due to loss of E-space.
- Arch circumference and width increase with growth of jaw bases.

- **Chewing pattern of child vs adult** = adult opens straight and then lateral/child moves laterally.

Natural bite opening: Occurs at 6, 12, 18 years of age, with eruption of permanent molars.

- 3 periods of bite opening (Schwarz).
- 6 years = when Ist molar erupts, 12 years = 2nd molar erupts, 18 years = 3rd molar erupts. It is due to that soft tissues covering the erupting molars touch each other and so patient feels pain and he keeps then in non-occlusion. So a gap is created anterior to them, in which the premolars are free to supra-erupt.
- U/L permanent incisors erupt lingual to primary teeth and move forward under tongue pressure as they erupt.
- 7-8 years age = critical period.
- Sudden change during the eruption of the CI and LI is shown by = **1.5 mm crowding** in both M and F. Average females recovers slightly better than males.
- No great relief of crowding in incisor region is expected after full eruption of LI.
  - Maxillary CI seem to erupt from LABIAL.
  - Mandibular CI, LI seem to erupt from LINGUAL.
  - Maxillary LI = no labial gingival bulge.
  - Maxillary second molar erupts D and F.
  - Maxillary third molar erupts D and B and outward.

DENTAL CARIES

(Also refer to the sections in oral pathology and in operative dentistry.)

3 theories of caries:

1. Proteolysis theory (Gottlieb and Frisbie).
2. Proteolytic chelation theory.
3. Acidogenic/chemo-parasitic theory (Miller).

Proteolytic chelation theory

First, organic component of enamel is attacked and then the breakdown products make chelates with the tooth minerals.

Acidogenic theory: Is most popular.

Acid produced from carbohydrates first causes the DECALCIFICATION OF inorganic part and then the DISINTEGRATION OF organic part of the tooth.

- **Main bacteria** = *S mutans; S sanguis; S salivarius.*
- *S mutans* is not present in oral cavity of infants at birth and is detected only after primary teeth begin to erupt.
- **Sucrose** is the main culprit sugars for caries.
- **PH** of acid produced = 5.5–5.2.
- 0.2% **chlorhexidine gluconate** is an anti-plaque, anti-bacterial and anti-septic agent.
- Acid diffuses in enamel surface through organic inter-prismatic material and starts demineralising outer edges of HA crystals.
- Outer surface of enamel is more resistant to demineralization so the greatest amount of demineralization is seen **10–15 microns** below the enamel surface. It forms **incipient subsurface** caries and is seen as **white spot.**
- Remineralization of subsurface incipient lesion is possible only if the surface layer is intact. Saliva and fluorides help in it.

Incipient caries

- Early lesion seen as white spot. Due to sub-surface demineralization.
- Intact surface layer; can be remineralized under saliva.

Occult/hidden caries

- These cannot be diagnosed clinically but detected by R/G, etc. only, e.g. bite wing or OPG.
- Associated with low caries rate due to F exposure; hidden lesions also known as fluoride bombs/or fluoride syndrome.

- Other methods of detection are FOTI (fiber optic trans-illumination); ERM (electrical resistance method).

Arrested caries

- i.e. progress of lesion is stopped; open to oral environment.
- Also known as **eburnation of dentin.**
- Yellowish brown colour.

3 peaks of new caries lesions are seen at = 4–8 yrs; 11–19 yrs; 55–65 yrs ages.

In **rampant caries** = lower incisors (teeth/parts of teeth considered to be resistant to caries) are attacked.

In **nursing bottle caries** = upper incisors esp **labial surfaces** are attacked; the milk gets collected in this area.

Linear enamel caries = also known as **odontoclasis;** it occurs in neonatal line of max anterior primary teeth.

Grading of root caries (acc. to Billings 1986)

Property	**Grade 1**	**Grade 2**	**Grade 3**	**Grade 4**
Surface texture	Soft	Soft, irregular	Soft	Deeply penetrated
Dental explorer	Penetrable	Penetrable	Penetrable	Deeply penetrated
Surface defect	No	< 0.5 mm deep	> 0.5 mm deep	Deeply penetrated
Pigmen-tation	Light tan to dark brown	Tan to dark brown	Light brown to dark brown	Brown to dark brown
Synonyms	Initial	Shallow	Cavitation	Pulpal

- First national oral health survey done by IDA was in = 1984.
- Since the enamel calcification at the time of eruption of teeth is incomplete and requires 2 years for its completion by saliva; so

the teeth are more susceptible to caries during 1st 2 years after eruption.

- Environmental factors have greater influence on caries than the genetic factors.

CARIES PROCESS

Demineralization = occurs at critical pH of 5.5 or below (5.2– 5.5).

Remineralization = can occur if pH is neutral by buffering action and ions, e.g. Ca and PO_4 in saliva can inhibit the process of demineralization by COMMON ION EFFECT.

Buffering action of saliva is due to = Ca and PO_4 ions.

3 primary factors (given by KEYES 1960) for initiation of caries are = susceptible tooth; microflora and the local substrate.

4th factor added to above list by Newbrun, 1982 = time.

Ions like Se, Cd, Pb, Mn, Ba = increase caries.

Caries susceptibility of primary teeth = EDCBA.

Caries **susceptibility** of permanent teeth = first molars are most and the lower 1, 2, 3 are least susceptible.

Sequence of caries attack in primary teeth is = mandibular molars; max molars; max anteriors.

D are the less susceptible to caries than E.

Mandibular 6 are more susceptible to caries than max 6.

CARIES ACTIVITY TESTS

1. **Lactobacillus count** = by dentocult test.

   If count is > 10,000 cfu/ml = high caries.

   If < 1,000 cfu/ml = low risk. (cfu = colony forming unit).

2. ***Strept mutans* count** = it is not a reliable test. Based on the fact that bacitracin inhibits growth of all other strept except *S mutans*.

3. **Cariogram** = 5 sectors of pie diagram have been noted as:

Color	**Significance**
Green	Chance to avoid caries
Dark blue	Diet
Red	Bacteria
Light blue	Susceptibility
Yellow	Circumstances

4. Snyder test = bromocresol green is used.
5. Salivary reductase test = diazoresorcinol dye is used.
6. Enamel solubility test.
7. Alban test.
8. *S mutans* adherence test.
9. *S mutans* screening test.
10. Buffer capacity test.
11. Dewar's test.
12. Fosdick calcium dissolution test.
13. Viscosity measurement.

Sugar substitutes

1. Caloric sweeteners = sugars and sugar alcohols.
2. Non-caloric sweeteners = aspartame; acesulfamate potassium; saccharin; sucrolose; neotame.
   - Glucose/dextrose; fructose/levulose and invert sugars are caloric sweeteners.
   - Sorbitol is less cariogenic than sucrose.
   - Xylitol has anti-microbial, anti-plaque properties; and is sugar substitute for diabetics.
   - Sucrose, maltose; fructose are cariogenic sugars.
   - Cane sugar contains which carbohydrate = ?

Diagnosis of caries: Besides clinical examination; exploration; radiographs, the latest methods are:

1. **FOTI, fibre optic trans-illumination** = decayed part of the tooth has a lower index of light transmission than the sound tooth part, it appears as darker shadow. It is good esp for the anterior teeth.
2. **Fluorescence** = in the carious teeth, the emission spectra shifts towards RED range, i.e. more than 540 nm under UV light. With argon laser light, carious tissue appears dark, fiery, orange, red. Diagnodent is based on fluorescence.
3. **ERM, electronic resistance measurement** = increased conductance or decreased resistance show the p.o. hypo or demineralization. It occurs due to increased pore volume in enamel.
4. **Ultrasonic** = i.e. using sound waves for caries detection. At the cavity site, a higher amplitude echo is produced.
5. **Dyes**
   - For enamel caries = calcein; zyglo ZL-22.
   - For dentin caries = fuschin, acid red system, 9-aminoacridine.

Nursing caries = maxillary anterior teeth are carious due to accumulation of milk.

Mandibular anterior teeth are spared due to tongue coverage and salivary action.

C/f = neck of the tooth is involved in a ring like pattern along the gum line.

Rampant caries = is an acute, wide spread caries with early pulpal involvement of the teeth, which are usually **immune to caries**. Massler defined it as suddenly appearing, rapidly burrowing, wide spread and uncontrollable caries causing early involvement of pulp and involves those teeth/surfaces, which are immune to caries.

Caries rate = 10 or more lesions per year.

Proximal surfaces of lower anteriors involved.

Esp mandibular incisors are affected.

Rapid appearance of new lesions occurs.

PIT AND FISSURE SEALANTS: (Details in sec on dental material also Vol. II and operative dentistry in Vol. III).

Proposed by Hyatt 1923.

Fissures are filled with silver or cement as soon as the teeth erupted.

Fissure eradication: Deep retentive fissures are converted in cleansable areas.

Mainly, **BIS-GMA** is the material used as sealants.

Types of fissures: V, U, I, K types (given by Nango 1960).

U, V types are wide and self-cleansable; non-invasive technique is used to remove them.

I, K types are narrow and caries prone, so invasive techniques are used.

Sealants can be of = self curing type and light curing types.

1st generation	Cured by UV light
2nd generation	Self cure
3rd generation	Visible light
4th generation	Fluoride releasing

Age at which P and F sealants are used:

3–4 yrs	For primary molars
6–7 yrs	For first permanent molars
11–13 yrs	For 2nd permanent molars

Viscosity of sealants should be less, so that it may penetrate the deep and narrow fissures and in etched surface micro-porosities by CAPILLARY ACTION.

FLUORIDES (Refer to Vol. II sec on Fluorides.)

History

Year	Investigator	Inference
1901	McKay enamel	**Colorado stains**; mottled
1933	Dean	**Shoe leather** survey
1939	Dean and McKay	Dental fluorosis
1944–1959	Knutson, Arnold	Grand Rapids = muskegon study of water fluoridation. Grand Rapids = experimental town; NaF added at 1 ppm level muskegon = control town

History (*Contd.*)

Year	Investigator	Inference
1946–1960	Blayney, Hill, Zimmerman	Evanston = Oak Park study 40% reduction in caries noted
1961	Backer Dirks, et. al.	Dutch study 88% decrease in smooth surface caries, 43% decrease in P and F caries
1965	Ludwig	New Zealand study 69% decrease in smooth surface caries, 43% decrease in P and F caries
1969	**WHO**	**Recommended 1 ppm F in drinking water**

- Maximum F concentration is in the first formed enamel, near the incisal edges and in the enamel layer located at or near the tooth surface.
- Maximum fluoride is accumulated in cementum.
- F conc is very less near CEJ. So in young children, the enamel is more susceptible to demineralization around the neck of tooth.
- So topical F Rx in young children is better for prevention and also for remineralization of incipient caries.
- F inhibits enz **enolase activity** in bacteria and so inhibits bacterial metabolism and acid formation.
- Tea = has 97 ppm F.
- Fishes = 84.5 ppm F.
- F is completely and passively absorbed from stomach.
- F absorption is inhibited by the p.o. calcium or Al compounds.
- Principal route of F excretion is urine.

- F is deposited in hard tissues of the body.
- In bone, it is deposited in the area of most active growth.
- In enamel, it forms fluorapatite and fluor-hydroxy apatite crystals, which are more resistant to acid attack.
- Highest F in dentin is adjacent to odontoblastic layers.
- In blood, 75% of F is in plasma and 25% in RBCs.
- In saliva, the F is = 0.02–0.03 ppm average.

Percentage of caries reduction with various forms of fluorides

Procedure	**% reduction in caries**
Community water fluoridation	50–60
Salt fluoridation	40
Dietary supplements	50–85
Fluoride dentifrices	20–30
Topical fluoride/professionally	30–40
Topical fluoride/self-application	20–50

METHODS OF FLUORIDE ADMINISTRATION

- F from saliva decreases acid production in plaque by **inhibiting the activity of enz glucosyl transferase** and so the metabolism of sucrose/glucose, etc.
- F at higher conc is bact E and so multiple F therapy should be done for each patient.
- **Fluoridation** = i.e. systemic application of F, e.g. through water fluoridation. NaF was the first compound used for water fluoridation.
- **Fluoridisation** = i.e. topical application of F.
- **Topical Fluoride application**

2% NaF	0.91 ppm F available
8% SnF_2	1.95 ppm F
1.23 % APF gel	?

Compound	Properties
SnF_2	Bad taste, stains arrested lesions stains silicate cements, but not harmful to procelain, low pH = 2.1–2.3; should be freshly prepared; applied for 4 min once/twice per year.
APF; as known as **Brudevold**	Does not stain or cause pigmentation, but damages the porcelain restorations applied for 4 min, 2 times/year. APF is a mix of NaF, HF acid, H_3PO_4 acid. PH = 3–3.5 more effective than NaF.
2% NaF	Neutral apH acceptable taste, does not damage/discolour the restorations, but multiple Rx are required. NaF was the **first compound used** for water fluoridation.
Knutson technique	NaF is used. Apply at 3, 7, 11, 13 yrs of age, as at these ages, the new teeth also erupt. Apply for 4 min. Applied 4 times at one week interval, so total 4 × 4, i.e. 16 applications.
Natural defense mechanism of saliva	Lysozymes and other antibacterial factors. Salivary pH to neutralize the acid, Ca and P contents of saliva.

- **Para-sympathetic stimulation** causes flow of watery and profuse saliva.
- **Sympathetic stimulation** causes flow of scanty and thick saliva.
- **Choking-off phenomenon** = after application of NaF, a layer of CaF_2 is formed which interferes with further diffusion of F ions in enamel surface.

- **Systemic fluorides** = get incorporated in developing enamel, also have topical effects as it gets secreted in saliva and gingival fluid.
- **Recommended dose** of F for children above 3 yrs of age is = 1 mg/day.
- F makes the P and F more shallow and self-cleansing.
- **Halo–effect or diffusion** = beverages bottled in fluoridated areas get supplied to other fluoride-deficient areas and pass on the beneficial effects.
- **Recommended level** of F ions in water according to WHO 1971 = 0.7–1.2 ppm; WHO 1994 = 0.5–1.0 ppm.
- **Calculation of F levels** = ppm F = 0.34 E; where E = 0.38 + 0.0062 × temp in F°. E is the estimated water intake by the residents of that area.
- **Salt fluoridation** = mostly KF (250 mg/kg salt) and NaF (225 mg/kg salt) are used.
- Only 6 countries have set specific policies for salt fluoridation = Belgium; France; Germany; Spain; Swiss; Hungary.
- **School-water fluoridation** = higher conc of F is required in school water, because children are there in school for small no. of hours and consume less water during that period. 4–6 times more conc of F than community water is used.

DIETARY Fluoride SUPPLEMENTS: (revised 1999)

Age yrs	**Conc of F in drinking water ppm**		
Yrs	**< 0.3 ppm**	**0.3–0.6 ppm**	**> 0.6 ppm**
0–6 months	–	–	–
6 months–3 yrs	0.25 mg/day	–	–
3–6 yrs	0.5 mg/day	–	–
6–16 yrs	1.0 mg/day	–	–

FLUORIDE VARNISHES

- e.g. bifluoride; duraphet (21000 ppm F); fluorprotector (7000 ppm F); fluoritop.
- Applied twice/ycar.
- Forms a water tight film on tooth surface, stays for many days and action of F occurs on the enamel surface.
- **Iontophoresis:** a small electric current helps to drive F ions into the enamel.
- **Fluoride dentifrices:** have 1000–1500 ppm F.

Age yrs	Use of F tooth paste
< 4 yrs	No
4–6 yrs	Once/day
6–12 yrs	Twice/day
> 12 yrs	Thrice/day

Safety features of F

Lethal dose	35–70 mg of F/kg body wt, i.e. • 5–10 gms of NaF for adult of 70 kg. • 1–2 gm of NaF for a child of 15 kg. • Rx = induce vomitting; gastric lavage; milk; hydroxides of Al/Mg/Ca; milk of magnesia. • Calcium gluconate i/v to prevent shock.
Certainly lethal dose CLD	5–10 gm of NaF or 32–64 mg F/kg body wt.
Safely tolerated dose STD	1/4th of CLD, i.e. 1.25 gm NaF or 8–16 mg F/kg body wt.

DEFLUORIDATION

- **Ion exchange method** = by using bauxite; zeolite; charcoal; clay; magnesite, etc.

- **Precipitation method** = by alum; alum and lime; calcium chloride, etc.
- **Membrane separation method** = i.e. by reverse osmosis.
- **Nalgonda technique** = uses lime and alum.
- Calcined magnesite and Nalgonda tech combined.
- **Prasanti technology.**

RECENT METHODS OF CARIES PREVENTION

1. **Anti-plaque agents** = interfere with enz. Glucosyl transferase.
2. **Altering surface morphology**/increasing tooth resistance = i.e. by using surface-active polymers, acidified calcium phosphate solution applied and then a fluoride solution is applied.
3. **Lasers** = CO_2 laser is used.
4. **Bacterial replacement Rx** = i.e. by genetic engineering of the bacteria, e.g. **Strept. Gordoni** are being produced which produce enz. Mutanase and decrease the acidogenic potential of *S mutans* and decrease plaque adhesion.
5. **Self-assembling polypeptides/SAP** = are protective; help in enamel remineralization.
6. **Chewing gums** = are sugar free; contain xylitol, lacititol; and urea.
7. **Tooth friendly sweets** = are non-cariogenic sweeteners, e.g. lacititol.
8. **Microdentistry.**
9. **Teledentistry.**
10. Indigenous products, e.g. neem; mango leaves; tea, etc.
11. **Caries vaccine** = can be given by either oral or systemic routes; oral route stimulates secretory IgA antibodies via MALT/GALT; systemic route is concerned with the production of IgG antibodies; these antibodies act vs *S mutans* and prevent its colonisation; they give secondary immune response.
12. **Genetically modified apple** = they contain a fragment of peptide which prevents the *S mutans* from sticking the teeth.

ROLE OF CHLORHEXIDINE AND ITS MOA IN DENTISTRY

0.2% of chlorhexidine gluconate is used.

It is bacteriostatic at low conc and bactericidal at high conc.

It is anti-plaque; antiseptic and antibacterial.

ROLE and MOA of ZOE (Also refer to the section of operative dentistry Vol. III.)

It arrests the progress of a disease.

Transforms soft; painful carious dentin into hard; leathery; arrested lesion under ZOE.

Decreases the bacterial count.

Has soothing effect on pulp and decreases inflammation.

Bacteriostatic and cariostatic.

ROLE and MOA of $Ca(OH)_2$ (Refer to the section of operative dentistry Vol. III.)

Moller's index for the dental caries (1966)

Grade	Smooth surface caries	Pit and fissure caries
0	Sound surface	Sound
1	White opaque areas with loss of luster catching of probe	Discoloration of P and F with slight or no
2	Slight discontinuity in enamel	Definite sticking of probe in P and F
3	A definite cavity with dentinal involvement	– do –
4	Probable pulp involvement	– do –

Moller's index for the dental caries (1966) (*Contd.*)

Grade	Smooth surface caries	Pit and fissure caries
Modification of moller's index		
5	Filled tooth	– do –
6	Tooth indicated for extraction	– do –
7	Tooth extracted due to caries	– do –
8	Unerupted tooth	– do –
9	Tooth missing due to other reasons	– do –

Dean's index for fluorosis

Index	Features
0	Normal enamel
0.5	**Questionable mottling** **Few white flecks**/spots
1	**Very mild mottling** Small opaque paper white areas scattered over the teeth involving < 25% tooth surfaces. Summit of cusps of premolars and 2nd molars are affected commonly.
2	**Mild mottling** More extensive **white, opaque areas** involving < 50% tooth surfaces
3	**Moderate mottling** All enamel surfaces affected **Attrition** with marked wear Brown staining

Dean's index for fluorosis (*Contd.*)

Index	Features
4	**Severe mottling** All enamel surfaces affected Marked enamel hypoplasia Discrete or confluent pitting **Corroded appearance** of tooth

Disclosing agents: e.g. erythrosin (FDC red); bismarc brown; mercurochrome; alpha-plac.

Disclosing solutions: (1) basic fuchsin + 95% ethanol; (2) KI + I_2 crystals + water + glycerine (3) wafers.

DENTIFRICES

Composition (Also refer to perio section in Vol. III.)

Abrasives	Dicalcium phosphate, ca—pyrophosphate, ca, mg carbonates, etc.
Foaming agents	Sodium laruryl sulfate.
Flavoring agents	Peppermint, spearmint, cinnamon, etc.
Humectants	Sorbitol, glycerol, propylene glycol, they prevent the hardening of pastes.
Binders	Natural gums, seaweed colloids, cellulose, etc. act as thickening agents.
Sweetening agents	Saccharine, sorbitol, etc.
Therapeutic agents	Fluorides.
Colouring agents	
Preservatives	
Anti-plaque agents	Triclosan, etc.
Medicines	Potassium nitrate as desensitising agents.

ORAL HYGIENE AIDS

Tooth brushes; floss; tooth picks; mouthwashes; dentifrices; datun; irrigation machines.

Types of tooth brushes: manual/powered; super soft/soft/medium/hard; straight/angled; small/medium/large; orthodontic brushes; interdental; proxa brush.

Style of bristles: pointed, straight, oblique, curved.

FLOSS: unitufted/multi-tufted, waxed/unwaxed.

METHODS OF TOOTH BRUSHING

According to 4 basic motions, there are:

1. Horizontal reciprocating = e.g. scrub method.
2. Vertical sweeping = e.g. roll and physiologic methods.
3. Circular motion = e.g. fones method.
4. Vibratory = Charters; Stillman; Bass methods.

A few **important points** regarding tooth brushing:

- Time taken for tooth brushing.
- Frequency of brushing.
- Force used during brushing.
- Most common and best method of brushing for a child.
- Surfaces to brush.
- No. of strokes.
- Age at which the child should see a dentist first.

Classification of children according to age.

- Infant
- Toddler
- Pre-school child
- Early school age child
- Pre-adolescent
- Adolescent

NUTRITIONAL ASPECTS

Weight gained during pregnancy.

1. 1 pound/month for first 3 months.
2. 1 pound/week for next 6 months.
3. Total weight gained = 25 lbs.
4. Average weight of infant at birth = 7.5 lbs.

- Alcohol intake during pregnancy causes fetal alcohol syndrome/ FAS.
- Ca and Mg interfere with Fe absorption.
- Most rapid period of growth in humans life = during first 6 months of life.
- Original birth weight of infant doubles at 6 months and triples at 1 yr of age.
- Breast feeding is best food till 4–6 months of age.
- Meat is best source of iron, as hemi iron.
- Milk is very poor in iron.
- Dietary calcium may protect against colon cancer.
- Carotene rich foods protect vs lung cancer.
- Hypertension is known as silent killer; it is associated with less calcium intake.
- Vitamin C = essential for collagen formation; decreases permeability of sulcular epithelium.
- Vitamin A = helps to maintain the integrity of epithelial tissues.
- Folic acid = required for the formation and maturation of RBCS and WBCs. It decreases permeability of sulcular epithelium and so decreases the inflammation.
- Vitamin E = acts as anti-oxidant; prevents free-radical formation; increases cell membrane resistance and inhibits prostaglandins formations.
- Calcium and phosphorus = adequate dietary ratio of Ca and P is 2:1.

- In hyper-parathyroidism = minerals get lost from bones, leading to osteroporosis and reduction in density and trabeculation of bones esp of alveolar bones.
- Periodontal disease may result from a low Ca or high P intake.
- Artificial sweeteners = e.g. saccharin; aspartame, etc.

LOCAL ANAESTHESIA (Refer to Vol. I also.)

- Local anaesthesia is defined as a loss of sensation in a circumscribed area of body caused by a depression of excitation in nerve endings or an inhibition of the conduction process in peripheral nerves.
- **Esters of benzoic acids** = e.g. butacaine, cocaine, ethyl amino benzoate, benzocaine, hexylcaine, piperocaine, tetracaine.
- **Esters of PABA** = chloroprocaine, prociane, propoxycaine, etc.
- **Amides** = articaine, bupivacaine, dibucaine, etidocaine, lidocaine, mepivacaine, prilocaine.
- **Quinolone** = centbucridine.
- LA prevents the normal passage of ions through the nerve membrane thus preventing the conduction of nerve impulses.
- Nerve membrane is a lipo-protein membrane; with resting potential at 70 mV.
- Intracellular fluid has mainly K^+ and extracellular fluid has Na^+ ions.
- Inside of resting nerve membrane is **negatively charged.**
- On stimulus, the trans-membrane potential increases to firing threshold, i.e. 40–55 mV, due to entry of Na^+ ions inside, and so **partial depolarization** occurs.
- LA stabilises the nerve membrane and blocks the normal passage of ions through the membrane.
- **Surface charge theory** = suggests that LA may increase binding of Ca^{++} to nerve membrane. Ca^{++} is normally displaced from membrane during impulse transmission allowing increased access of Na^+ ions.
- **Membrane expansion theory** = LA binds to receptors on membrane thus increasing membrane stability and prevents opening of channels for passage of electrolytes.

Configuration of LA molecule

- Hydrophilic amide part helps its diffusion through interstitial fluid to reach at the nerve.
- Lipophilic aromatic part helps LA diffusion in lipid rich nerve membrane.
- Intermediate chain determines it as an ester or amide.
- Amide LA are metabolised in liver.
- Ester LA are metabolized by enz. plasma cholinesterase.

Composition of LA

LA agent **Vasoconstrictor**	Adrenaline.
Reducing agents	Sodium metabisulphite; it protects vasoconstrictor from oxidation.
Preservatives	Methyl paraben, capryl hydrocuprieno-toxin, it stabilises the LA.
Fungicide	Thymol.
Vehicle	Ringer's solution.

- Methyl paraben may cause hypersensitivity/allergy.
- All LA except cocaine have vasodilating effect.
- Vasoconstrictors are contra-indicated in thyrotoxicosis.
- Prilocaine undergoes more rapid biotransformation than other amides.
- Warning against lip biting should be given immediately and repeated to the parents and patient before sending them off the clinic.

Theories of mechanism of action

1. Acethycholine theory	Discarded	Dett Barn 1967
2. Calcium displacement theory	Discarded	Goldman 1966
3. Surface repulsion theory	Not credible	Wei 1969
4. Membrane expansion theory	Esp for benzocaine	Lee 1976
5. Specific receptor theory	Most accepted	Strichartz 1987

Specific receptor theory: according to it, the LA binds on receptors present on Na^+ channels and prevents entry of Na^+ into the cell.

TECHNIQUES OF LA

Local infiltration

- Given supra-periosteal.
- Small nerve endings in area of surgery.
- 0.6–1.0 ml solution only is used.
- Can be used for deciduous molars also, because cortical plate is less dense in children than in adults.

Field block

- LA is given near the large terminal nerve branches.
- e.g. injections above the apex of the tooth in maxilla.

Nerve block

- LA is given near the main nerve trunk, e.g. inferior alveolar block.
- 1.8–2.0 ml solution is used.

Intraligamentary

- Used for a single tooth.
- LA is injected under high pressure.
- e.g. by peri-press or ligamaject syringes.

- 30 gauge needle is used.
- 0.2 ml solution is used.

Inter-septal

- Used to reinforce infiltration analgesia.
- Esp used for primary mandibular molars.
- 0.1 ml solution is used.

Intrapapillary

Intrapulpal

Intra-osseous

Topical anaesthesia = e.g. benzocaine; action is in within 30 sec.

Pressure injection/jet injection = e.g. syrijet; at 2000 psi pressure and 0.05–0.2 ml amount of LA injected; produces surface anesthesia.

Peri-press syringe = used for PDL injections; 0.14 ml solution is deposited; no vasoconstrictor is required in LA solution; useful in **bleeding disorders, e.g. hemophilia.**

Inferior alveolar injection

1. in < 5 yrs age child = 0.5 cm below the level of OP.
2. in 6 yrs child = at the level of OP.
3. in > 6 yrs age child = above the level of OP.
4. Terminal ends of inferior alveolar nerves cross the midline to opposite sides to provide the double innervation to the incisors; so local infiltration in that area is also required. Labial cortical plate in lower incisor area is very thin.

Mandibular conduction anesthesia = also known as **Gow Gates** technique.

- Here, extra-oral landmarks are used.
- LA is deposited at the base of neck of condyle.
- Wider area is anesthetised.

Nerve fibers of greater/anterior palatine nerves usually extend to the canine area.

In the area of max primary molars—there is a plexus formation of middle and posterior superior alveolar nerves.

Infiltration for primary teeth should be made closer to gingival margin as compared to permanent teeth, because roots of primary teeth are shorter.

RECENT METHODS

1. Iontophoresis = i.e. for surface anesthesia.
2. Intra-oral lignocaine patch.
3. Jet injection = surface anaesthesia.
4. Computer controlled injection system = e.g. wand LA system.
5. Electronic dental anesthesia = e.g. TENS.
6. **Topical anesthesia.**

Sprays	10% lignocaine	e.g. nummit spray
Oinments	5% lignocaine	
Emulsions/ jellys	2% lignocaine	
Ethyl chloride	Volatile	Produces anesthesia **by refrigeration**
Benzocaine	As topical LA; safest	Ethyl ester of PABA
EMLA	Eutectic mixture of LA; by Clark 1986	Has lignocaine and prilocaine mixture

ORAL SURGERY/EXTRACTIONS IN CHILDREN

- **Cowhorn forceps and elevators are C/I** in children to avoid damage to the permanent tooth buds.
- Young and elastic bone of child and incomplete root development makes extraction easy.
- Anterior primary teeth should be luxated to labial—because permanent tooth bud is present on its lingual side.
- Posterior teeth should be delivered to lingual.
- Fissural cysts are rare in children.

- Dentigerous cysts are most common.
- Traumatic cyst = no lining or soft tissue contents are found in the cyst cavity.
- Eruption cyst = occurs on the alveolar ridge.

PHARMACOLOGIC MANAGEMENT OF PATIENT BEHAVIOR

Conscious sedation

- Only patients who are ASA Class I or II are routinely acceptable for conscious sedation.

Inhalation sedation: Also known as **relative analgesia.**

- Most frequently used method.
- Nitrous oxide gas is used.
- Gas has a partition coefficient of 0.47 in blood.
- It must be coupled with > 20% oxygen during sedation.
- Absorbed from lung alveoli; no biotransformation; gets rapidly excreted by lungs, when conc gradient is reversed.
- May lead to **diffusion hypoxia** when the sedation is reversed, so patient should be maintained at 100% oxygen for 5–10 min at 5 liters/min and also keep N_2O conc as low as possible.
- It is a CNS depressant; causes altered state of awareness.
- Prolonged exposure may lead to spontaneous abortions, hepatic diseases, etc.
- It is stored in BLUE cylinders.

Plane I	Moderate sedation and analgesia	5–25% N_2O
Plane II	Dissociation sedation and analgesia	25–45% N_2O
Plane III	Total anesthesia/analgesia	45–65% N_2O
Plane IV	Light anesthesia/contact with the patient is lost	65–85% N_2O

DOSE CALCULATION FORMULAE

Young's formula	CD = age × AD/(age + 12)
Dilling's	CD = age × AD/20
Augsberger's	% of AD = 0.7 × wt in lbs of child
Clark's rule	CD = wt of child in lbs × AD/150
Individual dose	CD = wt in Kg × AD/70
Individual dose	CD = surface area × AD/1.7
Bastedo's	CD = AD × (child's age + 3)/30

(CD = Child's dose; AD = Adult dose)

Oral sedation drugs

- Midazolam; phenergan.
- Most universally accepted method and easiest.
- Effects are dependent on absorption of drugs in GIT.
- At least 30–45 min are required before the procedure.

Intramuscular

- Best area is upper outer quadrent on gluteal region.
- Anterior latereal aspect of thigh in vastus lateralis m.
- Middle of the postero-lateral aspect of deltoid m.

Rectal route

- Enterohepatic system is bye-passed.
- Drugs enter the circulation directly through intestinal mucosa.
- Drugs through this route are excreted slowly and so a longer duration of effect is there.

Intra-venous

Most rapid, most efficient and reliable and safest route.

Agents used.

GENERAL ANESTHESIA (See pharmacology section.)

- **Halothane** is the most common agent used of the inhaled halogenated anesthetics agents; others are N_2O, enflurane; isoflurane, etc.
- PAC, i.e. **pre-anesthetic check up** of the patient is a must to rule out any contra-indication.
- **Pre-anesthetic medications/PAM** to allay anxiety and fear of the patient; to relax him; to decrease the secretions; and to decrease unwanted autonomic reflexes.
- Anti-cholinergics = most commonly used is atropine and recently the glyco1pyrrolate.
- Sedatives = e.g. benzodiazepines; barbiturates; chloral hydrate and meperidine; midazolam, etc.
- Anti-emetic agents = hydroxyzine, metaclopramide.
- Fentanyl and droperidol are used.

Intra-venous induction

- Most common agent used is 2.5% thiopental sodium.
- Pre-oxygenation with 100% O_2 for 2–5 min is done.

Important points

- Maintenance of GA is by inhalational agents, e.g. diethyl ether; halogenated hydrocarbons; they are generally combined with N_2O gas.
- Semiclosed system is most commonly used technique for inhalational GA; other techniques are insufflation; semi-open; open and closed systems.
- An anesthetic's potency is defined as the concentration of the agent required to inhibit response to a standard surgical stimulus. It is expressed in terms of MAC, i.e. minimal alveolar concentration; MAC values are additive, when different agents are used in combination.

DENTAL MATERIALS

(Also refer to Vol. II for dental materials and operative in Vol. III.)

Etching patterns: Are of the 3 types, i.e.

1. Type I = generalised roughening of enamel surface occurs; hollowing of prism centers; intact peripheral regions of enamel rods, i.e. **honey-comb appearance** occurs.
2. Type 2 = prism peripheries removed or heavily damaged.
3. Type 3 = mixed type 1 and 2.

Etching in deciduous teeth

- A **longer etching time;** approx 120 sec, is required for primary teeth, because of the lower mineral content and higher internal pore volume and so a larger amount of exogenous organic material than in the permanent teeth.
- Retention of sealants is better in permanent teeth than the deciduous teeth, because deciduous teeth have some **prism-less enamel** mainly in cervical region and so no resin tags are formed.
- Layer of P and F sealants is felt by an instrument known as THYMOZIN or by a blunt probe after polymerisation.

Advantages of acid etching

- Increases the surface area by 200 times; depth of grooves formed is around 20–50 microns.
- Micro-mechanical bonding; stronger bond.
- Proper surface cleaning occurs.
- Decreased/zero micro-leakage.

Restorative dentistry

(Refer to the sections of dental material in Vol. II and to operative dentistry in Vol. III).

Chemical removal of caries

- By CARIDEX.
- N-monochloro-DL-2-aminobutyrate/NMAB.

Morphologic considerations of deciduous teeth

- Crowns of deciduous molars are bell-shaped, with a definite constriction in CEJ.
- Due to sharp constriction of neck of primary teeth = special precautions in forming the GINGIVAL FLOOR in class II cavity preparation.
- Pulp horns of deciduous teeth are sharper and longer, so deeper cavity should be made with precautions.
- Greater buccal and lingual extensions at cervical area is required in proximal box due to broad-flat contact areas of the deciduous molars and distinct buccal bulge in gingival 3rd.
- Width of isthmus should be = 1/3rd of inter-cuspal distance or less.
- Axio-pulpal line angle should be bevelled to avoid stresses in the material.
- Contact areas between primary molars are broader and flatter and situated gingivally; but on permanent molars these are present occlusally.
- Furcation of primary molars is towards cervical areas.
- Reparative dentin formation in primary teeth is more than the permanent teeth.
- Innervation in primary teeth is less, so primary teeth are less sensitive to operative procedures than the permanent teeth.
- Inorganic content of primary teeth is less in enamel and dentin.
- Primary cementum is abundant; secondary cementum is absent.

Cavity varnish = it is placed before placement of amalgam to help in.

- Prevents/Decreases marginal leakage.
- Decreases discoloration of dentin.
- Decreases sensitivity.

Functions of cavity liners

- Protects the pulp from thermal shock.
- Insulates vs galvanic actions.

- Inhibits mercury penetration in dentin.
- Anodyne effect on pulp.
- Anti-bacterial.
- Neutralizes acid of cements, e.g. of silicates; zinc phosphate.
- Decreases marginal leakage, etc.

Classification of rubber dam sheets

- Thin = 0.15 mm.
- Medium = 0.20 mm.
- Heavy = 0.25 mm.
- Extra-heavy = 0.30 mm.
- Rubber dam sheet size = 5 × 5 inches.
- Main clamp for a first permanent molar = ivory no. 7.
- For distal surfaces of canines-silver amalgam is the best choice, because it is a stress bearing contact area.
- If porcelain laminates are used—the inside surface of laminate is etched with HF acid and then coated with silane.

Bonding agents: i.e. primer.

- Contains thinned BIS-GMA resins without fillers; hence having lower viscosity.
- So penetrates the etched surface by **capillary action.**
- Produces good wetting.

Dentin bonding agents (Refer to section of operative dentistry in Vol. 3.)

- To bond with dentin, e.g. phosphorus esters of BIS-GMA; polyurethanes.
- GLUMA; 4-META, etc.

Black's concept of cavity designing

1. Outline form = the cavity should extend to 0.5 mm depth in dentin and 0.2–0.3 mm clearance from the adjacent tooth.
2. Resistance form.
3. Retention form.

4. Convenience form.
5. Removal of remaining carious dentin.
6. Finishing and detailing of cavity.

Recent concept of cavity making

- Minimal invasive technique.
- Remineralisation of early caries lesions.
- Reduction in cariogenic bacteria.
- Repair rather than replacement of existing restorations.
- Disease control.

How to avoid iatrogenic damage to the pulp?

Dehydration	Avoid it to prevent the displacement of the nuclei/cells of dentinal tubules.
Depth of cavity	Minimum of 2 mm thick dentin is required for pulp protection.
Heat production	Avoid it.
Nature of cutting	Use carbide burs with coolants esp water.
Polishing	Use wet field to avoid heat production. At temp > 46° C = stasis and thrombosis of blood occurs. At temp > 55° C = necrosis occurs.
Pressure	At low speed = < 4 oz. At high speed = < 12 oz.
Speed of rotation	> 1.5–2.5 lac rpm with coolant is safest.

Class II cavity design in primary molars: Typical points are:

- Gingival floor of proximal box is wide due to broader contact areas.
- Box converges occlusally.
- Isthmus should not be > 1/3rd the inter-cuspal distance.

- Axio-pulpal line angle should be bevelled and rounded to avoid the stress concentration.
- Gingival seat should not be bevelled because enamel rods in cervical areas are oriented occlusally.
- Axial wall should follow contour of the external surface to avoid the pulp exposure.
- Avoid the MB pulp horn in D tooth.
- Young permanent teeth esp first molars are not mineralized properly; the P and F are deeper and not united completely, so they are more susceptible to caries.
- Kinetic Cavity Preparation: It uses **fine abrasive particles** at high speed and pressure. Dimensions/type/material of particles and pressure and speed.
- Only materials with polyacrylic acid can adhere to the tooth, e.g. GIC, polycarboxylate cement.
- **GIC powder** is calcium fluoro alumino silicate glasses and GIC liquid is poly-alkenoic acid.
- Classification and generations of GIC, i.e. cermet; miracle mix; reinforced; water setting and light cure types.
- **Anhydrous GIC** = in it, liquid used is either clean water or dilute tartaric acid. Polyacrylic acid is incorporated in powder.
- **Resin–modified** = 15–25% of HEMA is incorporated in liquid and < 1% of photo-initiators are added.
- **GIC** is bonded chemically to enamel through ION-EXCHANGE METHOD.

COMPOMER = i.e. GIC + composite resin.

- Has dehydrated polyalkenoic acid also.
- Complete absence of water, so **no ion exchange** possible.
- In it, no fluoride uptake possible so compomer **is not a fluoride reservoir.**
- It adheres by **acid etch-resin bond system** to the tooth.
- Setting reaction of GIC is ACID-BASE TYPE, with the formation of calcium poly-acrylate chains through ion-exchange method.

- Before filling GIC in the cavity—the cavity should be conditioned with 10% poly-acrylic acid for 10 sec to remove the smear layer and to increase the surface energy.
- **SMEAR LAYER** (Refer to operative in Vol. III).
- Always prevent the setting GIC from water contamination and so use varnish to cover it. Otherwise the ions formed will get washed away with saliva, etc. and no adhesion with tooth will occur.
- GIC has a low pH.
- ABC of GIC = adhesion; biocompatible; anti-caries.
- GIC is biocompatible because poly-acrylic acid/poly-alkenoic acid has larger molecules with high m wt. and complex chains, which cannot penetrate the dentin and pulp.
- Also, free F prevents S. mutans to make the enamel surface resistant and harder.
- Also Ca and PO_4 ions exchange occurs and help in remineralization.

RECENT METHODS OF RESTORATIONS

1. Preventive resin restoration
2. **ART technique,** i.e. atraumatic restorative treatment.
   - Uses GIC.
   - Originated in Zimbabwe and Thailand.
   - Ion-exchange adhesion with walls of cavity.
   - Only hand instrumentation is used for removal of caries.
3. **Lamination technique—Sandwic technique**
   - GIC as base/dentin substitute = ion–exchange and adhesion to dentin.
   - CR as enamel substitute = for strength and esthetics; enamel and GI are acid etched with 37% phosphoric acid for 15 sec; fill and light cure for 40 sec; use increments if required to build up the restorations.
   - Light should be held close to the material without touching it.

4. Other latest and conservative methods for Class II cavity making are = tunnel cavity; slot cavity/minibox; proximal approach.
5. **BRAX-1 gene** = is responsible for the control of **enamel growth;** can be used as bio-mimetic dental material.

Important points

- Surface energy of enamel is low and fluoride decreases it even more; so the surface does not easily attract plaque and other molecules.
- Surface energy of all restorative materials especially the metallic ones is higher and so more debris accumulates; it may lead to marginal deterioration and secondary caries.
- Cavity varnish and etching can help decrease the micro-leakage.
- During restorations, the shade of resin should be selected before rubber dam placement, because dehydration of tooth causes it to appear lighter than normal.
- A calcium hydroxide liner should be placed on dentin before acid **etching.**

Cavity varnish

- It is a natural rosin/synthetic resin dissolved in a volatile solvent, e.g. chloroform, ether or acetone.
- Leaves a thin film on the surface of approx 4 micron thick.
- 2–3 applications are done for making continuous film.
- Reduces microleakage.
- It is not a thermal insulator.
- Prevents discoloration of teeth by preventing diffusion of metallic ions from amalgam into enamel and dentin.
- It prevents the acid from $ZnPO_4$ cement from penetrating the dentin.
- It should not be used with composite resins, as the resin gets softened and with ZOE cement as the eugenol prevents the polymerisation.

- Micro-leakage in amalgam decreases with age, due to accumulation of corrosion products in the interface between cavity and restoration.

Cement bases

- Main function is to replace the lost thickness of dentin.
- It promotes the recovery of injured pulp and its protection.
- Is a thermal insulator and barrier to acid penetration.
- **At least 0.5 mm thick** it should be, to properly bear the loads.
- It should support the condensation and masticatory load.
- **Material of choice** = GIC with its obvious advantages of biocompatibility; anti-caries and strength. Other materials used are $ZnPO_4$, Calcium hydroxide, etc.
- If zinc phosphate is used as a base, the varnish should be applied.
- If ZOE or Calcium hydroxide is used as base, then the varnish is used above the base.

Mercury toxicity

- M: A ratio = 6:5, i.e. Hg should be = 54.5%.
- Eame's technique or minimal Hg technique = Hg is approx 40% or in 1:1 ratio.
- Primary risk to a dental person is through INHALATION OF Hg VAPORS.
- Maximum safe level = 50 micro gm/cubic meter of air.

Preventive measures

1. Well ventilated operatory.
2. Waste Hg/amalgam should be stored in sealed container under sulphide solution.
3. If spilled, then clean as soon as possible.
4. Do not use vacuum cleaners.
5. Mercury suppressant powders.
6. Wash the skin with soap and water.

7. Use water spray and suction while grinding amalgam.
8. Do not use ultrasonic condensers.
9. Periodic monitoring of exposure levels.
10. Remove gold jewellery while using Hg.
11. Do not mull amalgam on palm as Hg may penetrate through skin.
12. Avoid heat generation during polishing; use coolants.

Delayed expansion

- It is seen after 4–5 days of placement; amount.
- In Zn containing alloys (Zn > 0.01%) amalgams.
- Moisture contamination, e.g. by saliva contamination or mulling on palm; leads to formation of H_2 gas and cause expansion.
- May lead to extrusion of fillings, margin breakage, voids and pain on mastication.
- Use Zn-free alloys to avoid it.
- Do not mull amalgam on palm.

Silicate cements

- It releases **fluoride;** which is an **enzyme-inhibitor** in carbohydrate metabolism and so anti-cariogenic; it increases enamel hardness.
- It gets stained and **disintegrated in oral environment.**
- Average life = 4 yrs.
- It is C/I in **mouth breathers.**
- Acidic pH even after a longer period of placement = leads to pulp irritation.
- Its strength is less.

Zinc phosphate cements

- Acidic pH so pulp irritation.
- Cool mixing slab and wider area of mixing is used.
- Incremental addition/6 increments of powder during mixing is done.

- Mixing time = 90 sec.
- Good strength, used as bases below amalgam restorations.
- Use varnish below it to prevent acid penetration towards pulp.
- Acid base reaction is **exothermic.**

TREATMENT OF DEEP CARIES

INDIRECT PULP THERAPY/indirect pulp capping:

- As known as gross caries removal.
- Teeth with deep caries, which are free of symptoms of pulpitis should be selected.
- A bactericidal dressing of Calcium hydroxide is placed at the base and cavity is closed with ZOE mix.
- Leads to sclerosis of dentin and formation of reparative dentin and arrested caries.

Uses of calcium hydroxide	Uses of ZOE
Indirect pulp capping	Provides healing atmosphere to pulp
Direct pulp capping	Decreases pulp inflammation/ anodyne effect
As base/liner in deep cavity	Decreases the bacterial count
Apexification	Germicidal
Intra-canal medicament	Neutralize irritants
Weeping canal Rx	Arrests caries
Apexogenesis	Reparative dentin formation
Perforated RC	Sclerosis of dentin
Pulpotomy	Decreases acid penetration towards pulp
Internal resorption	Has a very good marginal sealing ability of cavities and so prevents marginal leakage
Crown/root fracture Rx	
During the acid etching	
Can promote osteogenesis within 2 days	

- Kept for 6–8 weeks, the dentin formation starts after approx 21 days.
- Also helps in neutralizing the irritants and reducing the pulpal irritations.
- It decreases the risk of direct pulp exposure and preserves pulp vitality.

ROLE/MOA of Calcium hydroxide (Refer to sec on operative in Vol. III.)

Calcium hydroxide in contact with pulp immediately causes severe pulpal inflammatory response. It causes **4 stages:**

1. Localised necrosis of pulp.
2. Inflammatory cells come there.
3. Undifferentiated mesenchymal cells proliferated and form odontoblasts.
4. Dentin formation occurs.

DIRECT PULP CAPPING

- Should be done for pin-point, small accidental exposure of pulp during cavity preparation under isolated sterile conditions; it should not be of long duration.
- Exposure should be surrounded by sound dentin.
- Pain should be absent.
- No bleeding should be there.
- Calcium hydroxide is the material of choice for capping, e.g. dycal.

PULPOTOMY

- Removal of coronal pulp, which is inflammed.
- Vital normal pulp left in root canals for healing and growth of the roots.
- **Calcium hydroxide pulpotomy** = is used in the Rx of permanent teeth esp with immature root development for apical closure/ apexogenesis; there should not be any symptoms of painful pulpitis.

- **Formoa-cresol pulpotomy** = use in deciduous teeth; Calcium hydroxide should not be used in deciduous teeth as it cause internal resorption and so early exfoliation of teeth occurs. 1:5 conc of formoa-cresol is placed for 5 min only. It causes fixation of pulpal tissues. Seal the cavity with ZOE, etc.
- **If pulp** tissue of RC appears hyperemic then RCT is indicated, as it shows that the pulp inflammation has spread to RC also.
- Pulpotomy is done for **posterior teeth only,** because anterior teeth have **no sub-pulpal wall.**

Formoa-cresol has = 19% formaldehyde + 35% cresol in a solution of 15 % glycerine and water.

MOA of formoa-cresol

- It has germicidal action and fixation properties.
- It prevents tissue autolysis by bonding to proteins.
- Pulp becomes fixed and fibrous and acidophilic within few minutes of application.
- After a few days of application 3 zones are seen:
  1. Zone of fixation.
  2. Zone of atrophy/cells and fibers decrease.
  3. Zone of inflammatory cells diffusing to the apex.
- No reparative dentin formation occurs.

GLUTRALDEHYDE

- 2% glutraldehyde is better than formoa-cresol.
- Bactericidal; superior fixative properties
- **Better than formoa-cresol,** because
  - Its action is irreversible.
  - It has larger molecules which do not penetrate beyond apical foramen (self–limiting penetration).
  - It fixes the pulp instantly with lower doses.
  - Lesser amount is absorbed systemically.

- Initial zone of fixation of pulp does not migrate apically and so pulp remains normal and vital, below fixed zone.

Capping materials containing antibiotics

When mixed with calcium hydroxide:

- The anti-bacterial activity of penicillin is entirely destroyed.
- Chlortetracycline retards proliferation of fibroblasts and interferes with pulp healing.
- Vancomycin is compatible and helps in stimulating the formation of reparative dentin.

TRAUMATIC INJURIES

ELLIS' CLASSIFICATION

Class	Features
I	Fracture crown involving little or no dentin.
II	Fracture crown involving dentin but no pulp.
III	Fracture of crown involving pulp.
IV	Non vital tooth with/with out loss of crown structure.
V	Tooth loss due to trauma.
VI	Fracture of root with/without loss of crown structure.
VII	Displacement of tooth without fracture of crown/ root.
	VIII Fracture of crown en-masse.
IX	Injury to the deciduous tooth.

- ♦ **Contusion** = injury due to **blunt** trauma.
- ♦ **Abrasion** = injury due to **friction.**
- ♦ **Laceration** = injury which causes discontinuity in skin or mucous membrane.

- **Avulsion** = loss of tissue due to trauma.
- **Avulsion flap** = undermined laceration.

WHO CLASSIFICATION?

Classification by Andersen (1981)

A. Injuries to the hard dental tissues and pulp

1. Crown infraction (N 873.60): An incomplete fracture (Crack) of the enamel without loss of the tooth substance.
2. Uncomplicated crown fracture: A fracture contained to the enamel (N 873.60) or involving enamel and dentin, but not exposing the pulp (N 873.61).
3. Complicated crown fracture (N 873.62): A fracture involving enamel and dentin and exposing the pulp.
4. Uncomplicated crown root fracture (N 873.64): A fracture involving enamel, dentin and cementum but not involving the pulp.
5. Complicated crown-root fracture (N 873.64): A fracture involving enamel, dentin and cementum and exposing pulp.
6. Root fracture (N 873.63): A fracture involving dentin, cementum and the pulp.

B. Injuries to the periodontal tissues

1. Concussion (N 873.66): An injury to the tooth supporting structures without abnormal loosening or displacement of the tooth, but with warded reaction to percussion.
2. Sub luxation (N 873.66): An injury to the tooth supporting structures with abnormal loosening, but without displacement of the tooth.
3. Intrusive luxation (central dislocation) (N 873.67): Displacement of the tooth into the alveolar bone. This injury is accompanied by communication or fracture of the alveolar socket.
4. Extrusive luxation (peripheral dislocation) partial avulsion (N 873.66): Partial displacement of the tooth out of its socket.

5. Lateral luxation (N 873.66): Displacement of the tooth in a direction other than axially. This is accompanied by communication or fracture of the alveolar socket.

6. Exarticulation (complete avulsion) (N 873.68): Completed displacement of the tooth out of its socket.

C. Injuries of the supporting bone

1. Communication of alveolar socket (mandible N 802.20, maxilla 802.40): Crushing and compression of the alveolar socket. This condition is found together with intrusive and lateral luxation.

2. Fracture of the alveolar socket wall (mandible N 802.20, maxilla N 802.40): A fracture contained to the facial or lingual socket wall.

3. Fracture of the alveolar process (mandible N 802.20, maxilla N 802.40): A fracture of the alveolar process which may or may not involve the alveolar socket.

4. Fracture of the mandible and maxilla (mandibular N 802.21, maxilla N 802.42): A fracture involving base of the mandible or maxilla and often the alveolar process/jaw fracture). The fracture may or may not involve the alveolar socket.

D. Injuries to gingiva or oral mucosa

1. Laceration of gingiva or oral mucosa (N 873.69): A shallow or deep wound in the mucosa resulting from a tear and usually produced by a sharp object.

2. Contusion of gingiva or oral mucosa (N 902.XO): A bruise usually produced by an impact from a blunt object and not accompanied by a break of the continuity in the mucosa, causing sub-mucosal haemorrhage.

3. Abrasion of gingiva or oral mucosa (N 910.00): A superficial wound produced by rubbing or scraping of the mucosa leaving a raw bleeding surface.

Injuries to hard dental tissue and pulp		**Injuries to PDL tissues**	
N 873.60	Crown infarction	N 873.66	Concussion
N 873.60	Uncomplicated crown fracture/ enamel	N 873.66	Subluxation
N 873.61	Uncomplicated crown fracture/ dentin	N 873.67	Intrusive luxation
N 873.62	Complicated crown fracture/pulp	N 873.66	Extrusive luxation
N 873.64	Uncomplicated crown-root fracture	N 873.66	Lateral luxation
N 873.64	Complicated crown-root fracture	N 873.68	Exarticulation
N 873.63	Root fracture		

Injuries of the supporting bone		**Injuries to gingiva oral mm**	
Comminution of alveolar socket	Md = N 802.20 Mx = N 802.40	Laceration	N 873.69
Fracture of alveolar socket wall	Md = N 802.20 Mx = N 802.40	Contusion	N 902.x0
Fracture of alveolar process	Md = N 802.20 Mx = N 802.40	Abrasion	N 910.00
Fracture of max and mandibular	Md = N 802.21 Mx = N 802.42		

Vitality tests

1. Heat test with gutta percha stick.
2. Ethyl chloride spray, conc., pressure, time.
3. Ice.
4. EPT.
5. CO_2 snow.

Electric pulp test EPT (Also refer the section of endodontics in Vol. I and operative in Vol. III.)

- A negative response is not reliable indicator soon after the injury, because the tooth is in a state of shock and may recover vitality after some time.
- If injured tooth requires more current than normal tooth—it shows that pulp is undergoing degeneration.
- If less current is required—it shows pulpal inflammation.
- EPT is frequently unreliable on normal teeth also with open apices.

Thermal tests: More details/temp/time/response, etc. (Also refer the section of endodontics in Vol. I and operative in Vol. III.)

- It is more reliable in testing primary incisors in young children.
- Failure of tooth to respond to heat shows pulpal necrosis.
- If less heat is required—it shows pulpal inflammation.
- More painful response to ice shows pulpal pathosis.
- A traumatized tooth may be in a state of shock and may not respond immediately. So tooth must be re-tested in 7–10 days for vitality.

Pulp capping/direct pulp therapy

- Done within 1–2 hrs of injury and the vital pulp and the exposure is small.
- Calcium hydroxide is the material of choice.
- Adequate seal against leakage is must.

- Exposure should be < 1 mm, i.e. minimal exposure, with minimum haemorrhage; and of < 24 hrs duration.
- Agents used = calcium hydroxide is the best; isobutyl cyanoacrylate; resin bonding agent; hybridization; e.g. by 4-META; laser (CO_2), etc.

Pulpotomy

- **Apexogenesis,** i.e. physiologic root end closure/development and formation.
- If pulp exposure is larger and the tooth is permanent with open apices; and/or root fracture.
- Done for a injury after several hrs-days, i.e. 72 hrs.
- Calcium hydroxide is the material of choice.
- Formoa-cresol can also be used.
- It helps in normal root end closure of an immature tooth, because pulp in the root canals is vital.
- Access to RCs is easier with formoa-cresol pulpotomy as compared to calcium pulpotomy.
- Best for Class III and IV fractures of young permanent teeth with vital pulps and open apices.
- Laser pulpotomy = by Nd–YAG laser.
- Electro-surgical pulpotomy = it carbonizes and the heat denatures the pulp and bacterial contamination.

Pulpectomy = i.e. complete removal of pulp from the tooth; as known as root canal treatment.

Blunder-buss canals = i.e. RC is funnel-shaped; the lumen of RC is largest at the apex and smallest at the cervical part. These are very difficult to obturate esp in children, as there is no apical base against which the obturation can be done.

Apexification: Suggested by Frank.

- Is the process of stimulating the root growth/apical closure after pulpal necrosis in young permanent teeth.

- Based on normal physiologic root development pattern to help apical development.
- Often a calcific bridge develops just coronal to the apex, against which obturation can be done.
- Calcium hydroxide is the material of choice, mixed with CMCP.
- At least 6 months time is required.
- Rxed teeth are brittle due to non-vitality and thin dentinal walls of the roots.

RC obturating materials for deciduous teeth

- ZOE paste = it is resorbable with the root resorption of deciduous teeth.
- Calcium hydroxide.
- KRI paste.
- Iodoform paste.
- Vitapex.
- Gutta-percha is C/I in deciduous teeth as it does not resorb with the deciduous tooth roots.

External root resorption

Starts from without and pulp may not be involved. It is of **3 types:**

1. Inflammatory.
2. Traumatic.
3. Replacement = leads to ankylosis.

Internal resorption = also known as **pink tooth of Mummery.**

- Starts within the pulp.
- It requires **3 factors** for perusal, i.e. constant source of irritation/ vital pulp/denudation of dentin, i.e. removal of predentin layer.
- If any of the above 3 factors is removed, then it can be stopped.
- Rx = RCT.
- Calcium hydroxide is the material of choice.

TIME OF STABILISATION

Injury type	Period of stabilisation
Avulsion	1 week
Subluxation	2 weeks
Extrusion	2–3 weeks
Intrusion	6–8 weeks
Lateral luxation	6–8 weeks
Root fracture	2–3 months
Periodic follow up	Every 6 months

INTRUSION OF DECIDUOUS TEETH: It may cause:

- Damage to labial surface of permanent tooth known as Turner's hypoplasia, because the permanent tooth bud lies lingual to the deciduous tooth.
- It may deflect the path of eruption of permanent tooth.
- May cause dilaceration of root of permanent tooth.
- Intruded deciduous teeth are watched as they tend to re-erupt in 3–4 weeks. No attempt is made to reposition them.
- Root resorption and pulp necrosis are most common sequalae of intrusion.
- Deciduous teeth which are displaced but not intruded should be repositioned.

INTRUSION OF PERMANENT TEETH

- The prognosis of pulp is more favorable if root formation is incomplete.
- Teeth with complete root formation undergo root resorption more rapidly than with incomplete root formation.
- Root resorption if occurs is more extensive and progressed rapidly in incomplete root developed teeth.
- Have poor prognosis than deciduous teeth. The Rx is gradual orthodontic repositioning in 3–4 weeks and then stabilising them for 3–4 weeks.

- RCT within 2–3 weeks should be done to prevent inflammatory root resorption.
- Immature teeth RCT should be done with calcium hydroxide.

AVULSION

- Rx is replantation as soon as possible.
- Root resorption of the tooth occurs.
- Ankylosis may occur; also known as replacement resorption.
- Success of replanted tooth depends on length of the time the tooth was out of the socket.
- For success, the PDL should be viable and undamaged.
- Most common tooth = maxillary CI especially in Class II div 1 m.o., and Class I type 2 m.o., it is more common in boys.
- If time gap is < 30 min the prognosis is more favorable.
- If open apex, the prognosis for revitality is more favorable; the RCT should be done if closed apex.
- **Storage media** = for transportation, the best medium is ISOTONIC SALINE; or milk; the acceptable medium is saliva, buccal sulcus of the patient. It helps to keep the PDL vital and prevents the dehydration of the PDL. **Heck's medium** is one of the best synthetic medium for storage and carrying the avulsed tooth.
- Cleaning = wash with isotonic saline or milk.
- Socket wall should not be scraped.
- Root of the tooth/PDL should not be abraded.
- Proper stabilisation 7–14 days during healing is required; it should allow some mobility of implanted tooth.
- Rigid stabilisation leads to ankylosis.
- RCT should be done during 1st week of injury and RC should be filled with calcium hydroxide only. It helps to avoid root resorption.

ROOT FRACTURE

- Is uncommon in deciduous teeth due to more pliable alveolar bone.
- Pulp in permanent tooth with root fracture as better chance to recover than non-fracture. It is because the force of trauma gets distributed during root fracture.
- Fracture in apical half gets repaired with good prognosis. Fracture in cervical part has poorest prognosis.
- **4 types of healing** is expected after root fracture.
  - Healing with calcified tissue = most favorable.
  - Healing with interposition of connective tissue.
  - Healing with interposition of connective tissue and bone.
  - Interposition of granulation tissue = it is least favorable.
  - It requires 2–3 months of rigid stabilisation for healing.
  - RCT with placement of intra-canal implants is a good procedure for treatment.

IMPORTANT POINTS

1. Periodic follow up of traumatized tooth = every 6 months.
2. RCT is must for displaced teeth.
3. Calcium hydroxide is the material of choice for RC fillings for at least 1 yr after, which obturation with gutta-percha is done.
4. Calcium hydroxide prevents the root resorption in traumatized teeth.
5. Calcium hydroxide helps apexification in immature teeth.

Speech sounds

Sibilants	S, Z
Linguo palatal	T, D
Labio-dental	F, V
Linguo-dental fricatives	TH, CH, SH
Linguo-alveolar continuants	L

MEDICAL CONDITIONS RELATED TO DENTAL CONDITIONS

DISABLED CHILD

Horizontal scrub method of brushing is recommended.

Fluoride rinsing.

Topical vancomycin = is plaque reducing agent.

Mental retardation

- Idiot IQ < 25.
- Imbecile IQ 25–50.
- Moron IQ 50–70.

Downs syndrome

- Head is brachycephalic.
- Tongue = macroglossia; scrotal tongue.
- Teeth = microdontia; over-retained deciduous teeth; oligodontia.
- Short stature.
- **Class III m.o**; maxillary hypoplasia.
- **Brushfield spots** are present in eyes as the specking of iris.
- Incidence of **leukemia** is 10–20 times more than the normal patient.
- Septal cardiac defects.
- Incidence = 1.5:1000; more in older females.

With a Deaf patient

1. Speak at natural pace and directly to the patient.
2. Do not use exagerated facial expressions.
3. Use tell-show-do approach or/and sight-taste-touch approach.

Cerebral palsy = patient has motor disability as a loss of impairment of voluntary ms control.

Intra-oral findings = caries; PD diseases; malocclusion; bruxism.

1. Monoplegia = involvement of one limb only.
2. Hemiplegia = involvement of one side of body.

3. Paraplegia = involvement of both legs only.
4. Diplegia = involvement of both legs with minimal involvement of both arms.
5. Quadriplegia = involvement of all 4 limbs.

1. **Spastic cerebral palsy** = 70% cases.
   - Involvement of **cerebral cortex.**
   - Increased motor tone, **stiffness** and difficulty in moving limbs.
   - Lack of control of neck ms/**head roll.**
   - Difficulty to maintain upright posture.
2. **Athetosis/dyskinetic** = 15%.
   - Involvement of **basal ganglia.**
   - Uncontrolled voluntary ms contraction.
   - Hypertonic neck ms; open mouth; **protruded tongue;** hypotonic perioral ms.
   - **BRUXISM.**
3. **Ataxia** = 5%.
   - **Cerebellar** involvement.
   - Involved ms **unable to contract** completely.
   - Lack of balance and staggering gait.

RHEUMATIC FEVER

- It is due to group A streptococcal pharyngeal infections.
- Most common in 6–15 yrs age group.

Jone's criteria

Major criteria	Minor criteria
• Carditis	• Fever
• Poly-arthritis	• Arthralgia
• Chorea	• Prolonged PR interval in ECG
• Subcutaneous nodules	• Increased ESR; + ve CRP test
• Erythema marginatum	• Previous history of Rheumatic fever

INFECTIVE BACTERIAL ENDOCARDITIS

- Is a microbial infection of heart valves/endocardium.
- Acute form = by staph; group A strept; *pneumonococcus.*
- Subacute form = by **strept viridans.**
- Embolization is a characteristic feature due to bacterial vegetation.
- Transient bacteremia is important cause of SABE.
- Prophylactic antibiotics Rx is must before any invasive procedure to control bacteremia esp in prosthetic heart valves.
- RCT in esp deciduous teeth and/or permanent teeth should not be done.

HEMOPHILIA

- **Hemophilia A** = factor 8 deficiency/classical hemophilia.
  - X-linked recessive.
  - In males only.
  - Females are carriers.
- **Hemophilia B** = factor 9 deficiency/Christmas' disease.
  - In hemophilia, there is **normal fibrinolytic mechanism,** but thrombin production is inadequate.
  - Also inhibitor antibodies are formed vs the host clotting factors and so patient has decreased ability to respond to replacement therapy.
  - DDAVP/**desmopressin** is an extremely useful adjunct for hemostasis in mild hemophilia–A.
  - Oral intubation is preferred oven nasal if GA is required.
  - **Von-willebrand** disease = is autosomal dominant.
  - Pt have decreased factor 8 activity and abnormal platelet functions.
  - **Hallmark of hemophilia** = haemorrhage in joints and ms.

Hemophilia classification

Degree	**% of factor 8 or 9**
Severe	< 1 %
Moderate	1–5 %
Mild	5–35 %

Treatment

- Factor replacement therapy = purified concentrates of missing factors are given.
- Epsilon-amino caproic acid.
- I/v DDAVP = desmopressin acectate in mild hemophilia is given. It is an anti-diuretic hormone and it increases the factor 8 activity and releases endogenoús factors normally bound to vascular basement membrane.
- Cryoprecipitate transfusion.

During extractions

- Intraligamentary LA injections can be given.
- Local infiltration can be given when hemostatic level is > 25–30%.
- **Block anesthesia should never be given**, as if bleeding occurs in deeper tissues, it is difficult to control by pressure.
- **Replacement therapy** should be given before sub-gingival scaling.
- Conventional **RCT is preferred** over extraction.
- **Intrapulpal injections** are safer.
- **Electro-surgical procedure is not recommended** in the absence of replacement Rx. It may cause spontaneous bleeding after several days due to clot lysis.
- **No suturing** should be done.
- **Minimal traumatic** procedure should be used.

Local hemostatic agents

- Pressure pack.
- Bovine thrombin/avitene.

- Chromostat; adrenaline pack.
- Stomadhesive = local intra-oral bandage.
- Oxidised cellulose.

Haemorrhage associated with lacerations of mucosa

- Single dose of factor concentrates to increase the levels to 50%.
- E-ACA infusions continued till epithelialisation is complete.
- No need of more infusion of factor concentrates.

Lacerations requiring suturing

- Repeated doses of factor concentrate.
- Level = 25% of normal is maintained.
- EACA continued to healing of wound.

For extraction of deciduous/permanent teeth

- Factor 8 levels required = approx 100%.
- Loading dose of EACA.
- Maintenance dose of EACA for 7–10 days post-operative.
- Extraction should be atraumatic.
- Avoid suturing.

LEUKEMIA: (Also refer oral pathology in Vol I.)

- Proliferation of abnormal leukocytes, which appear in blood as immature and undifferentiated blasts cells.
- ALL = most common in children.
- Common in Downs Syndrome and Bloom synd.
- Commonest in 2–5 yrs age.
- AML = bone marrow transplantation is the Rx of choice.
- **Erythro-leukemia** = is as known as **DiGuglielmo.**
- S/s = pt has anemia; thrombocytopenia and granulocytopenia, tachycardia, hepatosplenomegaly, petechia, gingival bleeding, infections, vague bone pains.

Chemotherapy = multiple drugs given.

- First phase know as induction = given for 4 weeks.
- Cranial vault and testes are irradiated at 28th day to prevent relapse.
- Anti-leukemic drugs do not cross blood-brain barrier, so intrathecal methotrexate is given; it is know as CNS-intensification stage.
- 3rd stage = maintenance; for 2–2.5 yrs.
- Follow up every 3rd month by bone marrow aspiration.
- Prognosis of non-lymphocytic leukemia is poor.

Oral S/S

- Gingival bleeding and **hypertrophy;** common in non-lymphocytic leukemia.
- Cranial N palsies; jaw pains.
- Regional lymph-adeno-pathy (LAP).
- Petechiae and ecchymosis = common in ALL.
- Stasis in small vessels lead to anoxia and ulcerations and necrosis.
- Thrombocytopenia = vascular integrity decreases and so petechia/ecchymosis occur.
- **Gingival hyperplasia** = due to infiltration of leukemic cells.
- **Strangulation of pulp and necrosis and pus** formation.
- **Necrosis of PDL** = loosening of teeth.
- Generalized osteoporosis due to enlargement of Haversian canals and Volkmann's canals.
- Osteolytic lesions due to focal areas of necrosis and haemorrhages.
- **Generalised loss of trabeculations,** loss of lamina dura; widening of PDL; destruction of crypts of developing teeth.

Dental Rx

1. Preventive Rx = is the best.
2. All elective procedures should be deferred in an uncontrolled or relapse case.

3. Pulp Rx of deciduous teeth is C/I.
4. RCT of permanent teeth of a chronic granulocytic suppressed patient is C/I.
5. A platelet count of 1,00,000/cubic mm is adequate.
6. If platelets are < 20,000/cubic mm, no elective dental Rx given, as there is a high risk of bleeding.
7. If absolute granulocytic count is < 1000/cubic mm, then all elective dental Rx should be deferred.
8. Infections is the **primary cause of death** in leukemia.
9. **Most common cause of death** after bone marrow transplantation = infections.
10. Immature WBCs cannot fight infections and signs of inflammation are also suppressed.
11. **Candidiasis** is very common due to immuno-suppression. Its Rx is nystatin (dose = 1 lac units/ml).
12. **Avoid aspirin** (anti-platelet functions).
13. Use soft nylon brushings.

ANEMIAS

Iron deficiency anemia	Microcytic, hypochromic anemia
Vitamin B_{12} deficiency anemia	Macrocytic anemia; seen in strict vegetarians
Folate deficiency anemia	Macrocytic anemia: Found in malabsorption syndrome Lack of folic acid intrinsic factor
Pernicious anemia	Due to lack of Vitamin B_{12} intrinsic factor Atrophy of filiform papillae Hunter's glossitis Beefy red tongue Painful glossy tongue

ANEMIAS (*Contd.*)

Hemolytic anemia	Premature destruction of RBCs Rx = by **splenectomy**; folic acid
Aplastic anemia	Due to bone marrow dysfunction Fanconi's anemia is of congenital type Neutropenia causes infections Rx = by antibiotics; bone marrow transplantation;immuno-suppressive drugs, etc.
Sickle cell anemia	**Autosomal recessive** Abnormal Hb is +nt known as Hb–S Occurs in reduced O_2—tension. Sickel shaped RBCs can lead to infarctions and tissue damage due to vaso-occlusion. Skeletal deformities Jaw pains, labial anesthesia Hypercementosis; dense lamina dura. Osteoporosis due to bone marrow hyperplasia Hypomeneralised dentin; calcifications in pulp. Multiple systems get involved. **Dental Rx** = antibiotics to prevent infections. If GA is used, then at least 30% O_2 is required inhalation sedation is safe. **Desferrioxamine mesylate** S/C and **hydroxyurea** given to increase the levels of HbF and to avoid vaso-occlusive crisis. Conservative and stress-free methods.

ANEMIAS (*Contd.*)

Thalassemia	An autosomal recessive trait **Decreased synthesis of alpha/beta globin** chains. **Decreased Hb** production. **Hypochromic, microcytic** anemia **Thalassemia–major is most common form**.S/S = appear **within first yr** of life. Hepatosplenomegaly, folate deficiency; and growth retardation. Hemosiderosis due to iron overload. **Oral S/S = chipmunk facies** = enlargement of maxilla and spacing of teeth and increased overjet. **Chicken wire appearance** of alveolar bone. **Hair-on-end appearance** of skull Large medullary cavities, thin cortices and generalized osteoporosis.

CLEFT LIP AND PALATE

(Also refer to the section of oral surgery in Vol. III; and orthodontic and oral pathology in Vol. I).

Causes are = multifactorial; polygenic; hereditary; rubella infections; Downs syndrome, Treacher-Collins syndrome, Pierre, Robin syndrome; fetal alcohol syndrome, etc.

Primary palate = includes philtrum and alveolus bearing 4 incisors and palate anterior to incisive foramen. It develops from fusion of MNP and maxillary process b/w 4–7 weeks of IUL.

Secondary palate = fusion of palatal shelves from maxillary process; occurs b/w 7–12 weeks of IUL.

Cleft lip = failure of fusion of MNP and maxillary process.

Cleft palate = non fusion of palatal shelves.

Incidence = CLP more in males.

Isolated CP more in females.

Unilateral is more common than bilateral.

Left side is more than right side.

Classifications: Veau's system:

- Group I = cleft of soft palate only.
- Group II = cleft of hard and soft palates till incisive foramen.
- Group III = unilateral complete cleft lip and palate.
- Group IV = bilateral complete cleft lip and palate.

Facial growth in unrepaired cleft cases

- Occurs normal.
- Only local bony defect is present.
- Abnormal development of dento-alveolar segment near cleft lip due to absence of normal lip pressure.

Facial growth after CL repair

Maxillary growth in anterior direction is inhibited by tight upper lip scar and so maxillary hypoplasia and skeletal Class III relation.

Mandible is free to grow due to anterior crossbite and so unimpeded mandibular growth may cause mandibular prognathism.

Effect of CP repair

Scar causes contracted maxilla and so posterior cross bite.

Scar has red elastic tissue, which leads to relapse of orthodontic Rx/expansion.

Problems associated with CLP

1. Speech problems and nasal twang = especially BDKPTG consonants are affected.
2. Middle ear infections.
3. Nasal regurgitation and feeding problems.

4. Esthetics.
5. Psychological.
6. Respiratory.
7. Asymmetry and deviations.
8. Malocclusions and periodontal problems.
9. Velopharyngeal incompetence.

Management

By inter-disciplinary approach.

Feeding advice and feeding plates.

Pre-surgical orthopedics in only selected cases.

CL repair = rule of 10, i.e.

- 10 gm % Hb.
- 10 week age.
- 10 lbs wt.
- 10,000 WBCs.

CP repair

For adequate speech development.

Controls nasal regurgitation and feeding.

Early repair = maxillary growth is retarded.

Late repair = 4–5 yrs age; speech problems develop; but can be controlled by giving obturators to the patients to cover the defect.

Alveolar graft = at 9–10 yrs age; provide bony medium for the proper eruption of maxillary canines.

Management

Stage I = maxillary orthopedic stage; 0–18 months.

1. **Obturator** = to improve feeding problems; cross-cut nipple is used; orthopedic molding of cleft segment is done.
2. **Premaxillary orthopedics** = 0–4–5 months; esp bilateral CLP with premaxillary protruded; and posterior segments collapsed. It helps in preventing lip dehiscence after surgery.

3. **Chieloplasty** = surgical lip repair; helps in suckling; improves esthetics; has molding action on maxilla.
4. **Maxillary orthopedics** = 3–9 months; obturator; prevents constriction effect of lip closure; patient is ready for primary cleft bone graft at 6–9 months.
5. **Bone grafting**

Primary bone graft	In patients < 2 yrs of age
Early secondary bone graft	B/w 2–4 yrs
Secondary bone graft	B/w 6–15 yrs
Late secondary bone graft	In adults

But, primary bone graft leads to antero-posterior deficiency of maxilla and crossbite; limitation of maxillary growth.

6. **Palatoplasty** = surgical palatal closure; at 1–2 yrs age; helps in deve opment of normal speech; but scar formed interferes with the ransverse growth of maxilla and so narrow maxillary arch; posterior crossbite; red elastic scar tissue leads to relapse of expansion.

Stage II = primary dentition stage; no particular Rx required except crossbites; growth assessment; oral hygiene; speech development; obturator can be given if palatal defect.

Stage III = mixed dentition period; very crucial stage; skeletal and dental conditions Rx is required; crossbite treated by expansion. Delaire's face mask and chin cap for control of skeletal conditions.

Secondary alveolar graft = gives medium for the erupting maxiuary canine; gives bony support to lip and ala of nose; placed at 9–11 yrs age when canines root is 1/4–1/2 formed. Expand the arches before grafting so that adequate bone graft may be placed and to avoid future defects problems during expansion if done later.

Stage IV = permanent dentition; 12–18 yrs; surgical option for skeletal discrepancy; cosmetic surgeries.

Over-denture = is a complete or partial removable denture supported by retained roots to provide support, stability and tactile and proprioception and to reduce ridge resorption.

Types = immediate over-denture; transitional over-denture; remote over-denture.

Immediate denture = which are constructed before all the remaining teeth have been removed and is inserted immediately after removal of remaining teeth.

Obturator = which is used to close a congenital or acquired opening in palate.

Types = feeding Obturator/surgical Obturator/interior Obturator/hollow Obturator/metal base Obturator/palatal Obturator/speech bulb type Obturator.

SPACE MANAGEMENT

- **Best space maintainer** = natural tooth.
- Loss of space may lead to = malocclusions; impaction of the erupting tooth, etc.
- Maximum amount of space loss occurs = during first 6 months after extractions.
- Untreated proximal caries may also cause space loss due to drifting of the teeth.
- Premature loss of primary tooth may cause impaction/retarded eruption of its counterpart permanent tooth; so use the space maintainer.
- At an average, 4–5 months are required to move through 1 mm of bone. If more bone is present, a tooth will take more time to erupt through it.
- Arch length decreases during eruption of permanent teeth due to loss of E-space/leeway space.
- If deep COS is present; a 1 mm linear space is required per side for every mm of depth of COS to level it.
- Space m/m is imp in posterior area of deciduous dentition than in anterior area.
- Early loss of mandibular E may lead to mesial drifting of mandibular 6, and thus loss of space. So guiding appliances are used, i.e. distal shoe/Roche's/Willet's appliance is inserted.

- If bilateral loss of teeth is to be prevented then use lingual holding arch or Nance palatal arch.
- If natural spacing is present in primary incisor area, then no space maintainer is required.
- Loss of first permanent molar before eruption of 2nd permanent molar at the age of 8–9 yrs causes bodily shift of 7 in place of 6.
- But if 6 is lost at a later age, i.e. during eruption of 7 or after eruption of 7 then mesial tipping of 7 occurs.
- Loss of primary canine can lead to distal tipping of incisors in the space. It may hamper with the inter-canine width increase in U/L arches. It may lead to midline shift.

Space analysis: (Refer to section of orthodontics for cast/space analyses.)

Appraisal	Mm	Clinical significance
Large space excess	+ 3 mm	Long term planning
Space excess	< + 3–0	Wait and watch; do nothing
Equivalency	0	Watch carefully
Deficiency	< 0 to –2 mm	Use mandibular lingual holding arch
Deficiency	– 3 to – 6 mm	Space regain/expansion
Large deficiency	> – 6 mm	Space regain/expansion/ extractions

Different methods of space analysis

- Nance's method
- Carey's analysis
- Johnston-Tanaka analysis
- Profitt's analysis
- Tweed's method
- Moyer's analysis

Classification of space maintainers

- Fixed/removable/semi-fixed
- Active/passive
- Functional/non-functional
- Banded/bonded
- Unilateral/bilateral
- Maxillary/mandibular
- e.g. band and loop, band and bar, Trans-Palatal Arch, Lingual Holding Arch, Lingual Holding Arch with U-loops in premolar regions, Nance Palatal Arch, RPD, distal loop appliance, lip bumper, etc.

HYPOTHYROIDISM: Delayed eruption of teeth.

Cretinism = i.e. congenital hyperthyroidism. It is present at birth; short arms and legs; i.e. dwarf. Jaws are smaller and so crowding is there. Delayed primary/pmt dentition; MACROGLOSSIA is there and so anterior openbite is there.

HYPOPITUITARISM : It does not appear before 4 yrs age; there is delayed dentition. Decreased or retarded growth; due to decreased GH; prolonged reunion of primary teeh.

ACHONDROPLASIA : Growth of limbs is limited due to lack of calcifications in cartilages of long bones. Head size is large; nasa bridge and maxilla are deficien; skeletal class III m.o. here is deficient growth of cranial base due to early closure of synchondroses; it is related to increased father age.

DELAYED ERUPTION: Is also seen in fibromatosis gingiva; rickets; Gardener syndrome; chondro–ectodermal dysplasia; Ellis-van Creveld syndrome.

SUGAR SUBSTITUTES

1. Caloric sweeteners = sugars and sugar alcohols.
2. Non-caloric sweeteners = e.g. aspartame; acesulfamate potassium; saccharin; sucrolose; neotame.

Glucose / dextrose, fructose / levulose and invert sugars are caloric sweeteners.

Sorbitol is less cariogenic than sucrose.

Xylitol has antimicrobial, antiplaque properties and is a sugar substitute for diabeties.

Sucrose, maltose, fructose are cariogenic sugars.

Cane sugar contains which carbohydrate.

DENTAL CARIES

3 THEORIES of caries:

1. Proteolysis theory by Gottlieb and Frisbie.
2. Proteolytic–chelation theory.
3. Acidogenic/chemico-parasitic theory by Miller.

Proteolytic chelation theory

- According to this concept, first organic component of enamel is attacked and then, the breakdown products chelates with the tooth minerals.

Acidogenic theory = it is the most popular theory.

- The acid produced from carbohydrate first causes the **decalcification of inorganic** part and then the **disintegration of organic** part of the tooth.
- Main bacteria = are *Strept. mutans; Strept sanguis; Strept salivarius.*
- Sucrose is the main cariogenic sugar.
- *S. mutans* is not present in oral cavity of infants at birth and is detected only after primary teeth begin to erupt.
- pH of acid produced = 5.5–5.2.
- 0.2% Chlorhexidine gluconate si anti-plaque agent. Details from article.
- Acids diffuse in enamel surface through organic inter-prismatic material and start demineralising outer edges of HA crystals.
- Outer surface of enamel is more resistant to demineralization, so the greatest amount of demineralization is seen 10–15 microns below the enamel surface. It forms the INCIPIENT subsurface CARIES lesion and is seen as the white spot.

- Remineralisation of subsurface lesion is possible only if the surface is intact, with the help of saliva. Fluoride is also helpful.
- 3 peaks of new caries lesions are seen at = 4–8 yrs; 11–19 yrs; 55–65 yrs.
- Since the enamel calcification at the time of eruption is incomplete, and it requires 2 yrs for its completion under saliva, so the teeth are more susceptible to caries during 1st 2 yrs of eruption. The pits and fissures are deeper in immature teeth.
- Environmental factors have greater influence on caries than the genetic factors.

Definitions

1. Incipient caries = it is the early lesion, seen as the white spot on the enamel surface, without continuity defect. There is subsurface demineralization. It can undergo remineralization.
2. Occult caries / hidden caries; these cannot be identified clinically but detected on R/G only, e.g. bite wing, OPG. Latest methods, e.g. FOTI (fiber optic trans-illumination) and ERM (electrical resistance method). It is associated with low caries rate due to

GRADING OF ROOT CARIES (According to Billings 1986)

Property	Grade 1	Grade 2	Grade 3	Grade 4
Surface texture	Soft	Soft, irregular	Soft	Deeply penetrated
Dental explorer	Penetrable	Penetrable	Penetrable	Deeply penetrated
Surface defects	No	< 0.5 mm deep	> 0.5 mm deep	Deeply penetrated
Pigmentation	Light tan to brown	Tan to dark brown	Light brown to dark brown	Brown to dark brown
Synonyms	Initial	Shallow	Cavitation	Pulpal

fluoride exposure; the hidden lesions as known as FLUORIDE BOMBS / FLUORIDE SYNDROME.

3. Arrested caries = i.e. progress of lesion is stopped; it is as known as eburnation of dentin.
4. In rampant caries= lower incisors are attacked.
5. In nursing caries = upper incisors are attacked, because milk gets pooled around these teeth.
6. Linear enamel caries = as known as odontoclasia; it occurs in neonatal line of max anterior primary teeth.

First national oral health survey conducted by IDA = was in 1984

About IDA.

CARIES PROCESS

- Demineralization = it occurs at a critical pH of 5.2–5.5 or below.
- Remineralization = can occur if pH is neutral by buffering and Ca and PO_4 ions in saliva can inhibit the process of dissolution by COMMON ION EFFECT.
- Buffer action of saliva is due to = PO_4 and CO_3 ions.
- 3 Primary factors for caries (given by KEYS, 1960) are susceptible host, i.e. tooth; microflora and local substrate.
- 4th factor, i.e. TIME was added by newborn 1982.
- Irradiations, enamel hypoplasia; vitamin deficiency; diabetes; protein deficiency during the dental development increase the chances of caries.
- Ions, e.g. Se, Cd, Pb, Mn, Ba = increase caries.
- Caries susceptibility of deci teeth is = EDCBA.
- Caries susceptibility of pmt teeth is = 6 are most susceptible and lower 1, 2, 3 are least susceptible teeth.
- Sequence of caries attack in deci teeth is = mand molars; max molars; max anteriors.
- D are less susceptible to caries than E.
- Mand 6 are more susceptible to caries than max 6.

CARIES ACTIVITY TESTS: Amina's seminar also:

1. Lactobacillus count = by dentocult test, i.e.

   if count > 10,000 cfu /ml = high activity.

   if count < 1,000 cfu /ml = low (CFU = colony forming units).

2. *Strept. mutans* count: It is not a very reliable test. It is based on the fact that bacitracin inhibits growth of all other strept except *S mutans*.

3. Cariogram = There are 5 sectors of pie diagram, i.e.

Green	Chance to avoid caries
Dark blue	Diet
Red	Bacteria
Light blue	Susceptibility
Yellow	Circumstances

4. Snyder test = bromocresol dye is used.
5. Salivary reductase test = diazo-resorcinol dye is used.
6. Enamel solubility test.
7. Alban test.
8. *S. mutans* adherence test.
9. *S. mutans* screening test.
10. Buffer capacity test.
11. Dewar's test.
12. Fosdick calcium dissolution test.
13. Viscosity measurement.

DIAGNOSIS OF CARIES: Exoloration; R/G

Among the latest methods are:

1. FOTI = decayed part of tooth has a lower index of light transmission than the sound tooth part, it appears as darker shadow; it is good esp for anterior teeth.

2. Fluorescence = in carious teeth, the emission spectra shift towards red range, i.e. more than 540 nm under UV light. With argon laser light, carious tissue appears dark, fiery, orange-red. DIAGNODENT is based on fluorescence.
3. Electronic resistance measurements/ERM = increased conductance or decreased resistance shows the p.o. hypo- or demineralization. It occurs due to increased pore volume in the enamel.
4. Ultrasonic = i.e. using sound waves for caries detection; a higher amplitude echo is produced at the cavity site.
5. Dyes = for enamel caries = calcein; zyglo ZL–22. For dentin caries, fuschin, acid red system, 9–aminoacridine.

NURSING AND RAMPANT CARIES

Nursing caries = max anterior teeth are carious due to milk pooling there.

Mand anterior teeth are spared due to tongue covering and salivary pooling there.

s/s = neck of the tooth is involved in a ring–like pattern, along the gumline.

Rampant caries = is an acute, widespread caries with early pulpal involvement of teeth which are usually immune to decay, e.g. mand incisors, cusp–tips, etc. are affected most. Here rapid appearance of new lesions occurs.

Massler defined rampant caries as: Suddenly-appearing, rapidly burrowing, wide spread and uncontrollable caries causing early involvement of pulp and involves those teeth/surfaces regarded as immune to caries.

Caries rate is = 10 or more lesions/yr.

Proximal surfaces of lower anteriors involved.

9

MCQs in Orthodontics and Pedodontics

1. Which of the following is most important to the orthodontist with regard to the time treatment should begin?
A. The chronologic age of the patient
B. The physiologic age of the patient
C. Dental age of the patient
D. None of the above

2. Continuous heavy orthodontic forces may cause:
A. The PDL to become crushed
B. Resorption of cementum
C. Resorption of the alveolar bone
D. All of the above

3. Which cusp listed below of the maxillary first permanent molar serves as a reference point in identifying Angle's Class I, II and III occlusions?
A. Distobuccal
B. Mesiobuccal
C. Mesiolingual
D. Distolingual

4. Which space maintainer is most often used when the primary first molar needs to be prematurely extracted?
A. "Band and loop" space maintainer
B. "Distal shoe" space maintainer

C. "Lingual arch" appliance
D. "Nance" appliance

5. A child with a pulpally involved primary tooth comes into your office. Which of the following ideally is the best space maintainer for this child?
A. A "band and loop" space maintainer
B. A "distal shoe" space maintainer
C. The pulpally involved primary tooth
D. A "lingual arch" space maintainer

6. Displacement of a tooth from the socket in the direction of eruption is referred to as:
A. Tipping
B. Translation
C. Extrusion
D. Intrusion
E. Torque
F. Rotation

7. Which of the following determines the effect of a facebow headgear on the molars to which it is attached?
A. The relation of the outer bow to the center of resistance of the tooth
B. The direction of pull of the headgear strap
C. The length and position of the outer bow in relation to the inner bow
D. All of the above

8. Serial extraction procedures involve:
A. The orderly removal of selected permanent teeth only in a predetermined sequence
B. The orderly removal of selected primary teeth only in a predetermined sequence
C. The orderly removal of selected primary and permanent teeth in a predetermined sequence
D. The orderly removal of selected wisdom teeth only

9. Which appliance listed below is probably the most widely used today by orthodontists?
A. The universal appliance

B. The edgewise appliance
C. Begg's appliance
D. Removal appliance
E. Neither of the above

10. Which of the following alloys are used for archwires in orthodontics?

A. Stainless steel
B. Chromium-cobalt
C. Nickle—Titanium
D. All of the above

11. Which of the following are common characteristics of a Class II, Division 2 malocclusion?

A. The maxillary centrals are near normal anteroposteriorly or slightly in linguoversion
B. The maxillary lateral incisors are usually labiomesially flared and overlap the central incisors
C. Impinging overbite
D. All of the above

12. Conditions that may complicate molar uprighting include:

A. A high mandibular plane and open bite
B. Poor crown-to-root ratio and/or short roots
C. A severe lingual inclination of the tooth in addition to the mesial tipping
D. Occlusal plane disharmony (i.e. extruded maxillary and mandibular molars)
E. All of the above

13. A seven year old child with an otherwise good occlusion has a lingually locked maxillary permanent central incisor. There is sufficient overbite. What should be done?

A. Wait until all permanent teeth have erupted
B. Surgically reposition the central incisor
C. Correct the condition immediately with a simple appliance
D. None of the above

14. A diastema between erupting permanent maxillary incisors may indicate which of the following?

A. A normal stage of development before eruption of canines

B. It may be related to tooth size discrepancy or a mesiodens
C. It may indicate an abnormal frenum attachment
D. All of the above

15. A steep mandibular plane angle correlates with a:
A. Short anterior facial vertical dimensions and anterior open bite malocclusion
B. Long anterior facial vertical dimensions and anterior open bite malocclusion
C. Short anterior facial vertical dimensions and anterior deep bite malocclusion
D. Long anterior facial vertical dimensions and anterior deep bite malocclusion

16. A 13-year old patient has all teeth present and normal occlusion, molar root apices are not totally closed. The mandibular left first molar has been extracted. The ideal treatment at this time is what?
A. Place a fixed bridge
B. Place a space maintainer
C. Place a removable partial denture
D. Do nothing and observe

17. In a young child, which structure listed below grows in height and length to accommodate the developing dentition?
A. The tuberosity
B. The ramus
C. The condyles
D. The alveolar process

18. Class III malocclusion is also referred to as:
A. Retrognathism
B. Prognathism
C. Proclination
D. Neither of the above

19. A severe malocclusion may compromise which of the following aspects of oral function?
A. Mastication
B. Swallowing

C. Speech
D. All of the above

20. Displaced teeth related to functional shifts are usually seen in which two of the following circumstances?
A. Posterior crossbite after prolonged thumb sucking
B. Class II, Division I malocclusion
C. Anterior crossbite in mildly prognathic children
D. An anterior open bite after prolonged thumb sucking

21. An appropriate candidate for post-orthodontic circumferential supracrestal fibrotomy is:
A. An intruded mandibular second molar
B. A rotated maxillary lateral incisor
C. An extruded maxillary second premolar
D. A mandibular first molar that is in crossbite

22. The flat bones of the skull and part of the clavicle are formed by:
A. Intramembranous ossification
B. Endochondral ossification
C. Erythropoiesis
D. Epiphyseal formation

23. Relative to the primary mandibular canines, the permanent mandibular canines erupt:
A. Lingually
B. Facially
C. Distally
D. Mesially

24. Class I malocclusions share what basic characteristic?
A. The midface is concave
B. A harmonious skeletal profile
C. The midface is convex
D. None of the above

25. Which of the following are uses of cephalometrics in orthodontics?
A. Diagnosis
B. Analysis of treatment results

C. Longitudinal study of growth
D. All of the above

26. An anterior crossbite in the primary dentition is often indicative of which two of the following?
A. Impacted permanent maxillary canines
B. A skeletal growth problem
C. A developing Class II malocclusion
D. A developing Class III malocclusion

27. Bone deposition in which region listed below is responsible for the lengthening of the maxillary arch?
A. Palate
B. Tuberosity
C. Incisor
D. Zygomatic

28. In which direction do the permanent teeth move during eruption?
A. Mesially and occlusally
B. Occlusally and buccally
C. Buccally and mesially
D. Occlusally and lingually

29. Malocclusion is most often:
A. Acquired from a friend
B. Hereditary
C. Caused by antibiotics
D. Caused by bad habits

30. Ectopic eruption of a permanent maxillary first molar is frequently treated by:
A. Disking the distal of the primary first molar
B. An appliance incorporating a finger spring to move the primary second molar mesially
C. A brass wire placed between the primary second molar and permanent first molar
D. Extraction of the primary second molar

31. Which of the following statements are true concerning a mixed dentition analysis?
A. It is used to predict the amount of crowding after the permanent teeth come in
B. It is performed during the mixed dentition
C. It is performed with a boley gauge, study models and prediction table
D. All of the above statements are true

32. Which of the following is the most common removable retainer used in orthodontics?
A. Tooth positioner
B. Hawley retainer
C. Functional retainer
D. Anterior spring retainer

33. All of the following are fixed orthodontic appliances except:
A. Lingual archwire
B. Palate-separating devices
C. Lip bumpers
D. Edgewise mechanisms
E. Light-wire appliances

34. Which of the following is the best method for tipping proximally maxillary and mandibular anterior teeth?
A. Finger springs
B. Z-springs
C. Canine retractors
D. All are equally efficient

35. Class II malocclusion is also referred to as:
A. Retrognathism
B. Prognathism
C. Both of the above
D. Neither of the above

36. A major site of growth of the mandible is the:
A. Angle
B. Condyle
C. Ramus
D. Chin

37. Which of the following are true concerning a posterior crossbite in the mixed dentition?

A. It should be corrected as soon as possible

B. It should be thoroughly diagnosed as to whether it is of a dental, functional or skeletal origin

C. May be corrected with palatal expansion

D. May be associated with a mandibular shift

E. All of the above are true

38. "Primate spaces" in the primary dentition are found in which two locations?

A. In the maxillary arch, the primate space is located between the central incisors and lateral incisors

B. In the maxillary arch, the primate space is located between the lateral incisors and canines

C. In the mandibular arch, the primate space is located between the canines and first molars

D. In the mandibular arch, the primate space is located the lateral incisors and canines

39. In most Class II, Division I malocclusions, the body of the mandible and its superimposed dental arch are in a:

A. Mesial relationship to the maxilla and the maxillary incisors are usually in a labial axial inclination

B. Distal relationship to the maxilla and the maxillary incisors are usually in a lingual axial inclination

C. Mesial relationship to the maxilla and the maxillary incisors are usually in a lingual axial inclination

D. Distal relationship to the maxilla and the maxillary incisors are usually in a labial axial inclination

40. Which of the following would be indicative of maxillary retrognathism?

A. An SNB angle of approximately 82°

B. An SNA angle greater than 82°

C. An SNA angle less than 82°

D. An SNB angle less than 70°

41. There are many reasons why cross bites occur. Which one of the following is not one of them?
A. Jaw size
B. Heredity
C. Faulty restorations
D. Mouth breathing
E. Prolonged retention of primary teeth

42. Hyaline cartilage differs from bone in that hyaline cartilage may grow:
A. By appositional growth
B. By interstitial growth
C. Both of the above
D. Neither of the above

43. Which of the following theories most likely explains why there is a strong tendency for mandibular crowding in the late teens and early twenties?
A. Lack of leeway space
B. Pressure from third molars
C. Late mandibular growth
D. Late maxillary growth

44. The most commonly impacted teeth are:
A. Maxillary canines
B. Maxillary central incisors
C. Mandibular first premolars
D. Mandibular lateral incisors

45. Which of the following is the difference in the total of the mesiodistal widths between the primary canine, first molar and second molar, and the permanent canine, first premolar and second premolar?
A. Primate space
B. Leeway space
C. Moyer's space
D. Anatomic space

46. Which of the following facial profiles is usually accompanied by a Class II malocclusion?
A. An orthognathic profile

B. A retrognathic profile
C. A prognathic profile
D. None of the above

47. Which type of malocclusion listed below is most often associated with mouth breathing?
A. Dental open bite
B. Skeletal open bite
C. Dental cross bite
D. Skeletal cross bite

48. Which of the following types of headgear produces a distal and upward force on the maxillary teeth and maxilla?
A. Straight pull headgear
B. Reverse-pull headgear
C. Cervical-pull headgear
D. High-pull headgear

49. Which of the following is usually used as an etching agent before direct bonding of orthodontic bracket?
A. 10-15% unbuffered phosphoric acid
B. 35-50% unbuffered phosphoric acid
C. 75-85% unbuffered phosphoric acid
D. 100% unbuffered phosphoric acid

50. The most rapid losses in the perimeter of the arch usually are due to a:
A. Distal tipping and rotation of the permanent second molar after removal of the permanent third molar
B. Mesial tipping and rotation of the permanent first molar after removal of the primary second molar
C. Mesial tipping and rotation of the permanent canine after removal of the primary lateral incisor
D. Distal tipping and rotation of the permanent second premolar after removal of the permanent first molar

51. The rational for retention in orthodontics is to:
A. Allow for reorganization of the gingival and periodontal tissues
B. Minimize changes due to growth

C. Permit neuromuscular adaptation to the corrected tooth position
D. Maintain teeth in a stable conditions
E. All of the above

52. The time required to upright a molar can vary from:
A. 2-3 weeks
B. 1-2 months
C. 6-12 months
D. 2-3 years

53. A phase of dentition during which some of the teeth present in the oral cavity are permanent and some are primary is referred to as what?
A. Intermediate dentition
B. Succedaneous dentition
C. Mixed dentition
D. Non-succedaneous dentition

54. The existence of a forward shift of the mandible during closure is found in:
A. "True" Class III malocclusions
B. "Pseudo" Class III malocclusions
C. Class II div 2 malocclusion
D. Class II div 1 malocclusion

55. The most common site for a supernumerary tooth is:
A. Distal to the mandibular third molar (distomolar)
B. Between the maxillary premolars
C. Between the mandibular central incisors
D. Between the maxillary central incisors (mesiodens)

56. Which of the following can cause an open bite?
A. Tongue-thrusting
B. Thumb-sucking
C. Genetics
D. Speech impediments (i.e. lisping)
E. All of the above

57. Which of the following is the normal relationship of the primary molars in the deciduous dentition?
A. Distal step
B. Flush terminal plane
C. Mesial step
D. None of the above

58. Root fractures in which part of the tooth are more likely to undergo repair?
A. Coronal
B. Mid-root
C. Apical third of the root
D. Vertical fracture of tooth

59. The management of a child who must undergo dental extractions is based on which of the following factors?
A. The age and maturity of the child
B. The past medical and dental experiences that might influence the behavior of the child
C. The physical status of the child
D. The length of time and amount of manipulation necessary to accomplish the surgery
E. All of the above

60. Which of the following is a hereditary dental defect in which the enamel of the teeth is soft and undercalcified in context, yet normal in quantity?
A. Enamel hypoplasia
B. Enamel hypocalcification
C. Enamel hypomaturation
D. Fluorosis

61. What is the most reliable method to determine the pulp vitality in the case of a recently traumatized primary tooth?
A. Radiograph
B. Electric pulp test
C. Thorough intraoral examination
D. There is no reliable method

62. The pH of acidulated phosphate fluoride gels is in which of the following ranges?

A. 1 to 4
B. 4 to 7
C. 7 to 10
D. 10 to 12

63. Which pulpotomy technique listed below is recommended in the treatment of a permanent tooth with a carious exposure which also has immature root development?

A. Calcium hydroxide technique
B. Formocresol technique
C. Indirect pulp capping
D. Apexification

64. All of the following procedures have proved beneficial in treating a mentally retarded child except:

A. Speak slowly and in very simple terms
B. Listen carefully to the patient
C. Schedule long appointments
D. Ask the patient if there are any questions about anything you will be doing

65. Discolored primary teeth that are symptom-free and show no radiographic changes are best treated by:

A. No treatment
B. Extirpation of the pulp tissue followed by the placement of ZOE paste in the root canal space
C. Extraction
D. Pulpotomy

66. A condition characterized by an attention span that is less than expected for the age of the child, hyperactivity and impulsive behavior is called:

A. Epilepsy
B. Cerebral palsy
C. Attention deficit disorder
D. Muscular dystrophy

67. The hallmarks of cellulitis include:

A. Warmth
B. Erythema
C. Edema
D. Pain (tenderness)
E. All of the above

68. Which of the following is a primary center of calcification of a Tooth?

A. Ridges
B. Lobes
C. Grooves
D. Pearls

69. Ordinarily, a 6-year-old child would have what teeth clinically visible in the mouth?

A. All (20) primary teeth and 4 permanent first molars
B. 18 primary teeth and 2 permanent mandibular central incisors
C. 18 primary teeth, 2 permanent mandibular central incisors, and 4 permanent first molars
D. 16 primary teeth and 4 mandibular incisors

70. Which of the following drugs is widely used for pediatric sedation?

A. Meperidine
B. Chloral hydrate
C. Barbiturates
D. None of the above

71. Which of the following statements are true concerning cystic fibrosis?

A. Cystic fibrosis is an inherited disease of the exocrine glands, affecting approximately 30,000 children and adults.
B. Cystic fibrosis causes the body to produce an abnormally thick, sticky mucus, due to a faulty transport of sodium and chloride within cells lining organs such as the lungs and pancreas
C. Cystic fibrosis has a variety of symptoms. The most common of which are: a very salty tasting skin; persistent coughing,

wheezing or pneumonia; excessive appetite but poor weight gain; and bulky stools

D. An individual must inherit a defective copy of the CF gene-one from each parent to have cystic fibrosis

E. All of the above statements are true

72. All of the following statements concerning dental fluorosis are true except:

A. It is a diffuse, symmetric, hypomineralization disorder of ameloblasts

B. It is reversible

C. It only occurs with exposure to fluoride when enamel is developing (calcification period)

D. It is a toxic manifestation of chronic (low-dose, long-term) fluoride intake

73. Amelogenesis imperfecta is a condition in which:

A. The teeth have short roots and tend to wear rapidly

B. The teeth develop abnormally and many teeth are missing

C. The teeth are covered with thin, malformed enamel

D. Tooth buds are joined together during development and appear as macrodonts

74. All of the following statements concerning recurrent aphthous ulcers (canker sores) are true except:

A. They occur in women more than men

B. They may occur at any age, but usually first appear between the ages of 10 to 40

C. The cause is a coxsackie virus

D. They appear to be associated with stress

E. They usually appear on nonkeratinized oral mucosa including the inner surface of the cheeks and lips, tongue, soft palate and the base of the gingivae

75. An outstanding oral manifestation of both ectodermal dysplasia and cleidocranial dysplasia is:

A. Oversized crowns

B. Elongated roots

C. Enlarged mandible

D. Retained primary teeth

76. All of the following instances, except one, may make the use of a rubber dam impractical. Which is the exception?

A. The presence of fixed orthodontic appliances

B. A patient with congested nasal passages or other nasal obstruction

C. A very nervous or anxious patient

D. A recently erupted tooth that will not retain a clamp

77. The teeth joined together by cementum is diagnosed as:

A. Gemination

B. Fusion

C. Concresence

D. Dens in dente

78. Which of the following is true concerning a young epileptic who has a grand mal seizure in the dental office?

A. It is generally fatal

B. It is best treated by injecting insulin

C. They generally recover if restrained from self-injury and oxygen is maintained

D. It can be prevented with antibiotics

79. Type 1 diabetes:

A. It also called juvenile-onset or insulin dependent diabetes

B. Is the type of diabetes in which the body completely stops producing any insulin

C. Affects young adults

D. Is characterized by all of the above

80. Morphologically, the primary maxillary second molar strikingly resembles which tooth listed below?

A. Permanent maxillary third molar

B. Permanent maxillary second molar

C. Permanent maxillary first molar

D. Permanent mandibular second molar

81. If a child in your office requires antibiotic prophylaxis to prevent bacterial endocarditis, which regimen below is correct?

A. Amoxicillin 100 mg/kg 1 hr prior to dental appointment

B. Amoxicillin 75 mg/kg 2 hrs prior to dental appointment

C. Amoxicillin 50 mg/kg 1 hr prior to dental appointment
D. Amoxicillin 25 mg/kg 2 hr prior to dental appointment

82. The phenomenon of "strawberry tongue" is associated with:
A. Herpangina
B. Scarlet fever
C. Diphtheria
D. Mumps

83. Which of the following are true comparing the normal child periodontium to a normal adult periodontium?
A. There is greater blood and lymph supply
B. The alveolar crest is flatter
C. Gingival pocket depths are larger
D. Attached gingiva is not as wide
E. All of the above

84. Panoramic radiographs are excellent in demonstrating which of the following in a young patient?
A. Supernumerary teeth / Congenitally missing teeth
B. Axial inclinations of teeth / Apical development of the permanent teeth
C. Impacted teeth / Pathological lesions in the jaw
D. View of the mandibular condyles
E. All of the above

85. A veau's Class I cleft palate involves what structures?
A. Hard and soft palates
B. Soft palate only
C. Alveolar process only
D. Hard palate only

86. Cretinism is a deficiency disease, caused by the congenital absence of:
A. Insulin
B. Thyroxine
C. Calcitonin
D. Epinephrine

87. "Koplik's spots" are associated with:
A. Smallpox (Variola)

B. German measles (Rubella)
C. Mumps
D. Measles (Rubeola)

88. What is the minimum number of lobes from which any tooth may develop?
A. Two
B. Three
C. Four
D. Five

89. The permanent mandibular first molar has a morphology that closely resembles which primary tooth listed below?
A. Primary mandibular first molar
B. Primary mandibular second molar
C. Primary maxillary first molar
D. Primary maxillary second molar

90. Emergency treatment in the dental office for a child who has accidentally ingested a large amount of fluoride would include which of the following:
A. Induce vomiting mechanically or with the help of Ipecac syrup
B. Have patient drink large quantities of sodium bicarbonate
C. Have patients drink large quantities of milk
D. Crush ammonia vaparole under the patient's nose to keep the patient awake and conscious
E. Only a & c.

91. A child 19 months old will have how many teeth?
A. Four
B. Eight
C. Twelve
D. Sixteen
E. Twenty

92. Which of the following is the most common congenitally missing primary tooth?
A. Primary mandibular canine
B. Primary maxillary lateral incisor
C. Primary maxillary canine
D. Primary mandibular first molar

93. The primary mandibular second molar in a four year old has a large carious lesion with pulpal involvement. Radiographically there is periapical pathology on the distal root. There is furcation involvement and slight mobility. The treatment of choice is:

A. Direct pulp capping
B. Pulpotomy
C. Pulpectomy
D. Extraction

94. Upon oral examination, a three-year-old child is found to have intensely inflamed gingiva, a soar throat, fever, lymphadenopathy, and small fluid-filled vesicles on the mucosa of the lips, tongue and gingiva. The diagnosis is probably:

A. Chicken pox
B. Primary (acute) herpetic gingivostomatitis
C. Scarlet fever
D. Acute necrotizing ulcerative gingivitis (ANUG)

95. Which type of leukemia below is the most common pediatric cancer?

A. Acute myeloid leukemia
B. Chronic myelocytic leukemia
C. Acute lymphocytic leukemia
D. Chronic lymphocytic leukemia

96. What is the most effective method of reducing the dental caries problem in the general population?

A. School water fluoridation
B. Fluoridation of the communal water supply
C. Fluoride rinses at home
D. Frequent dental visits
E. Patient education

97. When placing a Class II amalgam in a primary tooth, the width of the isthmus should be:

A. About one-half the intercuspal width
B. About one-third the intercuspal width
C. About two-third the intercuspal width
D. About three-quarters the intercuspal width

98. Nursing-bottle caries is a widespread caries destruction of the deciduous teeth, which of the deciduous teeth are most commonly affected?

A. Mandibular incisors
B. Maxillary first molars
C. Mandibular first molars
D. Maxillary incisors

99. Gingivostomatitis is a condition that is:

A. Common particularly among elderly people
B. Common particularly among middle-aged adults
C. Common particularly among children
D. Uncommon

100. At the age of six years a child's head is what percentage of its adult size?

A. 30%
B. 50%
C. 80%
D. 90%

101. All of the following statements are true, except:

A. The primary teeth are darker in color than the permanent teeth
B. The pulp cavities are proportionately larger in the primary teeth
C. In general, the crowns of primary teeth are more bulbous and constricted than the permanent counterpart
D. The crown surfaces of all primary teeth are much smoother than the permanent teeth (in other words, there is less evidence of pits and grooves)

102. Preventive dentistry for adolescents may include which of the following?

A. Frequent dental office visits
B. Fluoride rinses at home
C. Fluoride tray applications
D. Brushing and flossing
E. Sealants

F. Fluoride tablets
G. All the above

103. All of the following statements are true except:
A. The occlusal anatomy of primary teeth is not as defined as that of permanent teeth therefore amalgam preps can be more conservative
B. Enamel and dentin are thicker in primary teeth, therefore amalgam preparations are deeper
C. The pulpal horns of primary teeth are longer and pointed, therefore amalgam preps must be conservative to avoid a pulpal exposure
D. Primary molars have an exaggerated cervical bulge that makes matrix adoption much more difficult

104. Which of the following is the first deciduous (primary) tooth to erupt?
A. Mandibular central
B. Mandibular first molar
C. Maxillary central
D. Maxillary first molar

105. Listed below are the usual events in the histogenesis of a tooth. Place them in their correct sequence (from what happens first to what happens last)
1. Deposition of the first layer of dentin
2. Differentiation of odontoblasts
3. Deposition of the first layer of enamel
4. Elongation of the inner enamel epithelial cells of the enamel organ
   A. 3,2,4,1
   B. 1,2,4,3
   C. 2,1,3,4
   D. 4,3,2,1

106. Which primary mandibular tooth listed below does not resemble any other primary or permanent tooth?
A. Primary mandibular canine
B. Primary mandibular lateral incisor

C. Primary mandibular first molar
D. Primary mandibular second molar

107. When do the permanent teeth begin to calcify?
A. At birth
B. One month
C. Four months
D. One year

108. Which stage in the life cycle of a tooth listed below includes final shaping of the tooth?
A. Initiation (Bud stage)
B. Proliferation (Cap stage)
C. Differentiation (Bell stage)
D. Apposition

109. Which of the following is the most frequently utilized route of administration for sedation in pediatric patients?
A. Oral
B. Inhalation
C. IV
D. IM

110. Which of the following cause delayed exfoliation of the primary teeth and delayed eruption of the permanent teeth?
A. Hypothyroidism
B. Hypopituitarism
C. Hypoparathyroidism
D. All of the above

111. The primary central incisors are usually exfoliated between what ages?
A. 6-8 years old
B. 7-9 years old
C. 9-10 years old
D. 10-12 years old

112. The primary maxillary canine differs from the permanent maxillary canine in which way listed below?
A. The cusp on the primary canine is much shorter and rounded
B. The mesial cusp ridge is longer than the distal cusp ridge

C. The mesial cusp ridge is shorter than the distal cusp ridge
D. None of the above

113. The greatest concentration of fluoride ions exists just beneath the enamel surface. During a routine prophylaxis it is possible that the use of abrasive polishing agents may remove the fluoride-rich layer of enamel.
A. Both statements are true
B. The first statements is true and the second statements false
C. The first statements is false and the second statement is true
D. Both statements are false

114. Which treatment listed below is the proper one for a Class II fracture of a permanent tooth with an immature apex?
A. Pulpectomy
B. Apply calcium hydroxide to exposed dentin and restore tooth with a permanent restoration
C. Pulpotomy
D. Observe

115. All of the following are dental characteristics of a Down syndrome child except:
A. A prominent thickened tongue
B. A high rate of caries
C. Delayed eruption of teeth
D. A high prevalence of malocclusion
E. Enamel dysplasia

116. The primary maxillary canine typically erupts around what age?
A. 7 months old
B. 10 months old
C. 18 months old
D. 24 months old

117. All of the following are the major features of Apert syndrome except:
A. Prematurely fused cranial sutures
B. A retruded midface
C. Fused fingers

D. Blindness
E. Fused toes

118. When treating a child who is obviously afraid, the dentist should:
A. Use restraint
B. Use the hand-over-mouth technique (HOME)
C. Permit the child to express his fear
D. Avoid all references to the child's fear

119. In most cases, the proper treatment for intruded primary anterior teeth is:
A. Repositioning
B. Extraction
C. Intermaxillary fixation
D. Administer no treatment

120. Which of the following are primary goals of indirect pulp capping?
A. To preserve the pulp vitality
B. To prevent pulp exposure
C. To save tooth structure
D. To arrest caries
E. To promote the formation of reparative dentin
F. All of the above

121. The process of shaping a patient's behaviour through appropriately timed feedback is called:
A. Tell-show-do
B. Voice control
C. Positive reinforcement
D. Distraction
E. Nonverbal communication

122. When operative or surgical procedures are performed on the mandibular primary or permanent teeth, which nerve listed below must be blocked?
A. Posterior superior alveolar nerve
B. Lingual nerve
C. Inferior alveolar nerve
D. Long buccal nerve

123. Which primary molar listed below is the most atypical of all the molars, primary and permanent, and appears to be intermediate in form and development between a premolar and a molar?

A. Primary mandibular first molar
B. Primary maxillary first molar
C. Primary mandibular second molar
D. Primary maxillary second molar

124. Which of the following is a beneficial effect of fluoride?

A. Interferes with plaque formation on teeth
B. Has antibacterial qualities
C. Remineralization is enhanced
D. Decreased enamel solubility
E. Inhibits glycolysis
F. All of the above

125. All of the following fluoride therapies should be recommended to a 13-year-old child who is prone to decay and lives in a community where the water is fluoridated at an appropriate level except?

A. Professionally applied fluoride every six months
B. Fluoride toothpaste
C. A low concentration fluoride mouth rinse
D. A high concentration fluoride mouth rinse

126. A simple fracture of the crown of a tooth involving little or no dentin would be classified as what?

A. Ellis Class I fracture
B. Ellis Class II fracture
C. Ellis Class III fracture
D. Ellis Class IV fracture

127. Which of the following are true concerning over-retained primary teeth in the mixed dentition?

A. They may prevent normal eruption of permanent teeth
B. This may be caused by abnormal root resorption of primary teeth
C. They are often treated by extraction
D. All of thc abovc

128. All of the following are contraindications of performing a direct pulp cap on a primary tooth except:

A. Spontaneous pain from the tooth
B. A pinpoint exposure with little or no hemorrhaging (bleeding)
C. A large exposure
D. Excessive hemorrhaging (bleeding)
E. Radiographic evidence of internal resorption

129. Which of the following is the main advantage of using 8% solution of stannous fluoride instead of a 2% solution of sodium fluoride for a topical fluoride treatment?

A. Will not stain
B. Better taste
C. Stable when kept in a polyethylene container
D. A single treatment may be given

130. Which pulpotomy technique listed below is recommended in the treatment of primary teeth with a carious exposure?

A. Calcium hydroxide technique
B. Formocresol technique
C. Zinc oxide eugenol technique
D. None of the above

131. The most common benign tumor of infants is:

A. A lymphangioma
B. A hemangioma
C. A neurofibroma
D. A pyogenic granuloma

132. All of the following are factors to consider when deciding whether a fluoride supplement should be prescribed to a child except:

A. The amount of fluoride in the child's drinking water
B. The age of the child
C. The type of topical fluoride applied professionally in the office
D. How responsible is the person who will be administering the supplement, whether it be the patient or the patient's parents

133. All of the following teeth are non-succedaneous, except:
A. The permanent maxillary and mandibular premolars
B. The permanent maxillary and mandibular first molars
C. The permanent maxillary and mandibular second molars
D. The permanent maxillary and mandibular third molars

134. An outstanding oral manifestation of achondroplasia is:
A. Rampant caries
B. Periodontal disease
C. Overcrowding of teeth
D. Supernumerary teeth

135. All of the following statements are true except:
A. Compared to the permanent maxillary central incisors, the incisal edge of the primary maxillary central incisors is straighter
B. No mamelons are present on the primary maxillary central incisors. There are mamelons present on the permanent maxillary central incisors
C. The crown of the primary maxillary central incisors is smaller Mesiodistally than the permanent maxillary central incisors
D. The crown of the primary maxillary central incisors has a shorter length inciso-cervically than the permanent maxillary central incisors

136. Interproximal caries on primary teeth may result in:
A. Eventual loss of the primary tooth
B. Loss of tooth structure
C. Arch length loss
D. All of the above

137. The most common of the craniofacial malformations is:
A. Bifid tongue
B. Macroglossia
C. Cleft palate and cleft lip
D. Anodontia

138. The sum of the mediodistal widths of the primary molars in any one quadrant is:
A. 5-10 mm greater than the permanent teeth that succeed them (premolars)

B. 2-5 mm less than the permanent teeth that succeed them (premolars)
C. 2-5 mm greater than the permanent teeth that succeed them (premolars)
D. 5-10 mm less than the permanent teeth that succeed them (premolars)

139. All of the following statements concerning acute necrotizing ulcerative gingivitis are true except:
A. It is also called Vincent's infection or "trench mouth"
B. It is a gingival disease characterized by painful hyperemic gingiva, punched out erosions of the interproximal papilla, covered by a gray pseudomembrane with an accompanying fetid odor
C. Risks include poor oral hygiene, poor nutrition, smoking, and emotional stress
D. It is usually affects children between the age of 5 to 10 years old

140. Which of the following is the most important technique of behavioral management in the pediatric dental patient?
A. Tell-show-do
B. Voice control
C. Positive reinforcement
D. Distraction
E. Nonverbal communication

141. Which primary mandibular molar has a prominent transverse ridge that unites the mesiobuccal and the mesiolingual cusps?
A. Primary mandibular first molar
B. Primary mandibular second molar
C. Both of the above
D. None of the above

142. A child eleven years old traumatized a permanent maxillary central incisor some time ago. The tooth in now painful and there is evidence of swelling. A periapical x-ray discloses a pathosis associated with the apex. The suggested treatment is:
A. Pulpotomy

B. Extraction
C. Pulpectomy
D. Observation

143. A 15-year -old female has lived in a non-fluoridated area all of her life. Which of the following is most likely to occur in this female when she moves to a community where the drinking water naturally contains 6 ppm of fluoride?
A. 50% reduction in dental caries
B. Moderate dental fluorosis
C. An increase in the amount of fluoride stored in her bones
D. Gastrointestinal problems

144. When preparing a primary tooth for a stainless steel crown, the cusps are reduced:
A. Approximately 1 to 1.5 mm
B. Approximately 5 to 6.5 mm
C. Approximately 10 mm
D. Approximately 15 mm

145. When do the primary teeth begin to form in utero?
A. One week
B. Three weeks
C. Six weeks
D. Ten weeks

146. Which two structures listed below join to form Hertwigs epithelial root sheath?
A. Stratum intermedium
B. Inner enamel epithelium
C. Stellate reticulum
D. Outer enamel epithelium
E. Stratum basale

147. Which two of the following decrease with age in the dental pulp?
A. Number of collagen fibers
B. Number of reticulin fibers
C. The size of the pulp
D. Calcifications within the pulp

148. No endodontic cases lend themselves to successful treatment without some degree of:
A. Irrigation
B. Debridement
C. Obturation
D. Medication

149. Which of the following irrigants is the most widely used in endodontics?
A. Sodium hypochlorite
B. Urea peroxide
C. Hydrogen peroxide
D. Saline

150. Which of the following appears to be the ideal storage media for a tooth that has been traumatically avulsed and will be out of its socket for more than an hour?
A. Soda
B. Sodium hypochlorite
C. Milk
D. Hydrogen peroxide

151. Which of the following are useful diagnostic aids that can be used to determine if a tooth has a vertical crown-root fracture?
A. Fiberoptic light for transillumination
B. Wedging the tooth in question and then taking an x-ray
C. Persistent periodontal defects in an otherwise healthy tooth
D. Having a patient bite forcefully on a bite stick
E. All of the above

152. Which of the following is generally believed to be the cause of internal resorption of a tooth?
A. Orthodontic treatment
B. Tooth fracture
C. The presence of a chronic pulpitis
D. Periodontal disease

153. Which of the following intracanal instruments is designed for the removal of pulp tissue, cotton pellet absorbent points and other soft materials, but not for canal enlargement?
A. Files

B. Reamers
C. Broaches
D. None of the above

154. Which of the following canals in a maxillary first molar is usually the most difficult to locate?
A. Palatal
B. Distobuccal
C. Mesiobuccal
D. All of the canals are relatively easy to find

155. The primary function of root canal sealers is:
A. To act as a lubricant, facilitating placement of the gutta-percha
B. To form a bond between the filling material and the dentin walls
C. To fill in the discrepancies between the filling material and the dentin walls
D. To exert antibacterial activity

156. Which material listed below has historically been the retrofilling material of choice?
A. Composite
B. Zinc-free amalgam
C. Gutta-percha
D. Methyl methacrylate

157. Which of the following will have a pulp chamber that will be triangular?
A. Permanent mandibular second premolars
B. Permanent mandibular molars
C. Permanent maxillary molars
D. Permanent maxillary lateral incisors

158. Which condition below is an apical lesion that develops as an acute exacerbation of a chronic apical abscess (also called a suppurative apical periodontitis)?
A. Cyst
B. Phoenix abscess
C. Granuloma
D. None of the above

159. Which of the following flap designs is preferred when performing endodontic surgery in the maxillary anterior region?
A. Vertical (single or double) flap
B. Scalloped (Leubke-Ochsenbein) flap
C. Curved (semilunar flap)
D. Palatal flap

160. Which condition listed below is the result of a pulpal infection that extends through the apical foramen to the periapical tissues?
A. Periodontal abscess
B. Gingival abscess
C. Periapical abscess
D. All of the above

161. Which mandibular premolar presents with more variations in root canal anatomy?
A. First premolar
B. Second premolar
C. Both of the above
D. None of the above

162. An apicoectomy is a resection:
A. Of the most coronal portion of the root
B. Of the coronal portion of the pulp horn
C. Of the most apical portion of the root
D. Of the entire pulp horn

163. Which of the following are chelating agents?
A. EDTA
B. RC-Prep
C. EDTAC
D. All of the above

164. According to the buccal object rule, when the x-ray tube is repositioned either at a more mesial or at a more distal angulation and a film is exposed, the root or canal farther from the film (the buccal) will
A. More in the opposite direction that the cone is directed
B. Move in the direction that the cone is directed

C. Not move at all
D. Moves up and down

165. Which of the following criteria must be met before a canal is considered ready to fill with gutta-percha?

A. The canal must be prepared in a manner that ensures optimum debridement and access to the apical area so that the filling material can be condensed to obliterate the entire preparation
B. The tooth must be asymptomatic
C. At the time of fill, the canal must be dry
D. If a bacteriologic culture test is being used, a negative culture must be obtained
E. All of the above

166. Anatomically, the dental pulp is divided into two portions, the coronal and radicular pulp. Which portion is located in the pulp chamber and pulp horns?

A. Coronal pulp
B. Radicular pulp
C. Pulp canal
D. Pulp cells

167. Which of the following are contraindications to the use of the electric pulp tester?

A. Inability to dry the tooth
B. Teeth that have crowns or are heavily restored
C. Tooth traumatized recently
D. Anesthetized teeth
E. Patient in severe pain
F. All of the above

168. Which tooth below will almost always have two canals?

A. Maxillary first premolar
B. Maxillary second premolar
C. Mandibular first premolar
D. Mandibular second premolar

169. Which of the following methods for using endodontic instruments involves no rotation of the instrument

whatsoever and relies on hard tissue removal on the outstroke only?

A. Filing
B. Reaming
C. Circumferential filing
D. All of the above

170. In all of the following conditions, the pulps of the involved teeth are likely to be non-vital except?

A. Apical scar
B. Radicular cyst
C. Traumatic bone cyst
D. Chronic dental abscess
E. Chronic periapical granuloma

171. In all of the following conditions, the pulps of the involved teeth are likely to be vital except?

A. Cementoma
B. Radicular cyst
C. Traumatic bone cyst
D. Globulomaxillary cyst

172. Which tooth listed below requires endodontic treatment most frequently?

A. Maxillary second molar
B. Mandibular first molar
C. Mandibular second bicuspid
D. Maxillary first bicuspid

173. Which of the following is the main function of the dental pulp?

A. Nutritive
B. Sensory
C. Protective
D. Formative

174. Which of the following is the procedures of choice when a broken endodontic instrument protrudes past the apex of a tooth?

A. Fxtract the tooth

B. The broken instrument is surgically removed, and then the entire canal is filled with gutta-percha
C. Fill the tooth with gutta-percha and observe
D. None of the above

175. Wearing gloves when using the electric pulp tester to test the vitality of a tooth may lead to a:
A. False-positive response
B. False-negative response
C. Both of the above
D. None of the above

176. Gutta-percha is freely soluble in which solvents listed below?
A. Alcohol
B. Chloroform
C. Xylol
D. Eugenol

177. The chronic apical abscess (CAA) is generally:
A. Very painful
B. Asymptomatic
C. Mildly painful
D. None of the above

178. Which of the following are contraindications to endodontic therapy?
A. A non-restorable tooth
B. A tooth with insufficient periodontal support
C. A tooth with a vertical root fracture
D. All of the above

179. Which two of the following situations offer better success for pulp capping?
A. Accidental exposure of the pulp
B. Pulp of a middle-aged person
C. Carious exposure of the pulp
D. Pulp of a young child

180. Which of the following is the most commonly used bleaching agent for endodontically treated teeth?
A. Ether

B. Superoxol
C. Chloroform
D. Sodium hypochlorite

181. Which condition listed below is characterized by pain that is spontaneous and has periods of cessation (intermittent in nature)?
A. Reversible pulpitis
B. Irreversible pulpitis
C. Chronic alveolar abscess
D. None of the above

182. The root canal for a mandibular canine is:
A. Wide Mesiodistally but thin labiolingually
B. Thin Mesiodistally but wide labiolingually
C. The same width Mesiodistally and labiolingually
D. Circular

183. Which type of external root resorption listed below may occur from combined injury to the PDL and cementum complicated by bacteria from an infected root canal space?
A. Surface resorption
B. Inflammatory resorption
C. Replacement resorption
D. None of the above

184. All of the following cells would be found in a hyperemic pulp after an exposure during caries removal, except:
A. Plasma cells
B. Lymphocytes
C. Goblet cells
D. Mast cells
E. Neutrophils (PMNs)

185. Which tooth listed below may have a pulp chamber that is somewhat triangular as opposed to oval?
A. Maxillary central incisor
B. Mandibular central incisor
C. Maxillary lateral incisor
D. Mandibular lateral incisor

186. Which of the following are considered to be the two objective of the access opening?

A. To provide patient comfort
B. To provide direct access to the apical portion of the canal
C. To facilitate visualization (location) of the canal
D. To remove all old restorative materials from the tooth

187. The earliest and most common symptom of an acute pulpitis is:

A. A dull throbbing sensation
B. Pain upon chewing
C. Thermal sensitivity
D. Discomfort, particularly on palpation

188. Which of the following teeth most often refer pain to the temporal region?

A. Mandibular molars
B. Maxillary incisors
C. Maxillary second premolars
D. Maxillary molars

189. The most common cause of acute osteomyelitis of the jaws is:

A. Unknown
B. Iatrogenic
C. Dental infection
D. Radiation

190. Which of the following are the two basic reasons for the use of post when restoring an endodontically treated tooth?

A. To strengthen the root
B. To retain the restoration
C. To protect the remaining tooth structure
D. To help in the fabrication of a crown

191. The most widely used material for apexification procedures is:

A. Gutta-percha
B. Calcium hydroxide
C. Zinc oxide
D. Eugenol

192. Which tooth listed below is most likely to have a curved root?

A. Maxillary central incisor
B. Maxillary lateral incisor
C. Maxillary canine
D. Mandibular central incisor

193. Which of the following factors are important to the success of intentional replantation?

A. A short extraoral time period (to maintain the viability of the periodontal ligament)
B. A healthy periodontium
C. A skillful extraction technique
D. All of the above

194. If an electric pulp tester is used to test a hyperemic tooth, the useful response will be which of the following?

A. The tooth will respond to less current than normal
B. The tooth will respond immediately to any current
C. The tooth will respond to higher current than normal
D. The tooth will not respond to any current

195. Which of the following are indications for performing a pulpotomy?

A. Treatment of pulp exposures in deciduous teeth
B. Treatment of pulp exposures in permanent teeth with undeveloped root apices
C. An alternative to extraction when endodontic therapy is unavailable
D. Temporary emergency treatment for an acute pulpitis
E. All of the above

196. When symptoms and clinical tests show the presence of pulpal pathosis in a posterior tooth and the radiograph shows no decay or restoration in any proximity to the pulp, this is virtually pathognomonic of:

A. Condensing osteitis
B. A vertical fracture of the tooth
C. Periodontal abscess
D. Secondary occlusal trauma

197. Avulsed primary/deciduous teeth:

A. Should be cleaned very well and replanted if within five hours of the injury

B. Are usually not replanted

C. Should be replanted immediately

D. Should have a pulpotomy performed on them prior to replantation

198. A reaming action produces a canal that is relatively:

A. Square in shape

B. Irregular in shape

C. Round in shape

D. Triangular in shape

199. When fitting the master cone in a properly prepared canal, the cone must:

A. Be 2 mm from the apex

B. Be within 1 mm of the working length and have a slight resistance to dislodgement

C. Fit to the exact apex

D. Be at least 1 mm past the apex

200. In most cases where there is endodontic-periodontic therapy indicated on a tooth, which is performed first?

A. Endodontic therapy

B. Periodontic therapy

C. Both should go simultaneously

D. None of the above

201. Orthodontic appliances can:

A. Cause irritation to the gingiva

B. Act as plaque harbors

C. Make proper oral hygiene difficult to perform

D. All of the above

Answer Key to MCQs in Orthodontics and Pedodontics

1	B	2	D	3	B	4	A
5	C	6	C	7	D	8	C
9	B	10	D	11	D	12	E
13	C	14	D	15	B	16	B
17	D	18	B	19	D	20	A, C
21	B	22	A	23	B	24	B
25	D	26	D, B	27	B	28	B
29	B	30	C	31	D	32	B
33	C	34	A	35	A	36	B
37	E	38	B, C	39	D	40	C
41	C	42	B	43	C	44	A
45	B	46	B	47	B	48	D
49	B	50	B	51	E	52	C
53	C	54	B	55	D	56	E
57	B	58	C	59	E	60	B
61	D	62	A	63	A	64	C
65	A	66	C	67	E	68	B
69	A	70	B	71	E	72	B
73	C	74	C	75	D	76	C
77	C	78	C	79	D	80	C
81	C	82	B	83	E	84	E
85	B	86	B	87	D	88	C
89	B	90	E	91	D	92	B
93	C	94	B	95	C	96	B
97	B	98	D	99	C	100	D
101	A	102	G	103	B	104	A
105	A	106	C	107	A	108	C
109	B	110	D	111	A	112	B
113	C	114	B	115	B	116	C
117	D	118	C	119	D	120	F
121	C	122	C	123	B	124	F
125	D	126	A	127	D	128	B
129	D	130	B	131	B	132	C
133	A	134	C	135	C	136	D
137	C	138	C	139	D	140	A

141	A	142	C	143	C	144	A
145	C	146	B, D	147	B, C	148	B
149	A	150	C	151	E	152	C
153	C	154	C	155	C	156	B
157	C	158	B	159	B	160	C
161	A	162	C	163	D	164	B
165	E	166	A	167	F	168	A
169	A	170	C	171	B	172	B
173	D	174	B	175	B	176	B, C
177	B	178	D	179	A, D	180	B
181	B	182	B	183	B	184	C
185	A	186	B, C	187	C	188	C
189	C	190	B, C	191	B	192	B
193	D	194	A	195	E	196	B
197	B	198	C	199	B	200	A
201	D						